The Acute Abdomen

Editor

RICHARD M. GORE

RADIOLOGIC CLINICS OF NORTH AMERICA

www.radiologic.theclinics.com

Consulting Editor
FRANK H. MILLER

November 2015 • Volume 53 • Number 6

ELSEVIER

1600 John F. Kennedy Boulevard • Suite 1800 • Philadelphia, Pennsylvania, 19103-2899

http://www.theclinics.com

RADIOLOGIC CLINICS OF NORTH AMERICA Volume 53, Number 6
November 2015 ISSN 0033-8389, ISBN 13: 978-0-323-41350-3

Editor: John Vassallo (j.vassallo@elsevier.com)
Developmental Editor: Donald Mumford

Radiologic Clinics of North America (ISSN 0033-8389) is published bimonthly by Elsevier Inc., 360 Park Avenue South, New York, NY 10010-1710. Months of issue are January, March, May, July, September, and November. Periodicals postage paid at New York, NY and additional mailing offices. Subscription prices are USD 460 per year for US individuals, USD 709 per year for US institutions, USD 220 per year for US students and residents, USD 535 per year for Canadian individuals, USD 905 per year for Canadian institutions, USD 660 per year for international individuals, USD 905 per year for international institutions, and USD 315 per year for Canadian and foreign students/residents. To receive student and resident rate, orders must be accompanied by name of affiliated institution, date of term and the signature of program/residency coordinatior on institution letterhead. Orders will be billed at individual rate until proof of status is received. Foreign air speed delivery is included in all *Clinics* subscription prices. All prices are subject to change without notice. **POSTMASTER:** Send address changes to *Radiologic Clinics of North America*, Elsevier Health Sciences Division, Subscription Customer Service, 3251 Riverport Lane, Maryland Heights, MO63043. **Customer Service: Telephone: 1-800-654-2452** (U.S. and Canada); **1-314-447-8871** (outside U.S. and Canada). **Fax: 1-314-447-8029. E-mail:** journalscustomerservice-usa@elsevier.com **(for print support);** journalsonlinesupport-usa@elsevier.com **(for online support).**

Reprints. For copies of 100 or more of articles in this publication, please contact the Commercial Reprints Department, Elsevier Inc., 360 Park Avenue South, New York, New York 10010-1710. Tel.: +1-212-633-3874; Fax: +1-212-633-3820; E-mail: reprints@elsevier.com.

Radiologic Clinics of North America also published in Greek Paschalidis Medical Publications, Athens, Greece.

Radiologic Clinics of North America is covered in *MEDLINE/PubMed (Index Medicus), EMBASE/Excerpta Medica, Current Contents/Life Sciences, Current Contents/Clinical Medicine, RSNA Index to Imaging Literature, BIOSIS, Science Citation Index,* and *ISI/BIOMED*.

Printed in the United States of America.

Contributors

CONSULTING EDITOR

FRANK H. MILLER, MD
Chief, Body Imaging Section and Fellowship
Program; Medical Director of MRI; Professor,
Department of Radiology, Northwestern
University Feinberg School of Medicine,
Chicago, Illinois

EDITOR

RICHARD M. GORE, MD
Chief, Gastrointestinal Radiology, North Shore
University Health System; Professor of
Radiology, University of Chicago, Evanston,
Illinois

AUTHORS

MARK E. BAKER, MD, FACR, FSAR, FSCBTMR
Staff Radiologist, Section of Abdominal
Imaging, Imaging Institute, Digestive Disease
Institute and Cancer Institute; Professor of
Radiology, Cleveland Clinic Lerner College of
Medicine of Case Western Reserve University,
Cleveland, Ohio

PETER BANNAS, MD
Department of Radiology, University of
Wisconsin-Madison, Madison, Wisconsin;
Department of Radiology, University Hospital
Hamburg-Eppendorf, Hamburg, Germany

SPENCER C. BEHR, MD
Department of Radiology and Biomedical
Imaging, University of California, San
Francisco, San Francisco, California

GENEVIEVE L. BENNETT, MD
Assistant Professor of Radiology, Abdominal
Imaging Division, Department of Radiology,
NYU Langone Medical Center, New York,
New York

JONATHAN W. BERLIN, MD
Professor of Radiology, University of Chicago
Pritzker School of Medicine; Department of
Radiology, Evanston Hospital, North
Shore University Health System, Evanston,
Illinois

NICHOLAS A. BODMER, MD
Department of Radiology, Advocate
Good Samaritan Hospital, Downers Grove,
Illinois

MARTINA DERME, MD
Specialist in Obstetrics and Gynecology,
Department of Gynecological, Obstetrical and
Urological Sciences, Sapienza University,
Rome, Italy

HARPREET S. DHATT, MD
Department of Radiology and
Biomedical Imaging, University of
California San Francisco, San Francisco,
California

CAROLYN K. DONALDSON, MD
Assistant Professor of Radiology,
University of Chicago Pritzker
School of Medicine; Department of
Radiology, NorthShore University
HealthSystem, Evanston, Illinois

JACOB S. ECANOW, MD
Clinical Assistant Professor of Radiology,
University of Chicago Pritzker School of
Medicine, Chicago; Department of Radiology,
North Shore University Health System,
Evanston, Illinois

MARIALUISA FRAMARINO-DEI-MALATESTA, MD
Specialist in Obstetrics and Gynecology,
Department of Gynecological, Obstetrical and
Urological Sciences, Sapienza University,
Rome, Italy

RAKHEE H. GOEL, MD
Abdominal Imaging Fellow, Imaging Institute,
Cleveland Clinic, Cleveland, Ohio

RICHARD M. GORE, MD
Chief, Gastrointestinal Radiology, North Shore
University Health System; Professor of
Radiology, University of Chicago, Evanston,
Illinois

GIANFRANCO GUALDI, MD
Specialist in Radiology, Radiology Department,
Umberto I Hospital, Sapienza University,
Rome, Italy

JAY P. HEIKEN, MD
Professor, Mallinckrodt Institute of Radiology,
Washington University School of Medicine,
St Louis, Missouri

FRANCESCA LAGHI, MD
Specialist in Radiology, Radiology Department,
Umberto I Hospital, Sapienza University,
Rome, Italy

GABRIELE MASSELLI, MD
Specialist in Radiology, Radiology Department,
Umberto I Hospital, Sapienza University,
Rome, Italy

UDAY K. MEHTA, MD
Assistant Professor of Radiology, University of
Chicago Pritzker School of Medicine;
Department of Radiology, Evanston Hospital,
North Shore University Health System,
Evanston, Illinois

VINCENT M. MELLNICK, MD
Assistant Professor, Mallinckrodt Institute of
Radiology, Washington University School of
Medicine, St Louis, Missouri

AARON MIRACLE, MD
Department of Radiology and
Biomedical Imaging, University of
California San Francisco, San Francisco,
California

GERALDINE M. NEWMARK, MD
Assistant Professor of Radiology,
University of Chicago Pritzker School
of Medicine; Department of Radiology,
Evanston Hospital, North Shore University
Health System, Evanston, Illinois

NEEL B. PATEL, MD
Jupiter Imaging Associates, Sheridan
Healthcorp, Jupiter, Florida

PERRY J. PICKHARDT, MD
Department of Radiology, University of
Wisconsin-Madison, Madison, Wisconsin

ERICK M. REMER, MD
Professor of Radiology; Director,
Abdominal Imaging Research, Imaging
Institute, Glickman Urological and
Kidney Institute, Cleveland Clinic,
Cleveland, Ohio

ROBERT I. SILVERS, MD
Assistant Professor of Radiology, University of
Chicago Pritzker School of Medicine;
Department of Radiology, Evanston Hospital,
North Shore University Health System,
Evanston, Illinois

KIRAN H. THAKRAR, MD
Assistant Professor of Radiology,
University of Chicago Pritzker School
of Medicine; Department of Radiology,
Evanston Hospital, North Shore
University Health System, Evanston,
Illinois

RUEDI F. THOENI, MD
Professor of Radiology (Retired),
Department of Radiology and Biomedical
Imaging, University of California,
San Francisco Medical School,
San Francisco, California

RAMAN UNNIKRISHNAN, MD
Urology Resident, Glickman Urological
and Kidney Institute, Cleveland Clinic,
Cleveland, Ohio

ZHEN JANE WANG, MD
Department of Radiology and Biomedical Imaging, University of California, San Francisco, San Francisco, California

DANIEL R. WENZKE, MD
Assistant Professor of Radiology, University of Chicago Pritzker School of Medicine; Department of Radiology, Evanston Hospital, North Shore University Health System, Evanston, Illinois

BENJAMIN M. YEH, MD
Department of Radiology and Biomedical Imaging, University of California San Francisco, San Francisco, California

Contents

acute setting. Although the clinical signs and symptoms of intestinal ischemia are nonspecific, computed tomography (CT) findings can be highly suggestive in the correct clinical setting. In our article, we review the CT diagnosis of arterial, venous, and nonocclusive intestinal ischemia. We discuss the vascular anatomy, pathophysiology of intestinal ischemia, CT techniques for optimal imaging, key and ancillary radiological findings, and differential diagnosis.

Infectious and inflammatory enterocolitides can present with an acute abdomen. The most common entities are ulcerative colitis, Crohn disease, and *Clostridium difficile* colitis. This article reviews the clinical and imaging findings of patients who present acutely with infectious and inflammatory enterocolitides. The acute abdomen can be defined as the sudden onset (generally <24 hours) of severe localized or generalized abdominal pain that prompts the patient to seek immediate medical assistance; most often a visit to the emergency department.

Acute urinary tract disorders often manifest as flank pain and are a common complaint of patients who present to the emergency department. The pain is often a vague, poorly localized sensation that may have a variety of causes. Laboratory and clinical findings, such as hematuria, are neither sensitive nor specific for determining the cause of the flank pain. Accordingly, imaging is an important tool in determining a diagnosis and management plan. Patients with acute urinary tract disorders who present with pain include those with calculi as well as renal infection, vascular disorders, and hemorrhage.

Premenopausal women with acute pelvic pain comprise a significant percentage of patients who present to the emergency room. Etiologies can be gynecologic, urologic, gastrointestinal, or vascular. Signs and symptoms are often nonspecific and overlapping. The choice of imaging modality is determined by the clinically suspected differential diagnosis. Ultrasound (US) is the preferred imaging modality for suspected obstetric or gynecologic disorders. CT is more useful when gastrointestinal or urinary tract pathology is likely. MR imaging is rarely used in the emergent setting, except to exclude appendicitis in pregnant women. This article presents a comprehensive review of imaging of acute gynecologic disorders.

Acute abdominal pain in pregnancy presents diagnostic and therapeutic challenges. Ultrasound remains the primary imaging investigation of the pregnant abdomen because of its availability, portability, and lack of ionizing radiation. MR imaging has been shown to be useful in the diagnosis of gynecologic and obstetric problems and in the setting of acute abdomen during pregnancy. MR imaging is often used when ultrasound is inconclusive. Computed tomography is the investigation of choice when there is a life-threatening situation and in case of traumatic injuries, when a rapid diagnosis is required.

Cross-sectional imaging plays a crucial role in the triage of patients with acute abdominal pain. Ionizing radiation exposure is a recognized drawback of computed tomography (CT), the primary imaging technique. MR imaging is a promising alternative to CT; it provides excellent image quality with high-contrast resolution without the disadvantages of ionizing radiation and iodinated contrast. This article provides a basic overview of the typical MR findings of the most frequent disease entities encountered in the setting of the nontraumatic acute abdomen, including direct comparison with CT findings to familiarize the readers with these same findings on MR.

PROGRAM OBJECTIVE

The objective of the *Radiologic Clinics of North America* is to keep practicing radiologists and radiology residents up to date with current clinical practice in radiology by providing timely articles reviewing the state of the art in patient care.

TARGET AUDIENCE

Practicing radiologists, radiology residents, and other health care professionals who provide patient care utilizing radiologic findings.

LEARNING OBJECTIVES

Upon completion of this activity, participants will be able to:
1. Review strategies in evaluating pain in each abdominal quadrant.
2. Discuss the evaluation of gastrointestinal disorders such as enterocolitis and bowel obstruction.
3. Recognize differences in the evaluation and treatment of acute gynecolgcal disorders between pregnant and non-pregnant patients.

ACCREDITATION

The Elsevier Office of Continuing Medical Education (EOCME) is accredited by the Accreditation Council for Continuing Medical Education (ACCME) to provide continuing medical education for physicians.

The EOCME designates this enduring material for a maximum of 15 *AMA PRA Category 1 Credit*(s)™. Physicians should claim only the credit commensurate with the extent of their participation in the activity.

All other health care professionals requesting continuing education credit for this enduring material will be issued a certificate of participation.

DISCLOSURE OF CONFLICTS OF INTEREST

The EOCME assesses conflict of interest with its instructors, faculty, planners, and other individuals who are in a position to control the content of CME activities. All relevant conflicts of interest that are identified are thoroughly vetted by EOCME for fair balance, scientific objectivity, and patient care recommendations. EOCME is committed to providing its learners with CME activities that promote improvements or quality in healthcare and not a specific proprietary business or a commercial interest.

The planning committee, staff, authors and editors listed below have identified no financial relationships or relationships to products or devices they or their spouse/life partner have with commercial interest related to the content of this CME activity:
Mark E. Baker, MD, FACR, FSAR, FSCBTMR; Peter Bannas, MD; Genevieve L. Bennett, MD; Jonathan W. Berlin, MD; Nicholas A. Bodmer, MD; Martina Derme, MD; Harpreet S. Dhatt, MD; Carolyn K. Donaldson, MD; Jacob S. Ecanow, MD; Anjali Fortna; Marialuisa Framarino-dei-Malatesta, MD; Rakhee H. Goel, MD; Richard M. Gore, MD; Gianfranco Gualdi, MD; Jay P. Heiken, MD; Francesca Laghi, MD; Gabriele Masselli, MD; Uday K. Mehta, MD; Vincent M. Mellnick, MD; Frank H. Miller, MD; Aaron Miracle, MD; Neel B. Patel, MD; Erick M. Remer, MD; Erin Scheckenbach; Robert I. Silvers, MD; Karthik Subramaniam; Kiran H. Thakrar, MD; Ruedi F. Thoeni, MD; Raman Unnikrishnan, MD; John Vassallo; Zhen Jane Wang, MD; Daniel R. Wenzke, MD.

The planning committee, staff, authors and editors listed below have identified financial relationships or relationships to products or devices they or their spouse/life partner have with commercial interest related to the content of this CME activity:
Spencer C. Behr, MD is a consultant/advisor for, with research support from, General Electric Company, and is a consultant/advisor for Grand Rounds.
Geraldine M. Newmark, MD has stock ownership in, and an employment affiliation with, Abbvie Inc. and OPKO Health Inc.
Perry J. Pickhardt, MD is a consultant/advisor for Check-Cap Ltd. and Bracco Diagnostics Inc., has stock ownership in Cellectar BioSciences, and is a co-founder of VirtuoCTC, LLC.
Benjamin M. Yeh, MD has stock ownership in Nextrast, Inc, research support from General Electric Company and the National Institutes of Health, and receives royalties/patents from Oxford University Press.

UNAPPROVED/OFF-LABEL USE DISCLOSURE

The EOCME requires CME faculty to disclose to the participants:
1. When products or procedures being discussed are off-label, unlabelled, experimental, and/or investigational (not US Food and Drug Administration [FDA] approved); and
2. Any limitations on the information presented, such as data that are preliminary or that represent ongoing research, interim analyses, and/or unsupported opinions. Faculty may discuss information about pharmaceutical agents that is outside of FDA-approved labelling. This information is intended solely for CME and is not intended to promote off-label use of these medications. If you have any questions, contact the medical affairs department of the manufacturer for the most recent prescribing information.

TO ENROLL

To enroll in the *Radiologic Clinics of North America* Continuing Medical Education program, call customer service at 1-800-654-2452 or sign up online at http://www.theclinics.com/home/cme. The CME program is available to subscribers for an additional annual fee of USD 315.

METHOD OF PARTICIPATION

In order to claim credit, participants must complete the following:

1. Complete enrolment as indicated above.
2. Read the activity.
3. Complete the CME Test and Evaluation. Participants must achieve a score of 70% on the test. All CME Tests and Evaluations must be completed online.

CME INQUIRIES/SPECIAL NEEDS

For all CME inquiries or special needs, please contact elsevierCME@elsevier.com.

RADIOLOGIC CLINICS OF NORTH AMERICA

ISSUE OF RELATED INTEREST

Magnetic Resonance Imaging Clinics, November 2015 (Vol. 23, Issue 4)
MR-Guided Interventions
Clare M. Tempany and Tina Kapur, *Editors*
http://www.mri.theclinics.com

THE CLINICS ARE AVAILABLE ONLINE!
Access your subscription at:
www.theclinics.com

Preface
Imaging of the Acute Abdomen

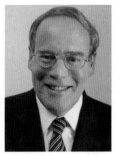

Richard M. Gore, MD
Editor

The term acute abdomen defines a clinical syndrome characterized by the sudden onset of severe abdominal pain requiring emergency medical or surgical treatment. It is one of the most frequent reasons for presentation of an adult to the emergency department, ranging from 4% to 10% of admissions. A prompt and accurate diagnosis is essential to minimize morbidity and mortality in these patients. The differential diagnosis includes a spectrum of infectious, inflammatory, ischemic, obstructive, hemorrhagic, and neoplastic disorders. The acute abdomen can also reflect extra-abdominal conditions, including cardiac, pulmonary, endocrine, or metabolic disorders.

The clinical diagnosis in patients with the acute abdomen is challenging because the clinical presentation as well as the results of physical examination and laboratory examination are often nonspecific and nondiagnostic. Sonography has developed a niche in evaluating the gallbladder in all patients and the appendix in children and pregnant women. MRI is being used with increasing frequency in pregnant women and children. MDCT has emerged as the premier imaging technique for the triage of most patients with the acute abdomen. MDCT has earned this role because of its ability to provide a global perspective of the gut, mesenteries, omenta, peritoneum, retroperitoneum, subperitoneum, and extraperitoneal spaces uninhibited by the presence of bowel gas and fat. Multiplanar reformatted images can be obtained with isotropic data sets facilitating accurate radiologic diagnosis.

In this issue of *Radiologic Clinics of North America*, the radiologic investigation of patients with the acute abdomen is presented using both a location-specific (eg, left upper quadrant pain) and a disease-specific (eg, bowel obstruction) approach. The organizing principle of this issue is the integration of rapidly changing information, common sense, and good judgement for the development of an expeditious approach to these often complicated patients. It is hoped that this issue provides a useful resource for guiding patient imaging in the setting of the acute abdomen.

Richard M. Gore, MD
Department of Radiology
Chief, Section of Gastrointestinal Radiology
North Shore University Health System
University of Chicago
Evanston Hospital
2650 Ridge Avenue
Evanston, IL 60201, USA

E-mail address:
rgore@uchicago.edu

Radiol Clin N Am 53 (2015) xv
http://dx.doi.org/10.1016/j.rcl.2015.08.010
0033-8389/15/$ – see front matter © 2015 Published by Elsevier Inc.

Evaluating Patients with Right Upper Quadrant Pain

Genevieve L. Bennett, MD

KEYWORDS

- Cholecystitis • Cholelithiasis • Choledocholithiasis • Gallstone ileus • Hepatitis
- Budd-Chiari syndrome • Portal vein thrombosis

KEY POINTS

- Many disorders of the liver, gallbladder, and biliary tree may cause right upper quadrant pain and clinical diagnosis may be challenging. Imaging plays a key role in establishing a prompt diagnosis and guiding appropriate management.
- Although ultrasonography is the initial imaging modality of choice for most hepatobiliary disorders, radionuclide imaging, computed tomography (CT), and MR imaging also play important roles.
- Acute cholecystitis may be associated with many complications, including gangrenous change, emphysematous and hemorrhagic cholecystitis, and perforation. These complications have characteristic imaging features that should be recognized.
- MR cholangiopancreatography achieves high accuracy in diagnosis of choledocholithiasis and allows for noninvasive imaging when ultrasonography and CT are indeterminate.

Right upper quadrant abdominal pain is 1 of the most common reasons for visits to the emergency department. Although acute cholecystitis is often the leading diagnostic consideration, there are many other causes of right upper quadrant pain and establishing a prompt and accurate diagnosis may be challenging. In this article, imaging evaluation of the most common causes of right upper quadrant abdominal pain is reviewed. Although abnormalities of the bowel or pancreas, such as peptic ulcer disease or pancreatitis, may be a cause of right upper quadrant pain, this article focuses on disorders of the liver, gallbladder, and biliary tract. In evaluation of these diseases, radiographs are generally of limited value. Ultrasonography is usually the initial imaging modality of choice for suspected hepatobiliary disease; however, there are also important roles for radionuclide hepatobiliary imaging, computed tomography (CT), and MR imaging. In this article, the complementary roles of these various imaging modalities in evaluation of the patient with right upper quadrant pain are discussed.

HEPATIC CAUSES OF ACUTE RIGHT UPPER QUADRANT PAIN

Hepatic diseases that may present with right upper quadrant pain include acute hepatitis, infection complicated by abscess formation, acute complications of chronic liver disease, and hepatic masses and vascular abnormalities.

Acute Hepatitis

Hepatitis is a nonspecific inflammatory response of the liver to a wide variety of agents that cause hepatobiliary injury. The leading cause of hepatitis, both acute and chronic, is viral infection. Other

Disclosures: The author has no disclosures.
Abdominal Imaging Division, Department of Radiology, NYU Langone Medical Center, 660 First Avenue, Room 332, New York, NY 10016, USA
E-mail address: genevieve.bennett@med.nyu.edu

Radiol Clin N Am 53 (2015) 1093–1130
http://dx.doi.org/10.1016/j.rcl.2015.06.002

causes include alcohol abuse, toxins, drug-induced injury, inherited metabolic disorders, ischemic injury, and autoimmune diseases.[1–3] Despite extensive evaluation, some cases remain indeterminate in cause. In addition to right upper quadrant pain, patients with hepatitis usually present with an enlarged, tender liver on physical examination, jaundice, and abnormal liver function tests.[4] Depending on the degree of hepatic dysfunction, there may be coagulopathy, ascites, encephalopathy, and ultimate progression to fulminant liver failure. Chronically, there may also be progression to fibrosis and cirrhosis. Clinical history, hepatitis serologies, and serum toxin levels help to establish the diagnosis. An important role of imaging in this setting is to exclude other conditions that may produce similar clinical and laboratory abnormalities, including extrahepatic cholestasis and diffuse metastatic disease.

The incidence of viral infection as a cause of acute liver failure shows wide geographic variation and depends on local prevalence of hepatotropic infections.[1] Hepatitis A and hepatitis E are transmitted via the fecal-oral route, most commonly through contaminated food and water. Acute infection may be self-limited or more fulminant, resulting in acute liver failure in less than 1% of affected patients.[1] Hepatitis B virus and hepatitis C virus are transmitted vertically or horizontally through exposure to contaminated blood or other body fluids via parenteral or mucosal exposure. Fewer than 4% of cases of acute viral hepatitis B lead to liver failure but mortality is higher than with hepatitis A or E.[1] The acute phase of HCV is often asymptomatic or very mild, and chronic hepatitis C infection is more common than fulminant infection in Western countries.[2] Less common viral causes of hepatitis include herpes simplex virus types 1 and 2, varicella zoster virus, Epstein-Barr virus, cytomegalovirus, and parvovirus B19.[1,5]

The imaging findings of the different causes of acute hepatitis are nonspecific and overlap. Hepatomegaly and periportal edema are common findings. At sonography, the edematous, inflamed liver is notable for decreased echogenicity of the parenchyma with increased prominence and brightness of the portal vein walls, which appear more echogenic in the background of the edematous liver.[6,7] This results in the so-called starry-night liver appearance (Fig. 1A); however, this pattern is nonspecific and may occasionally be observed in normal patients.[8] This appearance has also been seen in leukemia, lymphoma, and severe hepatic congestion.[9] Because of periportal edema in hepatitis, the gallbladder wall is often markedly thickened with an edematous and striated appearance[10–13] (see Fig. 1B). However, unlike acute cholecystitis, the gallbladder lumen in hepatitis is nondistended. Findings of acute hepatitis at CT include an enlarged liver with periportal edema that appears as low-attenuation tracking along the portal vessels, gallbladder wall thickening, and heterogeneous arterial-phase contrast enhancement[14–17] (Fig. 2). Reactive lymphadenopathy may be seen in the porta hepatis.

Gallbladder wall thickening may be observed in 51% to 91% of patients with acute hepatitis and a recent study suggested that the degree of gallbladder wall thickening may be a predictor of the severity of acute hepatitis or prolonged cholestasis.[18] On MR imaging, increased periportal T2 signal in the liver is compatible with periportal edema. Similar to CT, there is often patchy enhancement of the liver parenchyma on arterial-phase images that normalizes on later phases of enhancement, and gallbladder wall thickening.[16,17]

Alcoholic liver disease is one of the main causes of end-stage liver disease worldwide and encompasses a disease spectrum from steatosis, to steatohepatitis, in which there is steatosis,

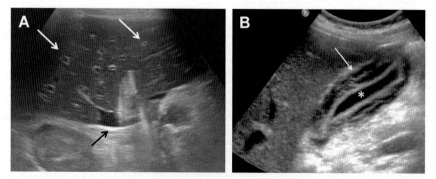

Fig. 1. Acute hepatitis: ultrasonography. (A) A 29-year-old man with acute hepatitis. There is increased prominence of the periportal echoes caused by periportal edema (white arrows), and a small amount of perihepatic ascites fluid (black arrow). (B) There is marked thickening and edema of the gallbladder wall (white arrow). The gallbladder lumen is collapsed (asterisk), helping to distinguish it from acute cholecystitis.

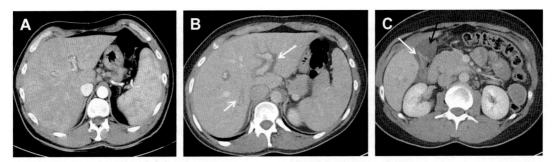

Fig. 2. Acute hepatitis: CT. (*A*) Image acquired during arterial phase of contrast enhancement shows patchy, heterogeneous enhancement of the liver caused by of edema. (*B*) Portal venous-phase image shows periportal low attenuation compatible with edema (*arrows*). (*C*) The gallbladder wall is markedly edematous and thickened (*black arrow*). The enhancing mucosa defines the collapsed lumen (*white arrow*).

inflammation, and fibrosis in the liver, and ultimately cirrhosis.[19] Alcoholic hepatitis is an acute form of alcohol-induced liver injury seen in patients who consume large quantities of alcohol for a prolonged period of time. There is a spectrum of severity that ranges from asymptomatic abnormality of liver function tests to fulminant liver failure and even death.[20] Patients with severe disease present with fever, jaundice, and abdominal tenderness, and there may be progression to multiorgan liver failure with reported short-term morbidity and mortality of 40% to 50%.[19] There are clinical scoring systems that assess the severity of alcoholic hepatitis, and liver biopsy may also be performed for staging of liver injury. Treatment of acute disease may include corticosteroids and anti–tumor necrosis factor alpha therapy.[21] Diagnosis of alcoholic hepatitis is generally established based on history, physical examination, and laboratory abnormalities.[20]

The hallmark of alcoholic liver disease on ultrasonography is hepatic steatosis. The liver is enlarged with increased echogenicity with associated acoustic attenuation and limited penetration,

resulting in decreased visualization of the portal and hepatic vein walls and diaphragm[16,22] (**Fig. 3**A). On CT, the liver is enlarged and shows decreased attenuation. Normal unenhanced liver parenchyma measures 45 to 65 Hounsfield units (HU) in density, generally more than 8 HU greater than that of the spleen. If density of the liver is 10 HU less than spleen on unenhanced scans or 25 HU less than the spleen on contrast-enhanced scan, this suggests steatosis[16,17] (see **Fig. 3**B). MR is the most sensitive and specific technique for detection of fat. Signal drop-out on opposed-phase chemical shift images or fat-suppressed MR sequences confirms the presence of fat[16,17] (see **Fig. 3**C). Similar findings may be observed in hepatic steatosis from other causes, including diabetes and obesity.

Hepatic Infection with Abscess Formation

Hepatic infections leading to abscess formation include pyogenic infection, amebiasis, and fungal and parasitic diseases. Infection of the liver can occur by hematogenous spread via the portal

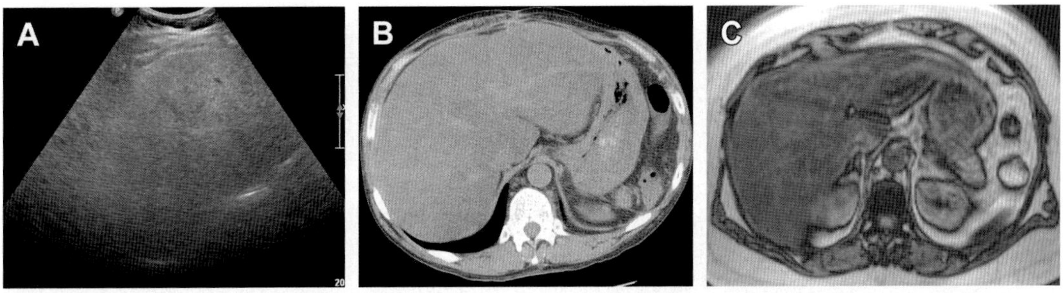

Fig. 3. Hepatic steatosis in the setting of alcoholic hepatitis. (*A*) Ultrasonography shows an enlarged liver with diffusely increased and heterogeneous echogenicity and acoustic attenuation. Portal vein radicles, hepatic veins, and diaphragm are not well visualized because of decreased penetration. (*B*) Unenhanced CT shows enlarged liver with decreased attenuation. There is increased attenuation of the hepatic vessels caused by the decreased density of the liver parenchyma. (*C*) Out-of-phase chemical shift MR imaging shows diffusely decreased signal in the liver compatible with the presence of fat.

vein or hepatic artery, ascending infection from the biliary tract, or from trauma. Throughout the world, *Entamoeba histolytica* is the most common cause of liver abscess, but, in developed countries, pyogenic liver abscess is more common.[23] Fungal infection most often occurs in immune suppressed patients, whereas parasitic infections generally occur after travel to endemic areas, such as Asia, Africa, and South America. Definitive diagnosis is made with history, serology, or culture from abscess, blood, or stool. Liver abscesses may be fatal if not promptly treated, often requiring a combination of both antibiotics and either surgical or percutaneous drainage.

Pyogenic liver abscesses most often result from biliary obstruction or hematogenous spread from a bowel source. In the past, it was thought that most hepatic abscesses were caused by *Escherichia coli* and originated from an infectious source in the bowel, such as diverticulitis; however, *Klebsiella pneumoniae* is now a more common cause of community-acquired pyogenic liver abscess.[22] In many instances, the infection is polymicrobial. Clinical symptoms include right upper quadrant pain, fever, and jaundice. Laboratory values show leukocytosis and abnormal liver function tests.

Imaging evaluation in suspected liver abscess usually begins with ultrasonography, with CT or MR imaging serving as helpful adjuncts if diagnosis is equivocal, for further evaluation before intervention, or to determine cause.[23–25] On sonography, the appearance of liver abscesses is variable; however, early in the evolution of abscess formation, before liquefaction, the abscess may have a solid appearance and mimic a mass or neoplasm, which is a potential pitfall[22] (Fig. 4A). Multifocal liver abscesses may mimic metastasis, and the clinical history and laboratory findings are critical in suggesting the correct diagnosis in

this setting. As necrosis and liquefaction progress, the abscess becomes increasingly cystic with a complex appearance with thick irregular wall, septations, and internal echoes and debris (Fig. 5A). Posterior acoustic enhancement confirms the fluid content. Doppler may show flow in the liver around the abscess and within the parenchymal septations. Markedly increased echogenicity with associated reverberation artifact suggests the presence of gas in the lesion.

On contrast-enhanced CT or MR, a low-density lesion with thick enhancing rim is the most common finding (see Figs. 4–6). The lesions may be single and nonloculated, or multiple and multiloculated.[26] Multiple small coalescing hypoattenuating lesions corresponding with the cluster sign is a typical appearance[27] (see Fig. 4C). The double-target sign corresponds with a low-attenuation central area surrounded by a high-attenuation inner ring and low-attenuation zone.[26] Occasionally, gas or a fluid-fluid level may be observed. Because of the inflammation and hyperemia in the adjacent liver parenchyma, there is often an associated transient hepatic-attenuation difference. Recently, the CT features of liver abscesses caused by *K pneumoniae* were described.[28] These features include a single abscess, unilobar involvement, solid appearance, association with thrombophlebitis, and hematogenous complications.

On MR imaging, early intensely enhancing abscess walls, which persist in thickness and intensity on delayed images, and prominent perilesional contrast enhancement are distinctive characteristics of liver abscesses (see Fig. 5C).[29] On MR imaging, abscesses and malignant lesions may have overlapping imaging features, including T1 hypointensity, T2 hyperintensity, and rim arterial enhancement. Recently, the added value of diffusion-weighted imaging has been shown in differentiating hepatic abscess from malignant

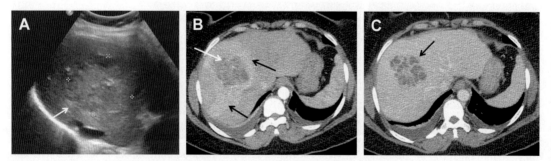

Fig. 4. Liver abscess. (*A*) Ultrasonography shows lesion of mixed echogenicity in the right hepatic lobe, mostly solid in appearance (*white arrow*). (*B*) Arterial phase of contrast-enhanced CT shows hypoattenuating lesion (*white arrow*) with associated increased perilesional enhancement caused by hyperemia from adjacent hepatic inflammation (*black arrows*). (*C*) Portal venous phase of contrast enhancement shows the abscess with multiple enhancing septations and loculations with a clustered appearance (*black arrow*).

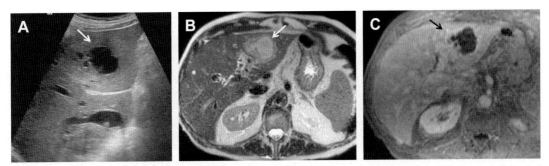

Fig. 5. Liver abscess ultrasonography and MR imaging. (*A*) Ultrasonography shows anechoic lesion in left hepatic lobe (*arrow*). (*B*) Single-shot fast spin-echo (SSFSE) MR image shows lesion with increased signal and thick, irregular wall (*arrow*). (*C*) Contrast-enhanced T1-weighted gradient-echo image shows thick enhancing wall (*arrow*).

mimickers.[30–32] These studies have shown that the center of an abscess may have lower apparent diffusion coefficient (ADC) values than that of a necrotic metastasis because of the presence of inflammatory cells, bacteria, necrotic tissue, and proteinaceous exudates, whereas the rim of an abscess shows higher ADC values because of decreased cellularity and increased extracellular fluid secondary to inflammation (**Fig. 7**). However, considerable overlap exists and the appearance of an abscess on diffusion-weighted imaging may vary depending on the stage of evolution.[33]

Amebic liver abscess is caused by the protozoa, *E histolytica*, and is spread by the fecal-oral route. Hepatic abscess results from ascending infection through the portal venous system. This infection is most prevalent in India, Africa, the Far East, and Central and South America; therefore, a history of recent travel to these areas is helpful in suggesting the diagnosis. Unlike pyogenic liver abscess, these abscesses tend to be solitary. Enzyme immunoassays specific for *E histolytica* circulating antibodies may aid in the diagnosis.

On sonography, there is a hypoechoic and homogeneous round or oval-shaped lesion with posterior acoustic enhancement, usually near or contiguous with the liver capsule. If there is disruption of the liver capsule, this is a highly suggestive finding.[23] On CT and MR, an amebic liver abscesses often appear as a round or oval low-attenuation mass that may contain septation.[23–25] The wall is generally 3 to 15 mm thick, enhances with contrast, and may be surrounded by a rim of edema (**Fig. 8**). If the abscess ruptures, lung abscess or pericardial effusion may be an associated complication. Medical treatment with nitroimidazole is effective in more than 90% of patients. Aspiration is only recommended if the patient fails to respond to treatment, if there is left lobe abscess, or if there is high risk of rupture.[23]

Fungal infection of the liver generally occurs in immune compromised patients and is most often seen in patients with prolonged neutropenia in the setting of leukemia and patients treated with chemotherapy. *Candida* is the most common organism, with *Aspergillus*, *Cryptococcus*, *Histoplasma*, and *Mucor* less frequently identified.[23–26]

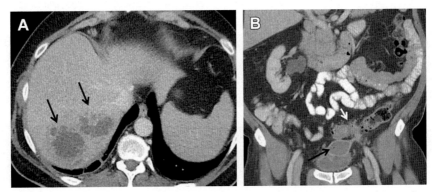

Fig. 6. Liver abscess secondary to diverticulitis in a 60-year-old man with right upper quadrant pain and fever. (*A*) Contrast-enhanced CT shows complex fluid-attenuation lesions with thickened, irregular walls (*arrows*) compatible with abscesses in the right hepatic lobe. (*B*) Coronal reformatted image of the pelvis shows sigmoid diverticulitis (*white arrow*) with abscess formation (*black arrow*) superior to the bladder.

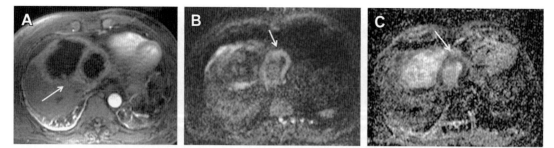

Fig. 7. Necrotic hepatic metastasis from squamous cell carcinoma. (*A*) Arterial-phase gradient-echo T1-weighted image shows 2 coalescing lesions with decreased signal intensity and rim enhancing wall (*arrow*). Appearance may mimic an abscess. (*B*) Diffusion-weighted image shows increased signal in the wall (*arrow*). (*C*) ADC map shows decreased signal in the wall (*arrow*) compatible with diffusion restriction, which is more consistent with a metastasis.

Lesions are typically small, measuring less than 1 cm. At ultrasonography, 4 different patterns have been described, including wheel-within-wheel appearance, bulls-eye appearance, hypoechoic lesions, and echogenic foci with variable posterior acoustic shadowing[34] (**Fig. 9**A). Typical CT findings include multiple small, round, low-attenuation lesions corresponding with microabscesses with ring enhancement on arterial-phase images (see **Fig. 9**B). Blood cultures in patients with candida infection are positive in only 20% of patients.[35] Diagnosis may be made on imaging, fine-needle biopsy, and response to antifungal therapy.

Parasitic diseases, including schistosomiasis, echinococcus, and toxocariasis may also result in hepatic abscess formation. Schistosomiasis is endemic to Africa, Asia, South America, and the Caribbean and is transmitted by freshwater snails. The most common species infecting humans include *Schistosoma mansoni*, *Schistosoma japonicum*, and *Schistosoma haematobium*. Schistosomes penetrate the human skin and move to the mesenteric veins. The eggs are subsequently carried by the portal vein to the liver.

Ultrasonography shows fibrous hyperechoic bands along the portal vein and branches caused by periportal fibrosis. CT findings of *S mansoni* include low-attenuation bands around the portal vein and branches in the central liver with contrast enhancement. Associated findings include hepatosplenomegaly, cirrhosis, ascites, collateral circulation, portal vein thrombosis, and varices.[36] With *S japonicum* infection, CT shows calcification along portal tracts in the periphery of the liver with a turtle-back appearance. Egg deposition and resultant calcification also occur along the subcapsular liver. There is contrast enhancement of periportal fibrosis and the thickened subcapsule.

Echinococcus, or hydatid disease, results from ingestion of food or water contaminated with echinococcal eggs. The eggs hatch in the duodenum, penetrate the intestinal mucosa, and enter the portal circulation, where they travel to the liver lungs and bone. *Echinococcus granulosus* is the most common form of infection and produces unilocular cysts and is endemic to Mediterranean countries, the Middle East, eastern Europe, Africa, Argentina, Chile, China, Australia, and New Zealand. *Echinococcus multilocularis* is found in the

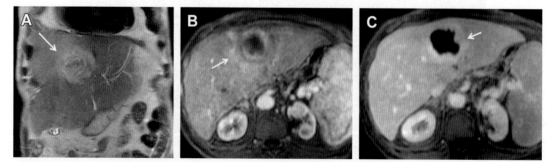

Fig. 8. Amebic liver abscess. (*A*) SSFSE image shows a single lesion of mixed signal with rim of edema (*arrow*). (*B*) Arterial-phase T1-weighted gradient-echo image shows single lesion with double-target sign rim enhancement and surrounding hyperemia (*arrow*). (*C*) Portal venous-phase T1-weighted gradient-echo image shows thick enhancing rim (*arrow*).

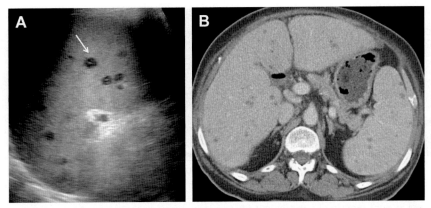

Fig. 9. Disseminated candidiasis in a patient with acute myelogenous leukemia. (*A*) Ultrasonography of the liver shows multiple small hypoechoic lesions (*arrow*). (*B*) Contrast-enhanced CT shows multiple small hypoattenuating lesions in the liver and spleen.

United States, Canada, and central and northern Eurasia, and produces multiloculated alveolar cysts. Patients with echinococcus may be asymptomatic for many years when the cyst is small. When the cyst enlarges, it may cause abdominal pain, palpable mass, and obstructive jaundice. Cyst rupture may result in anaphylaxis and spread to other parts of the body. Imaging is helpful in establishing the diagnosis because serology has variable sensitivity and specificity.[23–25] On ultrasonography, *E granulosus* cysts are thick walled with a double-line appearance and daughter cysts are frequently seen in the main cyst. The snowflake sign refers to the free-floating protoscoleces or hydatid sand that can be seen floating in the cyst. The water-lily sign refers to the detachment of the endocystic membranes that float in the cyst. Wall calcification may be thick and dense or thin.

On CT, *E granulosus* cysts are low attenuation and daughter cysts are observed in 75% of cases.[23] Daughter cysts show lower attenuation because of free-floating scolices in the main cyst. If there is mural calcification, this suggests absence of active infection (**Fig. 10**). Differential diagnosis includes other cystic lesions, including biliary cystadenoma, pyogenic liver abscess, and cystic metastasis. The presence of daughter cysts and curvilinear wall calcification in *E granulosus* and multiple small-clustered cystic and solid components with central ill-defined calcifications in *E multilocularis* help to suggest the diagnosis.[37] Antihelminthic drugs are the first-line therapy. For *E granulosus*, percutaneous drainage with instillation of a scolicidal agent may also be used. *E multilocularis* is highly invasive and wide local resection with hepatic lobectomy or liver transplant may be required.

Vascular Abnormalities of the Liver

Portal vein thrombosis

Portal vein thrombosis may occur in various settings, including cirrhosis, cholangitis, pancreatitis, appendicitis, diverticulitis, neoplasms such as hepatocellular carcinoma, pancreatic carcinoma, hypercoagulable states, and surgery, including liver transplantation.[38] In cirrhotic patients, bland thrombosis occurs in 11.2% to 15.8% of patients because of hypertension-related portal venous stasis.[39] Hepatocellular carcinoma may invade the portal vein directly in up to 44% of patients and this is a prominent feature of the diffusely infiltrative subtype[40] (**Fig. 11**). In these patients, thrombus often includes a combination of both bland and tumor thrombus. Pylephlebitis of the

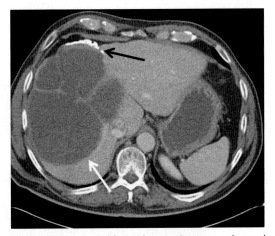

Fig. 10. Echinococcal liver abscess. Contrast-enhanced CT shows multiloculated cystic lesion (*white arrow*) with mural calcification (*black arrow*) compatible with chronic infection.

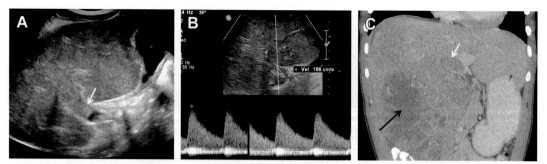

Fig. 11. Portal vein thrombosis caused by infiltrating hepatocellular carcinoma. (*A*) Gray-scale ultrasonography shows echogenic material in the main portal vein (*arrow*) compatible with thrombus. (*B*) Doppler image shows arterial flow in the thrombus compatible with tumor thrombus. (*C*) Coronal reformatted CT image shows large infiltrating mass in right lobe (*black arrow*) and filling defect expanding main portal vein (*white arrow*).

portal vein and associated thrombosis may result from a primary inflammatory process of the liver, such as hepatitis, or may propagate from the mesenteric veins in the setting of bowel inflammation, including diverticulitis and appendicitis (**Fig. 12**). Treatment of acute thrombosis includes both antibiotics and anticoagulation.

Ultrasonography depicts acute thrombosis as a dilated portal vein with absence of flow. Acute clot is often hypoechoic, whereas more chronic clot is hyperechoic.[38] Low-velocity flow may be seen in portal hypertension and must be differentiated from thrombosis using color, power, and spectral Doppler. Increased hepatic arterial flow is often observed. Arterial flow may be shown within the thrombus in the setting of tumor thrombus (see **Fig. 11B**). If ultrasonography is equivocal, or to better evaluate the extent of the thrombus, contrast-enhanced CT and MR imaging may be helpful. Again, acute thrombosis is usually associated with expansion and peripheral enhancement of the vein. Associated perfusional abnormality in the liver parenchyma is also observed with foci of increased enhancement on the arterial phase and decreased enhancement in the peripheral phase. Subacute and chronic thrombosis manifests as cavernous transformation of the portal vein, which refers to multiple tortuous venous collaterals at the porta hepatis that replace the portal vein.[41] There is also splenomegaly and portosystemic collateral formation. With malignant thrombus, arterial flow may be shown in the thrombus on Doppler ultrasonography and there may be enhancement at contrast-enhanced CT and MR. Acute thrombosis is treated with anticoagulation therapy. Thrombolysis and surgical thrombectomy may be required in certain cases.

Budd-Chiari Syndrome

Budd-Chiari syndrome (BCS) is defined as lobar or segmental hepatic venous outflow obstruction at any level from the small hepatic veins to the junction of the inferior vena cava (IVC) and the right atrium, regardless of the cause of the obstruction.[42] Hepatic venous outflow obstruction results in increase of sinusoidal pressure and diminished portal venous flow, resulting in centrilobular congestion and ultimately necrosis and atrophy.[43] In the acute form, there may be rapid development

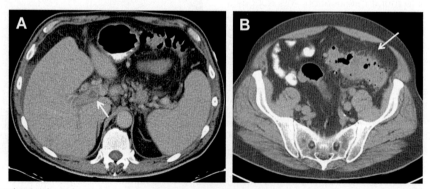

Fig. 12. Portal vein thrombosis caused by acute diverticulitis. (*A*) Contrast-enhanced CT shows filling defect in main portal vein (*arrow*). (*B*) Image through the pelvis shows diverticulitis of the sigmoid colon (*arrow*).

of hepatocellular necrosis, which is less common in the subacute or chronic forms. Most cases are acquired, with thrombus formation resulting in concentric thickening of the vein wall and subintimal fibrosis. There is a continuum from fresh thrombus to organized thrombus, fibrous tissue, recanalization, and calcification.[44] Many thrombotic disorders have been associated with BCS, including protein C and protein S deficiency, antiphospholipid syndrome, paroxysmal nocturnal hemoglobinuria, and myeloproliferative disorders.[45] In women, use of oral contraceptives, pregnancy, and the postpartum period have been associated with BCS.[46] Other causes include systemic lupus erythematosus, mixed connective tissue disease, Sjögren syndrome, nephrotic syndrome and protein-losing enteropathy, chemotherapy and radiation, bone marrow transplantation, and antineoplastic drug therapy.[42,43] Women are affected more than men and constituted 67% of patients in one series.[47]

Clinical presentation of BCS is variable and may be fulminant, acute, subacute, or chronic.[43] If fulminant, there may be rapid development of hepatic encephalopathy within 8 weeks after onset of jaundice. In the acute form, there is rapid onset of jaundice and ascites. The subacute or chronic form is more gradual and may be complicated by portal hypertension. Treatment is directed at the underlying cause with anticoagulant therapy for bland thrombus.

Ultrasonography, CT, and MR imaging may establish a diagnosis of BCS with absent venous flow the hallmark. Imaging manifestations depend on the stage of the disease. Doppler ultrasonography has a reported sensitivity of 87.5%.[48] Contrast-enhanced CT confirms the diagnosis with failure of contrast enhancement of the hepatic veins and inhomogeneous perfusion yielding a mottled appearance of the liver (**Fig. 13**). In the acute form, the liver is diffusely hypoattenuating and enlarged but morphologically normal, with narrowing of IVC and hepatic veins.[49] Signs of portal hypertension are often evident with splenomegaly and ascites. MR imaging shows similar findings (**Fig. 14**). Venous drainage of the caudate lobe is directly into the IVC and a compensatory increase in the venous drainage of this lobe occurs in BCS, resulting in hypertrophy of this lobe. In the acute phase, there is increased enhancement of the caudate lobe and central portion of the liver around the IVC with deceased peripheral enhancement. This pattern reverses in the portal venous phase with enhancement from capsular veins and washout from the central portion of the liver.[50] In the chronic phase, there is caudate lobe hypertrophy and atrophy of the peripheral segments with development of collateral circulatory pathways, including systemic, portosystemic, and intrahepatic vessels[49,51] (**Fig. 15**). Formation of benign hypervascular regenerative nodules is common in BCS and they range in size from 0.5 to 4 cm.[42] They are thought to result from compensatory hypertrophy of areas of the liver where arterial blood flow is preserved but portal inflow is reduced. These nodules generally show marked arterial-phase enhancement without washout in the portal venous phase, which helps to differentiate them from hepatocellular carcinoma[52] (see **Figs. 13A and 14A**). Large regenerative nodules may resemble focal nodular hyperplasia at imaging and histopathology.[53]

Cirrhosis is frequent but risk of hepatocellular carcinoma (HCC) in BCS is unknown. Biopsy of a suspicious or enlarging focal lesion, increase in alpha fetoprotein level, or resection of a suspicious nodule may confirm the diagnosis of HCC. Treatment involves treatment of the underlying disease followed by anticoagulation, vascular intervention, or liver transplantation.

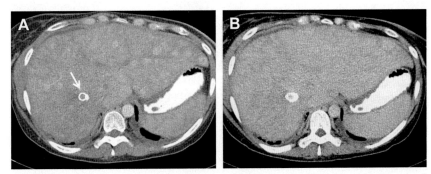

Fig. 13. BCS: CT findings. (*A*) Arterial-phase CT shows enlarged liver with multiple enhancing nodules. A transjugular intrahepatic portosystemic shunt (TIPS) is present (*arrow*). (*B*) Portal venous phase shows heterogeneous enhancement at periphery of liver with nonvisualization of the hepatic veins.

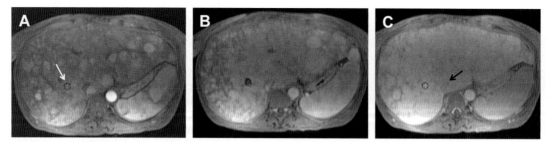

Fig. 14. BCS: MR findings. (*A*) Arterial-phase T1-weighted gradient-echo image shows multiple enhancing nodules. A TIPS (*arrow*) is present. (*B*) Early portal venous-phase image shows marked heterogeneous patchy enhancement, particularly at liver periphery. (*C*) Delayed portal venous phase shows persistent heterogeneous enhancement and lack of visualization of the hepatic veins. IVC is small in caliber (*black arrow*).

Hepatic Neoplasms

Primary and secondary hepatic neoplasms may be a cause of right upper quadrant pain if there are associated complications, most importantly hemorrhage and associated hepatic rupture. Hepatocellular carcinoma is the malignant tumor most often associated with this complication, whereas hepatic adenomas are the most frequent benign cause.[54] Hemoperitoneum caused by spontaneous rupture of hepatic metastases from primary tumors of the lung, pancreas, stomach, kidney, breast, prostate, testicle, gallbladder, melanoma, nasopharynx, choriocarcinoma, and hepatic lymphoma have been described. Hemorrhage and associated rupture are more likely to occur in a large lesion located at the periphery of the liver with lack of overlying normal hepatic parenchyma. This condition is a surgical emergency with an associated high mortality. Intrahepatic bleeding progresses to subcapsular hematoma and ultimately rupture through the hepatic capsule with intraperitoneal hemorrhage. CT is often performed in the emergent setting and confirms the presence

of a liver mass with disruption of the liver capsule and hemoperitoneum (**Fig. 16**). If there is active bleeding at the time of imaging, a contrast blush may be observed. Transcatheter arterial embolization is the most effective method of controlling bleeding. Hepatic resection may also be required. Rupture of an HCC should be suspected in any patient with a history of cirrhosis or HCC who presents with acute epigastric pain.

Perihepatic Inflammation

Perihepatitis refers to inflammation of the peritoneal capsule of the liver. This condition is classically associated with pelvic inflammatory disease and is referred to as Fitz-Hugh-Curtis syndrome.[55] The syndrome was proposed by Curtis[56] in 1930 as a fibrous adhesion, the so-called violin-string appearance, between the anterior surface of the liver and the abdominal wall in patients with gonococcal pelvic inflammatory disease, and by Fitz-Hugh[57] in 1934 as acute gonococcal peritonitis in the right upper quadrant abdomen. This condition is generally thought to result from the

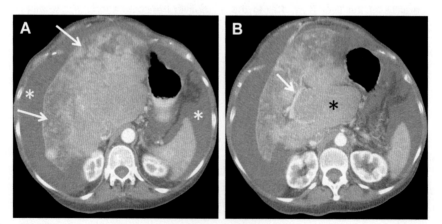

Fig. 15. Chronic Budd-Chiari: CT findings. (*A*) Small cirrhotic liver with enhancing nodule in the posterior right hepatic lobe, markedly heterogeneous peripheral enhancement (*white arrows*), ascites fluid (*asterisks*). (*B*) Enlargement of the caudate lobe (*asterisk*), small portal vein (*arrow*), hepatic veins not visualized.

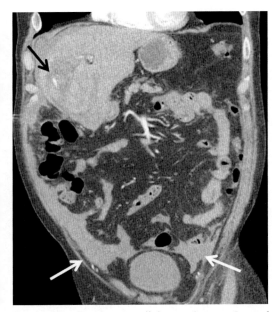

Fig. 16. Bleeding hepatocellular carcinoma. Coronal reformat from arterial phase of enhancement shows contrast blush (*black arrow*) compatible with active bleeding within a mass within the right hepatic lobe. There is moderate hemoperitoneum (*white arrows*).

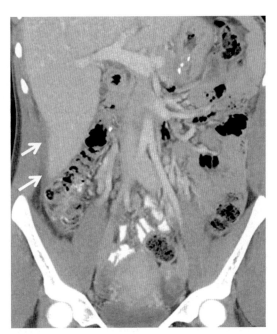

Fig. 17. Fitz-Hugh-Curtis syndrome in patient with pelvic inflammatory disease and right upper quadrant pain. There is spread of inflammation along the surface of the right hepatic lobe (*arrows*).

intraperitoneal spread of infection from the pelvic cavity; however, pathogenesis remains controversial and hematogenous and lymphatic spread of infection or an exaggerated immune response to infection has also been proposed. This perihepatic inflammation causes right upper quadrant pain that may mimic other causes, including acute cholecystitis. There are no specific findings at ultrasonography; however, ascites and adhesions between the liver capsule and the abdominal wall have been described.[58] At contrast-enhanced CT, there is an intense enhancement along the anterior surface of the liver, particularly during arterial phase of enhancement, caused by capsular inflammation.[59,60] Enhancement may persist on delayed phase, representing capsular fibrosis.[60] There may or may not be associated findings of pelvic inflammatory disease identified in the pelvis[60] but the diagnosis can be confirmed on a clinical basis (**Fig. 17**).

GALLBLADDER CAUSES OF RIGHT UPPER QUADRANT PAIN
Cholelithiasis

Gallstones are the most common abnormality of the gallbladder and are estimated to occur in approximately 20 to 25 million Americans, or 10% to 15% of the population.[61] Most patients with gallstones are asymptomatic. It is estimated that 10% to 18% of patients with gallstones develop biliary pain and 7% ultimately require operative intervention.[62] Complications include acute cholecystitis, and passage of stones into the biliary tree leading to gallstone pancreatitis or cholangitis.

Gallstones are composed mainly of cholesterol, bilirubin, and calcium salts, with smaller amounts of protein and other materials, including bile acids, fatty acids, and inorganic salts.[63] The development of gallstones is multifactorial. Risk factors include age, female gender, pregnancy, ethnicity (high in Native Americans and low in black and Asian compared with white people), family history, obesity, rapid weight loss, ileal disease, total parenteral nutrition, estrogen replacement therapy, diabetes mellitus, oral contraceptive use, and high serum triglyceride levels.[64] The type of gallstone and location in the biliary system vary depending on ethnicity. Most gallstones encountered in developed countries are cholesterol stones (about 80%), with a smaller number being pigmented stones. The pathogenesis is related to multiple factors, including cholesterol supersaturation in the bile, crystal nucleation, gallbladder dysmotility, and gallbladder absorption.[62] Pigmented stones are divided into black stones and brown stones. Black stones consist of calcium bilirubinate and mucin glycoproteins.[61] These stones are generally associated with hemolytic conditions or cirrhosis with increased levels of unconjugated bilirubin.[65] Brown stones are typically associated with bacterial infection, are more prevalent in Asian populations, and are usually located outside the gallbladder in the biliary tree.

Plain abdominal radiographs are of limited value in detection of gallstones because only 15% to 20% of gallstones are visible on abdominal radiographs.[66] Ultrasonography is the imaging modality of choice, with reported accuracy of 96% for detection of gallstones,[66–68] although this varies depending on equipment, technique, and stone size. On sonography, a gallstone appears as a highly reflective echo that is mobile with posterior acoustic shadowing (**Fig. 18**A, B). The features of mobility and shadowing help to differentiate them from other gallbladder abnormalities, including sludge, polyps, and masses. An aggregate of sludge may appear as a mobile echogenic nonshadowing focus. If the abnormality is adherent to the gallbladder wall, the identification of vascularity in the abnormality confirms a mass. Very small stones may only cast a shadow when imaged in aggregate (see **Fig. 18**C, D). In general, calculi larger than 2 mm should produce a shadow regardless of composition.[69,70] The demonstration of a posterior acoustic shadow also depends on transducer frequency. Grossman[71] showed that when a 5-MHz transducer was used, 0.2-cm to 0.3-cm stones were associated with shadowing, whereas, when a 2.25-MHz transducer was used, only stones that measured 0.4 cm cast a shadow. Greater detection of small stones is also achieved if the stone is in the center of the ultrasound beam.[70] A transducer of the highest possible frequency should be used with the focal zone placed at the level of the stone. Tissue harmonic imaging also increases detection.[72,73] In a study by Chintapelli and colleagues,[74] there was a false-negative rate of 1.3% for ultrasonography detection of stones in patients who went on to cholecystectomy. Missed stones were 5 mm or smaller in 10 patients and less than 1.0 cm in all 12 patients. If a stone is located in the gallbladder neck or trapped behind a fold it may be overlooked when the patient is only imaged in the supine position. Imaging in the upright or decubitus position may also help to identify these stones and increased shadowing of small stones when imaged in aggregate.

The wall-echo-shadow (WES) sign occurs when the gallbladder is contracted and the lumen is filled with shadowing stones. There is a high-amplitude echo that is linear or curvilinear in configuration with associated posterior acoustic shadowing.[75]

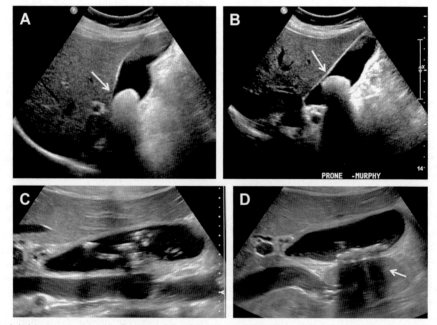

Fig. 18. Cholelithiasis: sonographic findings. (*A*) In the supine position, there is a stone located in the gallbladder neck, which casts a highly reflective shadow (*arrow*). (*B*) With the patient in the prone position, the stone moves into the gallbladder body (*arrow*), confirming that it is not impacted in the gallbladder neck. (*C*) Multiple small stones that individually do not shadow. (*D*) When the patient is imaged in the left lateral decubitus position, stones layer and cast a shadow (*arrow*).

There is perceivable gallbladder wall separate from the stones, which helps to differentiate it from calcification in the wall (porcelain gallbladder) (**Fig. 19**).

The identification of gallstones on CT depends on the differing density of the stone relative to bile.[76,77] The reported sensitivity for stone detection at CT is approximately 75%.[78] Calcified stones are the most readily identified (**Fig. 20A**). Stones with high concentrations of cholesterol may also be readily identified because these stones are less dense than bile (see **Fig. 20B**). When stones degenerate, nitrogen gas may collect in central fissures and create the Mercedes-Benz sign. This sign may be observed as a focal collection of gas in the nondependent gallbladder lumen. Noncalcified stones are soft tissue attenuation in density. Many stones are composed of a mixture of calcium, bile pigments, and cholesterol and may be similar in density to bile and not visible at CT. In one series, only 78.9% of stones identified at sonography had stones at CT.[79] A phantom study showed that the sensitivity of CT for detection of gallstones varies with kilovoltage peak (kVp), and is highest when CT is performed at 140 kVp rather than lower voltage settings.[80]

On T2-weighted MR images, gallstones appear as signal voids in the high-signal-intensity bile (**Fig. 21**). Signal intensity on T1-weighted images is variable depending on stone composition.[81–83] Other intraluminal filling defects that may mimic gallstones on T2-weighted images are blood clot, gas bubbles, and tumor.

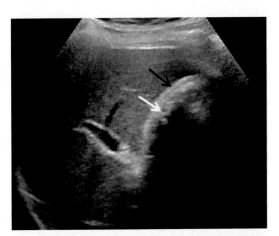

Fig. 19. Sonographic WES sign. Multiple stones filling the contracted gallbladder lumen create a curvilinear high-amplitude echo with associated posterior acoustic shadowing (*white arrow*). The gallbladder wall is identified as a separate curvilinear structure anterior to the stones (*black arrow*).

Biliary Sludge

Biliary sludge is a suspension of bile and particulate material in the gallbladder lumen.[84] There are various proportions of calcium bilirubinate, cholesterol monohydrate crystals, and gallbladder mucus. Sludge results from a combination of impaired gallbladder motility and alteration in nucleation factors.[85] Conditions that increase sludge formation include prolonged fasting, pregnancy, total parenteral nutrition, and critical illness. Patients with sludge may remain asymptomatic but may also develop biliary colic, cholecystitis, cholangitis, or pancreatitis.

On sonography, sludge generally appears as low-level echoes that layer dependently in the gallbladder lumen (**Fig. 22**). An appearance referred to as hepatization of the gallbladder occurs when the lumen is entirely filled with sludge and is similar in echotexture to the liver parenchyma. Occasionally, an aggregate of sludge (tumefactive sludge) may mimic an intraluminal mass. The use of Doppler in this setting is critical to evaluate for presence or absence of associated vascularity. Short-interval follow-up examination may also be necessary. MR imaging with contrast and subtraction imaging may be helpful in equivocal cases.

Acute Cholecystitis

Acute cholecystitis is the most frequent complication of gallstones and occurs with variable frequency in patient with gallstones, with reported frequency of up to 10% in symptomatic patients.[86] Most cases of cholecystitis occur when a stone impacts in the cystic duct or gallbladder neck, resulting in outflow obstruction of the gallbladder and associated luminal distention. Increasing gallbladder distention leads to increased intraluminal pressure, and venous and lymphatic congestion, followed by arterial stasis, mucosal sloughing, and ischemia.[62,87]

Inflammation of the gallbladder mucosa may result from chemical injury caused by bile salts and/or superimposed infection. If left untreated, there may be progression to necrosis, gangrene, and perforation. Most patients complain of persistent right upper quadrant pain, nausea, vomiting, anorexia, and fever. There is a positive Murphy sign corresponding with focal tenderness over the gallbladder on inspiration. There is leukocytosis, and liver enzyme and bilirubin levels may be mildly increased.[88] The symptoms may overlap with other causes of right upper quadrant pain. In a series of 52 patients with right upper quadrant pain and suspected cholecystitis, acute cholecystitis was confirmed in 34.6%, chronic cholecystitis in 32.7%, and 32.7% had normal gallbladders,[89]

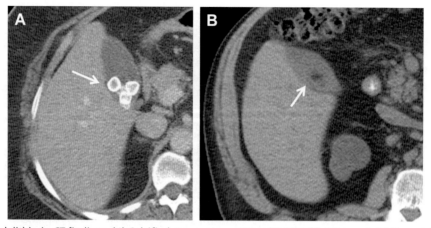

Fig. 20. Cholelithiasis: CT findings. (*A*) Calcified stones are most readily identified (*arrow*). (*B*) Noncalcified stones with lower density than bile may also be identified (*arrow*).

and imaging plays an important role in confirming the diagnosis.

Imaging

Ultrasonography is endorsed by the American College of Radiology (ACR) Appropriateness Criteria as the initial imaging study of choice for suspected acute cholecystitis in patients with fever, increased white blood cell count, and positive Murphy sign.[90] In a meta-analysis and systematic review of diagnostic performance of imaging in acute cholecystitis performed by Kiewert and colleagues,[91] 57 studies including 5859 patients were included. The sensitivity and specificity of cholescintigraphy were 96% and 90% compared with 81% and 83% for ultrasonography. However, ultrasonography provides the advantages of

being readily available and rapidly performed, involving no ionizing radiation, being able to confirm the presence of gallstones and detect complications of cholecystitis or biliary dilatation, and being able to provide an alternative diagnosis. In the ACR criteria, cholescintigraphy may be a useful adjunct to ultrasonography depending on the findings.

The ultrasonography findings in acute uncomplicated cholecystitis are well described and include gallstones, a positive sonographic Murphy sign, gallbladder distention, wall thickening, and pericholecystic fluid,[89,92–95] with the first 2 findings considered to be the most specific. In the study

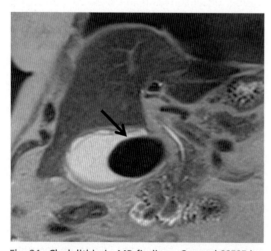

Fig. 21. Cholelithiasis: MR findings. Coronal SSFSE image shows large stone with low signal intensity in the gallbladder neck (*arrow*).

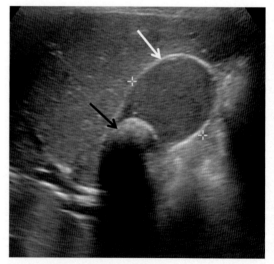

Fig. 22. Biliary sludge: sonographic findings. Sludge fills the lumen of the gallbladder (*white arrow*), which also has a large stone impacted in the neck (*black arrow*). The echotexture of the sludge is similar to that of the adjacent liver parenchyma.

by Ralls and colleagues,[96] a positive sonographic Murphy sign and the presence of gallstones had a positive predictive value of 92% for the diagnosis of acute cholecystitis. The sonographic Murphy sign may be unreliable if the patient has been administered pain medication before the examination and it also may be blunted in the setting of gangrenous cholecystitis. Identification of a stone impacted in the gallbladder neck or cystic duct increases the specificity of the examination (**Fig. 23**). In order to identify this, the patient should be evaluated in the upright or left lateral decubitus position to determine whether stones are mobile. Additional less specific findings include gallbladder distention, wall thickening, and pericholecystic fluid. Gallbladder distention may be limited if there is superimposed acute-on-chronic cholecystitis or if the gallbladder is perforated. Diffuse gallbladder wall thickening, greater than 3 mm, is observed in 50% to 75% of patients with acute cholecystitis[92] but may be associated with many other conditions, including chronic inflammation, liver disease, ascites, hypoalbuminemia congestive heart failure, human immunodeficiency virus infection, and sepsis.[11] Other causes include adenomyomatosis, and gallbladder neoplasm. If focal wall thickening is observed, complications such as gangrenous change or neoplasm should be considered. Pericholecystic fluid is also less specific, including in the setting of generalized ascites. The presence of sludge is another indication of gallbladder obstruction. Doppler evaluation may be an adjunct to gray-scale imaging.[97,98]

At hepatobiliary scintigraphy, the hepatic parenchyma is observed within 1 minute with peak activity at 10 to 15 minutes.[99] The bile ducts are usually visible within 10 minutes and the gallbladder should appear within 1 hour if there is patency of the cystic duct. If the gallbladder has not been visualized, imaging should be performed up to 4 hours. Prompt biliary excretion of the tracer without visualization of the gallbladder is the hallmark of acute cholecystitis[100] (**Fig. 24**). False-positive results may occur in patients with abnormal bile flow caused by liver disease or prolonged fasting with a distended sludge-filled gallbladder. Delayed filling may also occur in the setting of chronic cholecystitis. If the gallbladder is not visualized after 1 hour, intravenous morphine may be administered, which causes spasm of the sphincter of Oddi, increasing pressure within the bile ducts and increasing the likelihood of flow of bile into the gallbladder. If the patient has fasted for more than 24 hours, an oral fatty meal or intravenous cholecystokinin may be administered, resulting in gallbladder contraction so that the gallbladder can empty and then refill.

Although not the first-line imaging modality for evaluating patients with suspected cholecystitis, CT may initially be performed if this diagnosis is not suspected and the cause of the patient's pain is uncertain. CT is also a useful adjunct to ultrasonography when findings are equivocal and a complication is suspected. In a retrospective study at the author's institution, the overall sensitivity, specificity, and accuracy of CT for the diagnosis

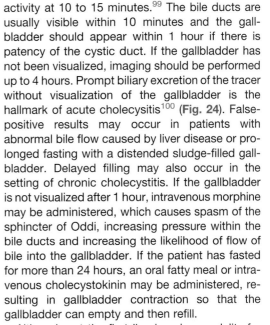

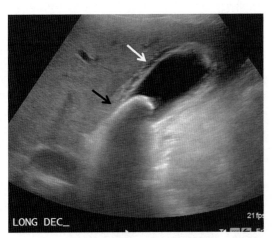

Fig. 23. Acute cholecystitis: ultrasonography. The gallbladder is distended and there is a large shadowing stone in the neck (*black arrow*). The wall is thickened and edematous (*white arrow*). A positive sonographic Murphy sign was elicited.

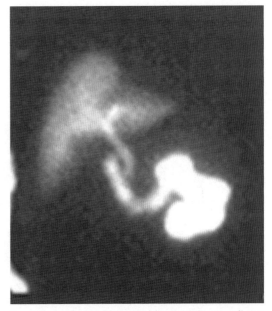

Fig. 24. Acute cholecystitis: hepatobiliary radionuclide scan. There is prompt biliary excretion of the tracer without visualization of the gallbladder.

of acute cholecystitis were 91.7%, 99.1%, and 94.3% respectively.[101] CT findings are similar to those observed at sonography and include a distended gallbladder, with or without stones; wall thickening; and pericholecystic fluid[78,94,95,101–104] (**Fig. 25**). Major and minor criteria have been described.[105] Major findings include calculi, mural thickening, pericholecystic fluid, and subserosal edema. Minor findings include gallbladder distention and sludge. Not all gallstones are visualized at CT; therefore, this is a limitation. The presence of pericholecystic inflammatory change is thought to be the most specific CT finding.[78,103] A finding that suggests gallbladder inflammation that may be observed at CT is increased contrast enhancement in the liver parenchyma adjacent to the gallbladder[106–108] (see **Fig. 25B**). This finding can help to establish the diagnosis when other findings are equivocal, and may be observed earlier than other CT findings.[109] Increased density of the gallbladder wall has been described as a finding on unenhanced CT in approximately 51% of patients with acute cholecystitis.[110] This increased density may be seen in the setting of mucosal hemorrhage and necrosis and may be a predictor of gangrenous change. A recent study evaluating the use of 64-slice multidetector CT (MDCT) for quantitative and qualitative assessment of acute cholecystitis found that pericholecystic fat stranding, mural stratification, pericholecystic hypervascularity, and spontaneous hyperattenuation of the gallbladder wall; short ($\leq$32 mm) and long ($\geq$74 mm) gallbladder axis enlargement; and gallbladder wall thickening ($\geq$3.6 mm) were the most discriminating and independent variables for the CT diagnosis of acute cholecystitis.[111] Comparative studies assessing accuracy of CT versus ultrasonography for the diagnosis of acute cholecystitis are limited and there is currently not enough evidence to support indiscriminate use of this modality in patients with suspected acute cholecystitis.[91]

MR is usually performed in the setting of suspected acute cholecystitis when other imaging findings are equivocal or the clinical picture is uncertain.[112–117] The excellent soft tissue contrast of MR imaging allows identification of inflammatory changes, provides detailed evaluation of the biliary tract, and is an alternative to CT when intravenous contrast is contraindicated. In the meta-analysis by Kiewiet and colleagues,[91] diagnostic accuracy of MR for diagnosis of acute cholecystitis was comparable with that of ultrasonography and MR is suggested as a helpful imaging modality when ultrasonography is technically limited. Detection of stones in the bile duct is important before laparoscopic cholecystectomy. Choledocholithiasis is present in 10% to 15% of cases of acute cholecystitis and MR cholangiopancreatography (MRCP) has a reported sensitivity of 89% to 100% and specificity of 83% to 100% for stones, although accuracy is worse for stones smaller than 3 mm[117] (discussed later). MR has also been shown to be superior to ultrasonography for detection of obstructing calculi in the gallbladder neck and the cystic duct.[118] In addition to detection of gallstones, MR readily shows gallbladder wall edema, which appears as high signal intensity on T2-weighted images (**Fig. 26**). In one series, pericholecystic high signal intensity on single-shot fast spin-echo (SSFSE) images had an overall accuracy of 89%, specificity of 79%, positive predictive value of 87%, and negative predictive value of 85% for detection of acute cholecystitis.[119] Contrast-enhanced T1-weighted images are also useful for diagnosis because degree of enhancement of the gallbladder wall may help to differentiate from chronic cholecystitis.[113] Transient increase in

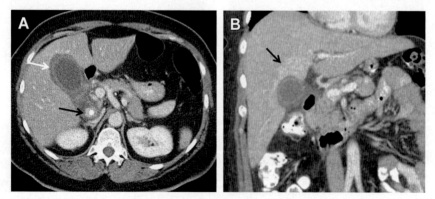

Fig. 25. Acute cholecystitis: CT features. (*A*) Axial contrast-enhanced image shows distended gallbladder with thickened wall (*white arrow*) and stone in the neck (*black arrow*). (*B*) Coronal reformatted image shows localized hyperemia around the gallbladder with increased contrast enhancement (*arrow*).

pericholecystic hepatic parenchymal enhancement may be seen in the arterial phase of enhancement, as with CT, and may be an important finding confirming the diatnosis[113,114] (see **Fig. 26B**). Increased gallbladder wall enhancement and increased transient pericholecystic hepatic enhancement have been shown to have the highest sensitivity and specificity for the diagnosis and differentiation from chronic cholecystitis.[120] MR imaging is also highly accurate in the detection of complications of acute cholecystitis, such as intramural necrosis, microabscesses, hemorrhage, wall discontinuity, perforation, and pericholecystic abscess. Recently, a potential role for T1-weighted MR cholangiography using agents that are both extracellular and hepatocyte specific with increased biliary excretion in the diagnosis of acute cholecystitis has been described.[121,122] This technique allows for functional evaluation as in hepatobiliary scintigraphy; however, further investigation in this application is needed.

Acute Acalculous Cholecystitis

Epidemiology and pathophysiology

Acute acalculous cholecystitis (AAC) is defined as an acute necroinflammatory disease of the gallbladder in the absence of cholelithiasis, and it accounts for approximately 10% of all cases of acute cholecystitis.[123] Histologic features include gallbladder wall inflammation, with necrosis of blood vessels in the muscularis and serosa of the gallbladder.[124] The most important risk factors for AAC are bile stasis, gallbladder ischemia, cystic duct obstruction, and systemic infection.[125,126] AAC occurs with increased incidence in patients who are critically ill or patients with prolonged illness, such as in the setting of trauma or after

prolonged stay in the intensive care unit (ICU). Other risk factors include major cardiovascular disorders, cardiopulmonary bypass, diabetes, autoimmune disease, bacterial and fungal sepsis, hyperalimentation, and AIDS. Rarely, the disease occurs de novo in the absence of these other risk factors in otherwise apparently healthy individuals.[127,128]

AAC is generally a more fulminant form of acute cholecystitis with higher morbidity and mortality and rapid progression to gangrene and perforation, with reported mortality as high as 65%.[129] Prompt diagnosis of AAC is important; however, the diagnosis often presents a challenge, particularly if there are no apparent risk factors. The diagnosis should be suspected in critically ill or injured patients who have fever or infection with no other apparent source.

Imaging

Ultrasonography

The sensitivity of ultrasonography for detection of AAC varies widely, from 36% to 92%[130] (**Fig. 27**). The diagnosis is often challenging because gallstones are not present and affected patients are often insensitive to pain because of altered mental status or medications, resulting in unreliable sonographic Murphy sign.[131] These patients also usually have coexisting abnormalities such as hypoalbuminemia, congestive heart failure, and long-standing parenteral nutrition, all of which are associated with gallbladder wall thickening, distention, and sludge. There is a great degree of overlap in ultrasonography findings of ICU patients with AAC and those without, with most ICU patients having some abnormality of the gallbladder.[132] Ultrasonography remains the initial

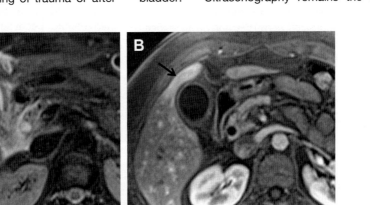

Fig. 26. Acute cholecystitis MR imaging findings. (*A*) T2-weighted image fat-suppressed image shows distended gallbladder with multiple stones, wall thickening, and pericholecystic fluid and inflammation. (*B*) Contrast-enhanced T1-weighted gradient-echo image shows localized hyperemia adjacent to gallbladder (*arrow*).

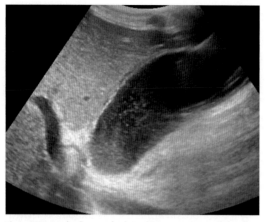

Fig. 27. Acalculous cholecystitis: sonographic features. The gallbladder is distended with sludge without stones. The wall is thickened. There was a positive sonographic Murphy sign.

imaging modality of choice because it can be performed portably at the bedside and ultrasonography is assigned the highest ranking for diagnosis of AAC in the ACR Appropriateness Criteria.[90] Cholescintigraphy is of limited value in the diagnosis of AAC, with a significant false-positive rate (nonvisualization of the gallbladder) of up to 40% in patients with hepatocellular dysfunction, prolonged fasting, or severe illness.[131,133] Although a negative study excludes acalculous cholecystitis, a positive study must be interpreted with caution. Specificity improves to 88% with the use of morphine.[134] A prospective study comparing ultrasonography and morphine cholescintigraphy (MC) in the diagnosis of AAC found that the sensitivities of ultrasonography and MC were 50% and 67%, specificities were 94% and 100%, positive predictive values were 86% and 100%, negative predictive values were 71% and 80%, and accuracies were 75% and 86%, respectively.[135] Combining both ultrasonography and cholescintigraphy may lead to greater diagnostic accuracy.

Computed Tomography/MR Imaging

CT or MR imaging may be helpful adjuncts to ultrasonography in the diagnosis of AAC. With the exception of absent gallstones, the CT and MR imaging findings of AAC are similar to those of calculous cholecystitis. The advantage of these modalities is that they may show pericholecystic inflammatory change and fluid and abnormalities of the gallbladder wall or adjacent hepatic parenchyma, which may not be identified on sonography, helping to confirm the diagnosis when ultrasonography is equivocal. Similar to

sonography, less specific findings that may also be observed include gallbladder distention, sludge, and wall thickening. However, a recent study showed that a normal gallbladder at CT is useful in excluding the diagnosis of AAC.[136]

Often patients with AAC are critically ill and cannot undergo cross-sectional imaging evaluation. If there is no other source of sepsis discovered, it may be prudent to proceed with percutaneous cholecystostomy, which can be performed at the bedside. Percutaneous cholecystostomy has been shown to be a safe and effective procedure in patients with acute cholecystitis who are not candidates for surgery.[137] Percutaneous cholecystostomy can be useful for both diagnosis and treatment in patients with sepsis of unknown cause and equivocal imaging findings of AAC.[138–140]

COMPLICATIONS OF ACUTE CHOLECYSTITIS
Gangrenous Cholecystitis

Gangrenous cholecystitis is a severe form of acute cholecystitis associated with vascular compromise and intramural hemorrhage, necrosis, and intramural abscess formation. This condition is most often the result of stone impaction in the cystic duct, with progressive distension of the gallbladder and ultimately ischemic necrosis of the wall.[141] The incidence of this complication ranges from approximately 2% to 30% in various surgical series.[142–144] There is a higher incidence in men, patients of advanced age, and those with cardiovascular disease. Treatment is generally emergency cholecystectomy to avoid life-threatening complications such as perforation. There is a higher rate of conversion to open cholecystectomy than in uncomplicated acute cholecystitis so it is important to make the diagnosis before surgical intervention because the approach may be altered.[145–147]

The ultrasonography features of gangrenous cholecystitis include the presence of heterogeneous, striated thickening and irregularity of the gallbladder wall, and intraluminal membranes resulting from desquamation of the gallbladder mucosa[148,149] (Fig. 28). Irregular or asymmetric thickening of the gallbladder wall likely results from ulceration, hemorrhage, necrosis, or microabscess formation. A striated appearance of the gallbladder wall was found in 40% of patients in the series by Teefey and colleagues.[148] However, in a more recent analysis by the same investigators, this finding was nonspecific for the presence of gangrenous cholecystitis and it can be found in nongangrenous cholecystitis and other conditions that cause gallbladder wall edema, such as

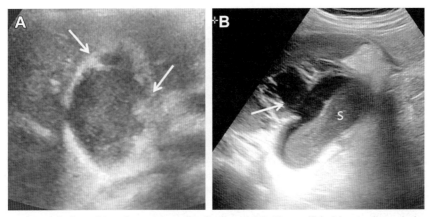

Fig. 28. Gangrenous cholecystitis: ultrasonography findings. (A) The gallbladder is distended and contains sludge. There was also a large stone in the neck (not shown). The wall is thickened and irregular in contour (arrows). (B) Different patient with markedly thickened and irregular gallbladder wall with focal discontinuity and intramural abscess (arrow). There is a large amount of sludge (s) in the gallbladder lumen.

hepatitis.[150] Intraluminal membranes are considered a more specific finding. Importantly, a sonographic Murphy sign may not be present in these patients because of associated denervation of the gallbladder wall. The sonographic Murphy sign was positive in only 33% of patients with gangrenous cholecystitis in the series by Simeone and colleagues.[151] Additional findings include intramural abscess and/or pericholecystic fluid collection or abscess formation caused by perforation of the gallbladder.

CT findings of gangrenous cholecystitis parallel the findings on sonography and include intraluminal membranes, intraluminal hemorrhage, irregularity or disruption of the gallbladder wall, and pericholecystic abscess formation.[78,101,103,152–154] An additional finding that may be identified at contrast enhanced CT is irregular or absent gallbladder wall enhancement[101,154] (Fig. 29). In a study by the author,[101] CT was highly specific for identifying acute gangrenous cholecystitis (96%) but had low sensitivity (29.3%). The most specific

CT findings of gangrenous cholecystitis were gas in the gallbladder wall or lumen, intraluminal membranes, irregularity or absence of the gallbladder wall, pericholecystic abscess, and lack of gallbladder wall enhancement. The presence of pericholecystic fluid, degree of gallbladder distention in the short axis, and degree of mural thickening were also predictive of the severity of gallbladder inflammation. In a more recent study by Wu and colleagues,[155] the presence of a perfusional defect of the gallbladder wall (discontinuity or decreased enhancement of the gallbladder wall), was associated with CT diagnosis of gangrenous cholecystitis with accuracy of 80%, sensitivity of 70.6%, specificity of 100%, and positive predictive value of 100%. These studies show that intravenous contrast should be administered if possible because this improves delineation of the wall and identification of lack of enhancement, intramural abscess, or focal disruption, all of which are important features of gangrenous cholecystitis. MR may show similar findings (Fig. 30).[115,117]

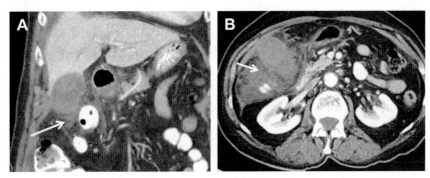

Fig. 29. Gangrenous cholecystitis: CT findings. Coronal (A) and axial (B) contrast-enhanced images show pericholecystic inflammatory change and fluid (arrow) and lack of gallbladder wall enhancement.

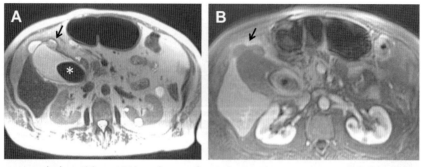

Fig. 30. Gangrenous cholecystitis on MR imaging: perforated necrotic gangrenous gallbladder. (A) Axial SSFSE image shows thickened and edematous wall of the gallbladder, which is irregular in contour with a focal area of wall discontinuity (*arrow*). There is a large stone in the gallbladder neck (*asterisk*). (B) Contrast-enhanced T1-weighted gradient-echo image shows pericholecystic abscess (*arrow*).

An important potential pitfall to keep in mind is that gallbladder carcinoma may be mimicked by the mural changes in acute cholecystitis, particularly gangrenous cholecystitis. If there is concern based on ultrasonography findings, CT may be of benefit in showing an enhancing gallbladder mass and detecting direct invasion of the liver and presence of liver metastases. Liang and colleagues[156] found that, in the differentiation of acute cholecystitis and gallbladder carcinoma, features that favored carcinoma included focal gallbladder wall thickening, intraluminal mass, nondistended gallbladder with diffuse wall thickening, and enlarged regional lymph nodes.

Hemorrhagic Cholecystitis

Hemorrhagic cholecystitis is an uncommon complication of acute cholecystitis and usually occurs in the setting of cholelithiasis and gangrenous cholecystitis. Transmural inflammation causes mural necrosis and ulceration, resulting in hemorrhage into the gallbladder lumen.[157–159] Intraluminal blood clots may become impacted in the cystic duct or common bile duct or pass into the small bowel. The clinical presentation may be identical to uncomplicated acute cholecystitis with fever and right upper quadrant pain, but may also include biliary colic, jaundice, hematemesis, and melena.[160] Massive upper gastrointestinal bleeding and hemoperitoneum rarely occur.[161] Prompt diagnosis is essential because of the associated high mortality.

On ultrasonography, blood in the gallbladder lumen can be recognized as hyperechoic material that is generally more hyperechoic than biliary sludge (**Fig. 31**A). Clotted blood may appear as a clump or mass adherent to the gallbladder wall or heterogeneous echogenic material, simulating a mass if organized.[162–164] In addition to other findings of cholecystitis, CT also shows increased density of bile[157] (see **Fig. 31**B). A fluid-fluid level may be observed with a high attenuation–dependent component simulating the hematocrit effect observed in acute hemorrhage.[160] Other causes of high-density bile include biliary excretion of iodinated contrast material or milk of calcium; these do not generally appear as echogenic on

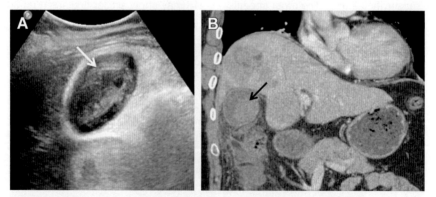

Fig. 31. Hemorrhagic cholecystitis: CT and ultrasonography findings. (A) Ultrasonography shows echogenic sludge in the gallbladder lumen (*arrow*). (B) Coronal reformatted CT shows high-attenuation material corresponding with blood clot (*arrow*) in the gallbladder lumen.

sonography and a fluid-fluid level is not observed. Hemoperitoneum is seen in the setting of associated gallbladder perforation with active contrast extravasation if there is active hemorrhage.[165] On MR imaging, blood products appear as high signal intensity within the gallbladder lumen on T1-weighted images and moderate to high heterogeneous signal intensity on T2-weighted images.[114]

Emphysematous Cholecystitis

Emphysematous cholecystitis is a rare, life-threatening, and rapidly progressive complication of acute cholecystitis that results from cystic artery compromise and allows the proliferation of gas-producing organisms in an anaerobic environment and penetration of gas into the gallbladder wall.[166,167] The organisms most commonly associated with emphysematous cholecystitis are *Clostridium welchii* and *E coli*.[167] This complication occurs with higher frequency in patients with diabetes (up to 50%) and male patients (up to 71%), and gallstones may be absent in up to one-third of patients.[168] There is a high risk of gangrene and a perforation rate 5 times higher than in acute uncomplicated cholecystitis.[168,169]

The mortality for emphysematous cholecystitis is 15%, compared with 4% in uncomplicated acute cholecystitis.[168] Prompt diagnosis is critical; however, the clinical presentation may be indistinguishable from uncomplicated acute cholecystitis. The diagnosis is particularly challenging in diabetic patients because severe symptoms may be absent. Before cross-sectional imaging, emphysematous cholecystitis was diagnosed on the abdominal radiograph and classically described in 3 stages. Stage 1 includes gas in the gallbladder lumen, stage 2 includes gas in the gallbladder wall, and stage 3 includes gas in the pericholecystic soft tissues. Ultrasonography and CT are now considered more sensitive in the detection of smaller amounts of gas. Ultrasonography findings vary depending on the amount and location of gas.[170,171] A small amount of gas in the gallbladder wall may appear as an echogenic focus with associated ring-down or comet-tail artifact. Larger amounts of intramural gas and intraluminal gas may appear as a curvilinear arc of increased echogenicity with associated so-called "dirty" posterior acoustic shadowing that obscures the gallbladder fossa (**Fig. 32**A). It may be difficult to differentiate emphysematous cholecystitis from a contracted gallbladder with stones or a porcelain gallbladder with calcified wall.[170]

CT has a higher sensitivity than sonography for the identification of emphysematous cholecystitis and plays an important complementary role to ultrasonography if this complication is suspected and ultrasonography findings are equivocal.[172] CT is also helpful when the gallbladder cannot be adequately visualized at sonography. CT findings include gas within the gallbladder wall or nondependent portion of the lumen[173–175] (see **Fig. 32**B). There may be extension of gas into the pericholecystic soft tissues. CT may also show additional complications, such as abscess formation and perforation. Free intraperitoneal gas indicates associated free gallbladder perforation and constitutes a surgical emergency.

The MR imaging features of emphysematous cholecystitis have not yet been well described; however, a recent report describing MR imaging features in a case of emphysematous cholecystitis included (1) a signal void in the nondependent portion of the gallbladder and intermediate signal intensity fluid in the dependent portion of the gallbladder, representing a gas-fluid level; (2) a low-signal-intensity rim surrounding the gallbladder,

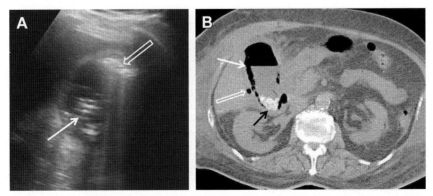

Fig. 32. Emphysematous cholecystitis. (*A*) Ultrasonography shows stones in the distended gallbladder (*white arrow*). The anterior wall of the gallbladder shows increased echogenicity (*open arrow*) with associated dirty posterior acoustic shadowing, compatible with gas. (*B*) CT shows gas in the gallbladder wall and lumen (*white arrow*) and focal area of perforation (*open arrow*). Stones are also noted (*black arrow*).

indicating gas in the gallbladder wall; and (3) regions of very low signal intensity in the pericholecystic soft tissues, indicating extraluminal gas caused by perforation.[176] Gas may be recognized as blooming artifact on gradient-echo and echoplanar sequences.

Gallbladder Perforation

Perforation of the gallbladder is most often a complication of severe acute cholecystitis, occurring in approximately 8% to 12% of cases, with associated mortality of up to 24.1%.[177,178] When the cystic duct is obstructed, progressive gallbladder distention and inflammation is followed by vascular compromise, gangrene, necrosis, and ultimately perforation.[178,179] The fundus is the most frequent site of perforation because of the poor blood supply in this area. Associated complications include bacteremia, septic shock, bile peritonitis, and abscess formation with mortalities ranging from 6% to 70%.[177,180–183]

Gallbladder perforation is subclassified into 3 types[180,181]: (1) acute free perforation into the peritoneal cavity, which is associated with the highest mortality; (2) subacute perforation with pericholecystic abscess, which is the most common; and (3) chronic perforation with cholecystoenteric fistula formation and possible progression to gallstone ileus. Abscess formation may be confined to the gallbladder fossa, spread into the peritoneal cavity, or involve the liver.[184,185]

Emergent cholecystectomy is the treatment of choice for perforated gallbladder. Clinical signs and symptoms may be nonspecific and may be indistinguishable from uncomplicated cholecystitis, particularly in diabetic patients, so imaging plays an important role in diagnosis.[186] On sonography, the gallbladder wall is irregular or ill defined with focal or global loss of the gallbladder wall's normal sonoreflectivity.[173] There is a large amount of pericholecystic fluid or a loculated pericholecystic collection.[179] A focal defect in the wall of the gallbladder is a more specific finding but may not always be visualized[187,188] (**Fig. 33**A).

CT may play an important role in diagnosis of suspected gallbladder perforation.[189–191] Interruption of the gallbladder wall or a focal mural defect may be more readily identified at CT than at ultrasonography. In a study comparing ultrasonography with CT in 13 patients with surgically proven gallbladder perforation, a mural defect was visualized in 7 patients (53.8%) at CT but in no patient on ultrasonography.[191] Associated CT findings include pericholecystic or intrahepatic abscess and spilled stones (see **Fig. 33**B). Free gallbladder perforation is identified when there is free intraperitoneal fluid, which represents bile often in association with a collapsed gallbladder. In these instances, presence of localized pericholecystic inflammatory change offers a diagnostic clue as to the cause of free fluid and peritoneal inflammatory changes. Because of its superior soft tissue resolution and multiplanar imaging capability, MR may also be a useful adjunct if ultrasonography and CT findings remain equivocal.

CHRONIC CHOLECYSTITIS
Pathogenesis and Epidemiology

Chronic cholecystitis is associated with gallstones in 95% of cases and may result from a single episode or multiple recurrent episodes of acute cholecystitis. The cause is related to intermittent obstruction of the cystic duct or neck as well as gallbladder dysmotility.[63] Chronic inflammatory changes cause the gallbladder wall to become thickened and fibrotic, and with increasing fibrosis the gallbladder eventually becomes shrunken and

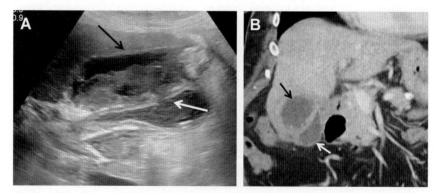

Fig. 33. Contained gallbladder perforation. (*A*) Ultrasonography shows focal defect in the anterior wall of the sludge-filled gallbladder (*white arrow*). There is a large pericholecystic abscess (*black arrow*). (*B*) CT shows the decompressed gallbladder (*white arrow*) and the pericholecystic abscess, which contains small stones (*black arrow*).

distorted. If there are coexisting acute and chronic inflammatory changes at pathology, the-term chronic active cholecystitis may be used.[192]

Imaging

A diagnosis of chronic cholecystitis may be difficult to establish at imaging and correlation with clinical history is required. Ultrasonography findings include gallstones and thickened gallbladder wall with contraction of the gallbladder that persists with fasting. On CT, pericholecystic inflammatory change may be absent. On MR, gallbladder wall thickening related to chronic inflammation shows low signal intensity, whereas acute cholecystitis is associated with edema in the wall, which shows increased signal intensity on T2-weighted images.[114] Also, the increased perihepatic contrast enhancement observed with acute cholecystitis can be helpful in differentiating acute from chronic inflammation.[113,114,120] Chronic acalculous cholecystitis caused by recurrent biliary colic in a patient without evidence of gallstones is particularly difficult to diagnose. In the absence of gallstones, it is often difficult to attribute patients' symptoms to gallbladder inflammation. However, these patients may benefit from cholecystectomy for relief of symptoms.[193] Diagnosis may require nuclear medicine evaluation, including evaluation of the gallbladder ejection fraction. A decrease in gallbladder ejection fraction is a common feature of both calculous and acalculous chronic cholecystitis.[194] Cholecystokinin cholescintigraphy with calculation of gallbladder ejection fraction has been shown to be a helpful predictor of symptomatic relief after cholecystectomy.[195]

GALLBLADDER TORSION

Torsion, or volvulus of the gallbladder, is a rare cause of right upper quadrant pain, occurring primarily in elderly patients and most commonly in women.[196] Rotation of the gallbladder at the hilum may be complete or incomplete ($\leq 180°$) and either clockwise or anticlockwise, and gallstones occur in up to 32%.[196] The cause is uncertain but may be attributed to age-related laxity of mesenteric attachments and anatomic variations that may lead to gallbladder hypermobility.[196,197] If not detected and treated, there is progression to gallbladder necrosis. The diagnosis may be suspected clinically in a patient with sudden onset of right upper quadrant pain, nausea and vomiting, leukocytosis, and palpable gallbladder.[198] Imaging findings may be nonspecific and overlap with acute cholecystitis. However, suggestive findings include a distended gallbladder with an abnormal orientation out of the gallbladder fossa in addition to findings of gallbladder inflammation.[197] A V-shaped distortion of the extrahepatic bile ducts and a twisted pedicle inferior to the liver may be observed on noncontrast CT, and poor enhancement of the gallbladder wall and twisting of the cystic artery with a whirl sign may be observed at contrast-enhanced CT.[198,199] Correlation with prior imaging studies may be helpful to suggest the abnormal positioning of the gallbladder (Fig. 34).

CHOLEDOCHOLITHIASIS
Pathogenesis and Epidemiology

Biliary calculi that form de novo within the biliary tract are referred to as primary stones, whereas those that migrate from the gallbladder through

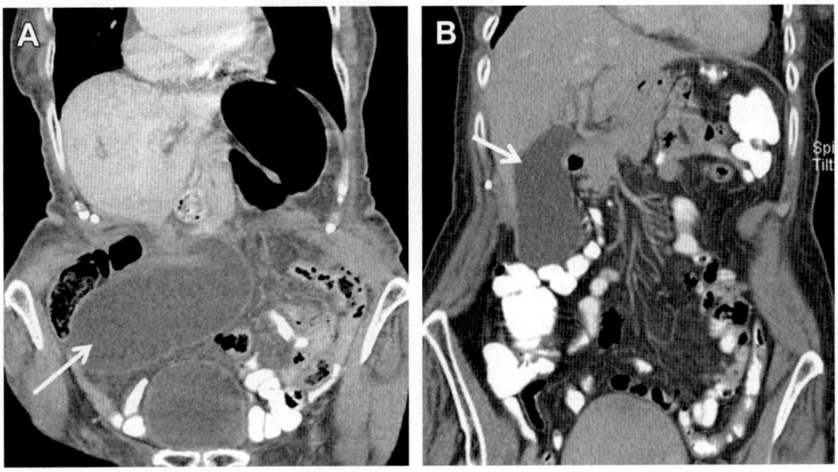

Fig. 34. Gallbladder volvulus. An 87-year-old woman with acute-onset right upper quadrant pain and palpable abdominal mass. (A) The gallbladder (arrow) is markedly distended and is in a horizontal lie located outside the gallbladder fossa. (B) Previous CT in same patient showed normal orientation of the gallbladder (arrow).

the cystic duct or a cholecystocholedochal fistula are referred to as secondary stones.[200] Most stones within the bile ducts are secondary stones. Migration of gallstones among asymptomatic patients occurs in approximately 3% to 5% of patients per year, with 1% to 2% of patients per year developing symptoms, including biliary colic or acute pancreatitis.[201,202] Between 7% and 20% of patients undergoing cholecystectomy have 1 or more stones in the common bile duct, which may be clinically silent.[203] From 20% to 30% of patients with gallstone pancreatitis have persistent common bile duct stones that fail to traverse the ampulla.[204] If a stone remains lodged in the common bile duct this can also lead to a potentially life-threatening associated ascending cholangitis.

Primary stones are classified according to their location within the biliary tract: intrahepatic, extrahepatic, or ampullary. These stones develop in the setting of bile stasis and colonization of the bile with enteric organisms. Obstruction of bile may be related to inflammatory or iatrogenic strictures, congenital strictures, or periampullary diverticula.[200] These stones are frequently associated with parasitic infections of the biliary tree, such as *Ascaris lumbricoides* when the stones become the nidus for stone and inflammatory stricture formation.

Imaging

Endoscopic retrograde cholangiopancreatography

Endoscopic retrograde cholangiopancreatography (ERCP) and percutaneous transhepatic cholangiography are highly accurate for the detection of choledocholithiasis and allow therapeutic intervention. However, these are invasive procedures with associated risks, including pancreatitis, sepsis, and hemorrhage. The reported complication rate of ERCP ranges from 3.0% to 5.5% and mortality from 0.2% to 1.0%.[205,206] Therefore, ERCP is generally reserved for patients who require intervention, including those with an impacted stone, or with a high probability of stones and negative prior examinations. Stones within the biliary tract may be readily detected with MRCP, and less accurately with ultrasonography and CT.

Ultrasonography

Ultrasonography is the primary imaging modality of choice for evaluation of right upper quadrant pain and is considered superior to CT in the initial imaging evaluation of biliary disease.[94,207] The reported sensitivity of ultrasonography is variable and ranges from 22% to 75% for common bile duct stones.[208–211] Limited sensitivity results in part from inability to completely visualize the common bile duct, particularly the distal duct, because of interposed bowel gas. In a study by Laing and colleagues,[212] 8 of 9 (89%) proximal and 16 of 23 (70%) distal common bile duct stones were visualized at sonography. Scanning the patient in the erect right posterior oblique or right lateral decubitus position minimizes gas in the gastric antrum and duodenum and improves visualization of the distal duct. Water may also be administered orally to provide an acoustic window in the gastric antrum or duodenum. Improved contrast enhancement and reduction of side lobe artifacts afforded by tissue harmonic imaging improves the sonographic detection of choledocholithiasis.[213] Common bile duct stones appear as echogenic foci, which may or may not cause posterior acoustic shadowing depending on size and composition (**Fig. 35**). As with cholelithiasis, nonshadowing stones may be difficult to differentiate from aggregates of sludge or soft tissue masses. Improved accuracy can be accomplished with the use of endoscopic ultrasonography,[214] but this is more invasive and operator dependent.

Computed Tomography

Unenhanced conventional CT has a reported sensitivity of 75% in the detection of choledocholithiasis.[215–217] Indirect signs such as ductal dilatation or abrupt termination of the duct may be useful but are not conclusive findings. MDCT has a higher sensitivity, ranging from 65% to 88%.[218–221] Multiplanar reformatted (MPR) coronal images through the common bile duct may

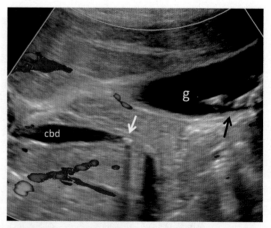

Fig. 35. Choledocholithiasis: sonographic appearance. Obstructing stone (*white arrow*) in the distal common bile duct (cbd) appears as echogenic focus with posterior acoustic shadowing. Additional stones (*black arrow*) are present in the gallbladder (g).

be useful in depicting stones (**Fig. 36**). When specifically evaluating for choledocholithiasis, water should be used to opacify the bowel because positive oral contrast material may obscure visualization of distal common bile duct stones and fill perivaterian duodenal diverticulae. In a study comparing MDCT and ERCP for the detection of common bile duct calculi, CT had a sensitivity of 88%, specificity of 97%, and accuracy of 94%.[218] Bile window settings (adjusting the window level setting to the mean attenuation of the common bile duct and the window width to 150 HU) improves visualization of noncalcified stones by creating better contrast between bile and soft tissues.

As with gallstones, the CT appearance of common bile duct stones is variable. Depending on their composition, stones may be calcified, soft tissue, or low density with respect to bile. Calcified stones are the most readily identified. Unenhanced images are better for detection because most stones are slightly hyperdense. Four CT criteria for detection of common bile duct stones have been described: (1) a target sign refers to a central density, corresponding with the stone, surrounded by hypoattenuating bile or ampullary soft tissue; (2) the rim sign corresponds with a faint rim of increased density along the margin of a low-density area; (3) the crescent sign refers to a calculus with increased density surrounded by a crescent of hypoattenuating bile; and (4) indirect signs include abrupt termination of a dilated distal common bile duct without visible surrounding mass or biliary dilatation. Abrupt termination of the common bile duct without soft tissue mass was most often associated with pancreatic carcinoma.[215]

CT cholangiography is an additional technique that may be used to visualize the biliary tract and choledocholithiasis. MDCT is performed after indirect opacification of the biliary tract with oral or intravenous iodinated cholangiographic agents.[222,223] Improved z-axis resolution is achieved with multidetector array scanners and high-resolution reconstructions of the biliary tract.[224] In one series, CT cholangiography provided excellent visualization of biliary anatomy and filling defects, with 95% sensitivity for choledocholithiasis.[225] Other more recent series also show promise of these techniques in evaluation of choledocholithiasis.[226–229] A major drawback of this technique is the associated risks of contrast-induced allergic reactions.[230] At the author's institution, this technique is currently used primarily to define donor biliary anatomy before liver transplantation and does not play a role in evaluation of the choledocholithiasis.

MR Imaging

MRCP was introduced in the 1990s as a noninvasive and low-risk technique to evaluate the biliary system and has high accuracy in the detection of common bile duct stones.[231,232] The reported sensitivity, specificity, and accuracy of MRCP for choledocholithiasis range from 85% to 100%, 90% to 90%, and 89% to 97%, respectively.[233,234] MRCP has been shown to be more sensitive for the detection of common bile duct stones than ultrasonography and CT[82] and is highly accurate for the detection of common bile duct stones in patients with symptomatic gallstones.[234]

MRCP sequences include heavily T2 weighted thin-slice (3–4mm) half-Fourier acquisition single-shot turbo spin echo (HASTE) or half-Fourier rapid acquisition relaxation enhancement (RARE) that allow rapid acquisition, with imaging of the biliary tract in a single breath hold, reducing motion

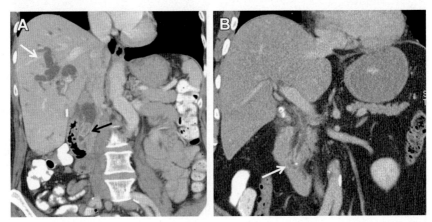

Fig. 36. Choledocholithiasis: CT appearance. (*A*) Coronal reformatted image shows large stone (*black arrow*) in the distal common bile duct with intrahepatic biliary dilatation (*white arrow*). (*B*) Small calcified stone (*arrow*) in the distal common bile duct not seen on ultrasonography.

artifact.[233,235,236] Conventional unenhanced T1-weighted and T2-weighted MR images are also usually performed. Gadolinium-enhanced images are helpful if neoplasm or inflammatory disease is suspected.[237,238] High-resolution fat-suppressed T1-weighted three-dimensional (3D) gradient-echo imaging provides high-resolution images of the biliary tree that can be reconstructed in any plane. The use of negative oral contrast agents including pineapple juice or iron oxide agents reduces overlapping T2 signal in the stomach and proximal small bowel.[233] Recently, 3D T2-weighted TSE imaging has shown promise and offers improved anatomic accuracy, higher signal/noise ratio, and thinner sections without gaps.[239–241] When combined with new techniques, such as the parallel acquisition technique, data acquisition time is shortened while retaining spatial resolution and contrast.[242,243] Faster gradients and navigator-based respiratory triggering also allow improved image quality.[233,243] A more recently investigated technique includes the use of intravenous contrast agents that are taken up by hepatocytes and excreted through the biliary system allowing for high-resolution, isotropic T1W three-dimensional GRE images of the biliary tract.[243]

On MRCP, stones generally appear as well-circumscribed low-signal-intensity filling defects in the biliary tract (**Fig. 37**). MRCP can detect stones as small as 2 mm[82] and may be a helpful adjunct to ultrasonography and CT when biliary calculi are suspected but not definitively visualized. MRCP may also be helpful if a noncalcified stone is difficult to differentiate from a soft tissue mass. Stones may also be identified as high-signal-intensity filling defects on T1-weighted images and these images can supplement MRCP images in equivocal cases. Diagnostic pitfalls include gas, blood, or other abnormality within the duct simulating stones, as well as signal loss caused by surgical clips after cholecystectomy. High signal from adjacent fluid collections, ascites, or edema may also interfere with biliary signal. Pseudo-obstruction of the extrahepatic bile duct may be caused by arterial pulsatile compression, most commonly at the common hepatic duct, caused by the right hepatic artery,[244] and flow artifacts may mimic filling defects.[245] It is important to review coronal source and axial T2-weighted images to avoid these pitfalls.

Cholangitis

Acute cholangitis results from biliary stasis and partial or complete obstruction of the biliary tract, and can also represent an acute-on-chronic process, such as in patients with chronic primary sclerosing cholangitis. Clinical presentation includes abdominal pain, fever, and jaundice. In acute suppurative cholangitis there is pus in the biliary tract with ultimate progression to biliary sepsis if untreated, with associated high morbidity and mortality. The most common bacteria in infected bile without prior instrumentation include *E coli*, *K pneumoniae*, *Enterococcus faecalis*, and *Streptococcus* species.[246]

In acute cholangitis, at ultrasonography, thickening of the common bile duct wall may be identified in addition to biliary dilatation. The most common CT finding is biliary obstruction, often with associated diffuse and concentric thickening and increased enhancement of the bile duct

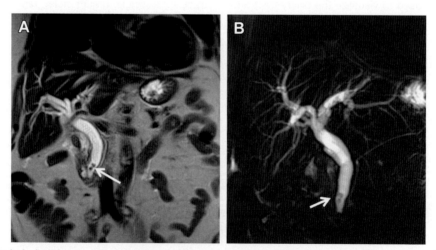

Fig. 37. Choledocholithiasis: MR and MRCP findings. (*A*) Coronal SSFSE image shows 2 stones as low-signal-intensity filling defects (*arrow*) in the dilated common bile duct. (*B*) MRCP in the same patient shows the 2 stones in the dilated common bile duct (*arrow*). Moderate intrahepatic biliary dilatation is also shown.

wall.[247] In arterial-phase enhancement, there is nodular, patchy, wedge-shaped, or geographic inhomogeneous hepatic parenchymal enhancement. These features are described in a CT scoring system.[248] At MR imaging, acute cholangitis is shown by periportal edema and distention of the biliary tree on T2-weighted sequences[243] (Fig. 38). There is progressive enhancement of the bile duct wall on fat-suppressed, contrast-enhanced T1-weighted sequences during the portal venous phases and delayed phases of enhancement.[238] On MRCP, in suppurative cholangitis, there is purulent material with low signal intensity on T2-weighted images, and/or intermediate signal intensity on T1-weighted images. MRCP is useful for detection of sites of obstruction and cause. Periportal inflammation is seen as areas of high signal intensity along the intrahepatic and extrahepatic biliary tree on T2-weighted images. Complications include pyogenic liver abscess, portal vein thrombosis from pylephlebitis and biliary peritonitis.[247] Treatment includes antibiotic therapy and biliary drainage with ERCP or percutaneous transhepatic drainage.

INTRAHEPATIC BILIARY CALCULI
Recurrent Pyogenic Cholangitis

Intrahepatic biliary calculi may occur in the setting of biliary strictures with long-standing obstruction, such as after biliary surgery or in the setting of Caroli disease.[249] In the Asian population, the most common entity associated with the formation of primary intrahepatic stones is recurrent pyogenic cholangitis, also referred to as oriental cholangiohepatitis. This disease is endemic in southeast Asia and is more frequently encountered in the United States because of increased immigration from Asia.[250,251] Features of this disorder include pigment stone formation within the intrahepatic and extrahepatic bile ducts, stricture development, and biliary dilatation. Clinically, this disorder

is characterized by recurrent attacks of fever, chills, jaundice, and abdominal pain. The cause of this disorder is not clear, although it is postulated that infection of the biliary tract with parasitic organisms such as *Clonorchis sinensis* results in biliary stasis and stone formation. Ultimately, there is progression to stricture formation, biliary obstruction, and hepatic cirrhosis with an increased risk of cholangiocarcinoma.

Imaging

Noninvasive cross-sectional imaging techniques, including CT, ultrasonography, and MR imaging, now play a more important role than invasive cholangiographic methods.[252–256] Ultrasonography shows intrahepatic and extrahepatic biliary dilatation, with intrahepatic stones that may or may not shadow. A nonshadowing stone may mimic an echogenic soft tissue mass. CT provides more complete evaluation of the full extent of disease and associated complications such as liver abscess and pancreatitis (Fig. 39A). CT can be particularly helpful if the patient has already undergone biliary enteric bypass surgery, in which case associated pneumobilia may obscure findings at sonography. Noncontrast images may be helpful to identified noncalcified pigment stones, which are soft tissue density. The use of intravenous contrast provides improved visualization of ductal wall and periductal enhancement indicating active infection/inflammation[254] as well as detection of abscesses. Findings of biliary dilatation and stone disease are often more prominent in the left lateral lobe and this is an important distinguishing feature of this disorder. Hepatic atrophy correlates with portal vein occlusion and is usually most prominent in the lateral segment of the left lobe.[257] MR and MRCP are also often useful in the identification of intrahepatic biliary calculi and associated parenchymal abnormalities[253] (Fig. 39B).

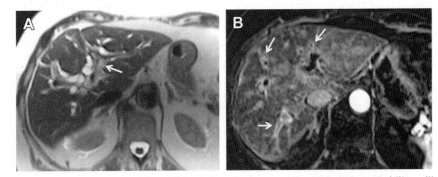

Fig. 38. Cholangitis: MR appearance. (*A*) Axial SSFSE image shows moderate intrahepatic biliary dilatation with periductal increased signal (*arrow*). (*B*) Postcontrast subtraction image shows increased periductal contrast enhancement (*arrows*).

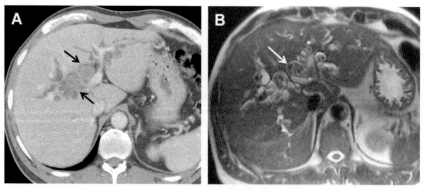

Fig. 39. Recurrent pyogenic cholangitis. (*A*) CT shows dilated intrahepatic bile ducts filled with soft tissue–attenuation material (*arrows*) compatible with pigment stones. (*B*) Axial SSFSE image shows the dilated intrahepatic bile ducts with multiple hypointense filling defects compatible with pigment stones (*arrow*).

OTHER CAUSES OF RIGHT UPPER QUADRANT PAIN RELATED TO GALLSTONES
Spilled Gallstones After Laparoscopic Cholecystectomy

Gallbladder perforation during laparoscopic cholecystectomy occurs in approximately 10% to 40% of cases, with associated spillage of gallstones occurring approximately 6% to 8% of the time.[258] This condition occurs most frequently during resection of an acutely inflamed gallbladder and may occur during dissection of the gallbladder from the hepatic bed or removal through the umbilical incision. Late abscess formation is rare, with an incidence of less than 1%,[259–261] and occurs most frequently when both bile and calculus spillage occur. Infectious complications are most likely to occur with bilirubinate stones because they contain viable bacteria that serve as a nidus of infection. The spilled stones most often remain in the peritoneal cavity adjacent to the liver and cause a subhepatic abscess or abscess in the retroperitoneum below the subhepatic space. However, because of pneumoperitoneum and peritoneal irrigation at the time of laparoscopy, stones may also migrate to distant sites. More unusual locations for abscess formation include the pleural space, abdominal wall at the trocar site, and within an incisional hernia. Because of the indolent nature of the infection, the time interval for presentation after surgery ranges from 1 month to 10 years, with a reported peak incidence around 4 months.[258] Patients usually present with vague constitutional symptoms such as nausea, anorexia, and low-grade fever. However, the patient may remain asymptomatic and the spilled stones are an incidental finding.

Ultrasonography, CT, and MR imaging are effective in identifying the abscess and associated dropped gallstones.[262] The abscess appears as a thick-walled fluid collection, most commonly located posterior to the right lobe of the liver. On ultrasonography, stones appear as echogenic foci and at CT as calcified densities (**Fig. 40**). At MR imaging, stones may be identified as low-signal-intensity foci on T2-weighted images. Recognizing the history of prior laparoscopic cholecystectomy and careful search for spilled stones, particularly when an abscess is identified in the subhepatic space, is important in establishing the diagnosis. The abscess may be misdiagnosed as tumor or abscess from another cause if the stones are not radiopaque or not recognized or located in a less typical location. If stones are found in other locations, such as the pelvis, the presence of clips in an otherwise empty gallbladder fossa may help to suggest the diagnosis. Surgical or percutaneous removal of the stones is necessary for complete cure because infected

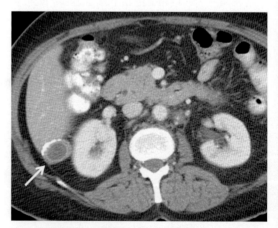

Fig. 40. Spilled gallstone after laparoscopic surgery. CT in patient with right upper quadrant pain and cholecystectomy 5 years prior shows large stone posterior to inferior right hepatic lobe (*arrow*).

stones cannot be sterilized with antibiotic therapy.[263,264]

Mirizzi Syndrome

Mirizzi syndrome refers to common hepatic or common bile duct obstruction from extrinsic compression by an impacted gallstone in the gallbladder neck or cystic duct or from associated inflammatory changes, and can be complicated by a cholecystocholedochal fistula.[265–267] Mirizzi syndrome is an uncommon complication of longstanding cholelithiasis and recurrent episodes of jaundice and cholangitis are the usual clinical presentation. This syndrome is reported in up to 2% of patients operated on for symptomatic gallstone disease.[268] Preoperative diagnosis is important because standard cholecystectomy technique is associated with an increased risk of extrahepatic bile duct injury secondary to dense fibrosis and edema around the hepatoduodenal ligament.[269]

Mirizzi syndrome may be diagnosed with ultrasonography, CT, or MR imaging.[270,271] The hallmark is intrahepatic biliary dilatation and dilatation of the common hepatic duct to the level of the porta hepatis with normal caliber of the distal common bile duct. A stone may be identified in the gallbladder neck or cystic duct (**Fig. 41**). MPR imaging with either CT or MR can be particularly helpful to identify the extrinsic nature of the obstruction. MR imaging has been proposed as most useful for showing dilatation of the intrahepatic ducts, the level of obstruction, and the location of gallstones.[271]

Gallstone Ileus

Gallstone ileus results from perforation of the gallbladder caused by chronic cholelithiasis and inflammation with fistula formation between the gallbladder and an adjacent viscus. Gallstones that have migrated from the gallbladder through the fistula then result in a mechanical bowel obstruction. Fistula formation most commonly occurs between the gallbladder and duodenum, followed by the colon and stomach.[208,272] Obstruction usually occurs in the small intestine when a gallstone larger than 2.5 cm lodges in the lumen. The most common sites of gallstone impaction are the ileum (54%–65%), the jejunum (27%), and the duodenum (1%–3%).[273] Bouveret syndrome describes a proximal gallstone impaction resulting in duodenal or pyloric obstruction and symptoms of gastric outlet obstruction. Gallstone ileus accounts for approximately 1% to 5% of all cases of nonmalignant small bowel obstruction, increasing up to 25% in patients more than 65 years of age.[273]

Less than half of patients presenting with gallstone ileus have a known history of preexisting gallbladder disease. Patients usually present with clinical symptoms of bowel obstruction and an abdominal radiograph may be the initial imaging study performed. The classic triad of findings on an abdominal radiograph, referred to as the Rigler triad[274] includes presence of bowel obstruction, pneumobilia, and the obstructing gallstone. However, this is visualized in only 30% to 35% of patients.[275] CT is frequently used to evaluate patients with bowel obstruction to confirm diagnosis, determine the cause of obstruction, and evaluate for complications. CT is superior to the plain abdominal radiograph for visualization of the obstructing gallstone and detection of small amounts of gas in the gallbladder and biliary tree[276–278] (**Fig. 42**). Diagnosis may be challenging if the gallstone is not calcified and is similar in density to the intraluminal bowel content. The cholecystoenteric fistula may also be identified, for which MPR images are helpful. Cholecystoenteric fistula may develop in the absence of gallstone ileus, usually resulting from chronic gallbladder inflammation. CT findings include a contracted gallbladder containing air, and visualization of a fistulous tract.

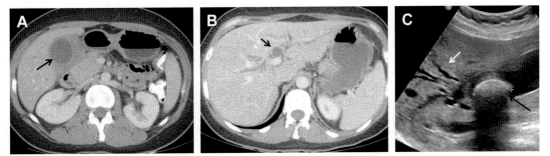

Fig. 41. Mirizzi syndrome. (*A*) Contrast-enhanced CT shows distended gallbladder with marked wall thickening (*arrow*). No radiodense stone was seen. (*B*) There is intrahepatic biliary dilatation (*arrow*). (*C*) Ultrasonography shows a large stone impacted in the gallbladder neck (*black arrow*). There is associated intrahepatic biliary dilatation (*white arrow*). The common bile duct was of normal caliber (not shown).

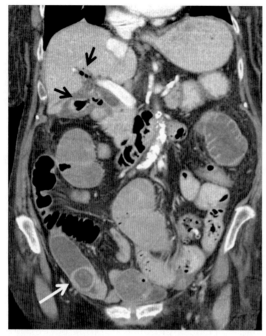

Fig. 42. Gallstone ileus. Coronal reformatted CT shows air in the gallbladder and intrahepatic biliary tree (*black arrows*). There are multiple dilated fluid-filled loops of small bowel compatible with small bowel obstruction. At the transition point, there is a large noncalcified gallstone in the lumen of the distal ileum in the right lower quadrant (*white arrow*).

REFERENCES

1. Bernal W, Auzinger G, Dhawan A, et al. Acute liver failure. Lancet 2010;376:190–201.
2. Schiodt FV, Lee WM. Fulminant liver disease. Clin Liver Dis 2003;7:331–49.
3. Mondelli MU, Cerino A, Cividini A. Acute hepatitis C: diagnosis and management. J Hepatol 2005; 42(Suppl):S108–14.
4. Privette TW, Carlisle MC, Palma JK. Emergencies of the liver, gallbladder and pancreas. Emerg Med Clin North Am 2011;29:293–317.
5. Jayakumar S, Chowdhury R, Ye C, et al. Fulminant viral hepatitis. Crit Care Clin 2013;29:677–97.
6. Kurtz AB, Rubin CS, Cooper HS, et al. Ultrasound findings in hepatitis. Radiology 1980;136:717–72.
7. Needleman L, Kurtz AB, Rifkin MD, et al. Sonography of diffuse benign liver disease: accuracy of pattern recognition and grading. AJR Am J Roentgenol 1986;146:1011–5.
8. Tchelepi H, Ralls PW, Radin R, et al. Sonography of diffuse liver disease. J Ultrasound Med 2002;21: 1023–32.
9. Spence SC, Teichgraeber D, Chandrasekhar C. Emergent right upper quadrant sonography. J Ultrasound Med 2009;28:479–96.
10. Maresca G, De Gaetano AM, Mirk P, et al. Sonographic patterns of the gallbladder in acute viral hepatitis. J Clin Ultrasound 1984;12:141–6.
11. van Breda Vriesman AC, Engelbrecht MR, Smithuis RH, et al. Diffuse gallbladder wall thickening: differential diagnosis. AJR Am J Roentgenol 2007;188:495–501.
12. Jüttner HU, Ralls PW, Quinn MF, et al. Thickening of the gallbladder wall in acute hepatitis: ultrasound demonstration. Radiology 1982;142:465–6.
13. Suk KT, Kim CH, Baik SK, et al. Gallbladder wall thickening in patients with acute hepatitis. J Clin Ultrasound 2009;37:144–8.
14. Yoo SM, Lee HY, Song IS, et al. Acute hepatitis A: correlation of CT findings with clinical phase. Hepatogastroenterology 2010;57:1208–14.
15. Kawamoto S, Soyer PA, Fishman EK, et al. Nonneoplastic liver disease: evaluation with CT and MR imaging. Radiographics 1998;18:827–48.
16. Mortele KJ, Ros PR. Imaging of diffuse liver disease. Semin Liver Dis 2001;21:195–212.
17. Rofsky NM, Fleishaker H. CT and MRI of diffuse liver disease. Semin Ultrasound CT MR 1995;16: 16–33.
18. Park SJ, Kim JD, Seo YS, et al. Computed tomography findings for predicting sever acute hepatitis with prolonged cholestasis. World J Gastroenterol 2013;19(16):2543–9.
19. Kim W, Kim DJ. Severe alcoholic hepatitis-current concepts, diagnosis and treatment options. World J Hepatol 2014;6(10):688–95.
20. Sohail U, Satapathy SK. Diagnosis and management of alcoholic hepatitis. Clin Liver Dis 2012;16: 717–36.
21. Lucey MR, Mathurin P, Morgan TR. Alcoholic hepatitis. N Engl J Med 2009;360:2758–69.
22. Shin DS, Jeffrey RB, Desser TS. Pearls and pitfalls in hepatic ultrasonography. Ultrasound Q 2010;26: 17–25.
23. Benedetti NJ, Desser TS, Jeffrey RB. Imaging of hepatic infections. Ultrasound Q 2008;24:267–78.
24. Doyle DJ, Hanbidge AE, O'Malley ME. Imaging of hepatic infections. Clin Radiol 2006;61:737–48.
25. Oto A, Akhan O, Ozman M. Focal inflammatory diseases of the liver. Eur J Radiol 1999;32:61–75.
26. Halvorsen RA, Korobkin M, Foster WL, et al. The variable CT appearance of hepatic abscesses. AJR Am J Roentgenol 1984;142(5):941–6.
27. Jeffrey RB Jr, Tolentino CS, Chang FC, et al. CT of small pyogenic hepatic abscesses: the cluster sign. AJR Am J Roentgenol 1988;151(3):487–9.
28. Alsaif HS, Venkatesh SK, Chan DS, et al. CT appearance of pyogenic liver abscesses caused by *Klebsiella pneumoniae*. Radiology 2011;260: 129–38.
29. Balci NC, Semelka RC, Noone TC, et al. Pyogenic hepatic abscess: MRI findings on T1 and T2

weighted and serial gadolinium-enhanced gradient-echo images. J Magn Reson Imaging 1999;9:285–90.

30. Chan JH, Tsui EY, Luk SH, et al. Diffusion-weighted MR imaging of the liver: distinguishing hepatic abscess from cystic or necrotic tumor. Abdom Imaging 2001;26:161–5.

31. Park HJ, Kim SH, Jang KM, et al. Differentiating hepatic abscess from malignant mimickers; value of diffusion-weighted imaging with an emphasis on the periphery of the lesion. J Magn Reson Imaging 2013;38:1333–41.

32. Schmid-Tannwald C, Schmid-Tannwald CM, Morelli JN, et al. Role of diffusion-weighted MRI in differentiation of hepatic abscesses from non-infected fluid collections. Clin Radiol 2014;69:687–94.

33. Lee NK, Kim S, Kim DU, et al. Diffusion-weighted magnetic resonance imaging for non-neoplastic conditions in the hepatobiliary and pancreatic regions: pearls and potential pitfalls in imaging interpretation. Abdom Imaging 2015;40:643–62.

34. Pastakia B, Shawker TH, Thaler M, et al. Hepatosplenic candidiasis: wheels within wheels. Radiology 1988;166(2):417–21.

35. Masood A, Sallah S. Chronic disseminated candidiasis in patients with acute leukemia: emphasis on diagnostic definition and treatment. Leuk Res 2005;29(5):493–501.

36. Manzella A, Ohtomo K, Monzawa S, et al. Schistosomiasis of the liver. Abdom Imaging 2008;33(2):144–50.

37. Czermak BV, Akhan O, Hiemetzberger R, et al. Echinococcosis of the liver. Abdom Imaging 2008;33(2):133–43.

38. Tirumani SH, Shanbhogue AK, Vikram R, et al. Imaging of the porta hepatis: spectrum of disease. Radiographics 2014;34:73–92.

39. Amitrano L, Guardascione MA, Brancaccio V, et al. Risk factors and clinical presentation of portal vein thrombosis in patients with liver cirrhosis. J Hepatol 2004;40(5):736–41.

40. Kanematsu M, Semelka RC, Leonardou P, et al. Hepatocellular carcinoma of diffuse type: MR imaging findings and clinical manifestations. J Magn Reson Imaging 2003;18(2):189–95.

41. Gallego C, Velasco M, Marcuello P, et al. Congenital and acquired anomalies of the portal venous system. Radiographics 2002;22(1):141–59.

42. MacNicholas R, Olliff S, Elias E, et al. An update on the diagnosis and management of Budd-Chiari syndrome. Expert Rev Gastroenterol Hepatol 2012;6:731–44.

43. Torabi M, Hosseinzadeh K, Federle MP. CT of nonneoplastic hepatic vascular and perfusion disorders. Radiographics 2008;28:1967–82.

44. Kage M, Arakawa M, Kojiro M, et al. Histopathology of membranous obstruction of the inferior vena cava in the Budd-Chiari syndrome. Gastroenterology 1992;102(6):2081–90.

45. Darwish Murad S, Plessier A, Hernandez-Guerra M, et al, EN-Vie (European Network for Vascular Disorders of the Liver). Etiology, management, and outcome of the Budd-Chiari syndrome. Ann Intern Med 2009;151(3):167–75.

46. Perarnau JM, Bacq Y. Hepatic vascular involvement related to pregnancy, oral contraceptives, and estrogen replacement therapy. Semin Liver Dis 2008;28(3):315–27.

47. Darwish Murad S, Valla DC, de Groen PC, et al. Determinants of survival and the effect of portosystemic shunting in patients with Budd-Chiari syndrome. Hepatology 2004;39(2):500–8.

48. Bolondi L, Gaiani S, Li B, et al. Diagnosis of Budd-Chiari syndrome by pulsed Doppler ultrasound. Gastroenterology 1991;100:1324–31.

49. Kim TK, Chung JW, Han JK, et al. Hepatic changes in benign obstruction of the hepatic inferior vena cava: CT findings. AJR Am J Roentgenol 1999; 173:1235–42.

50. Brancatelli G, Vilgrain V, Federle MP, et al. Budd Chiari syndrome: spectrum of imaging findings. AJR Am J Roentgenol 2007;188:W168–76.

51. Erden A. Budd-Chiari syndrome: a review of imaging findings. Eur J Radiol 2007;61:44–56.

52. Brancatelli G, Federle MP, Grazioli L, et al. Benign regenerative nodules in Budd Chiari syndrome and other vascular disorders of the liver: radiologic-pathologic and clinical correlation. Radiographics 2002;22:847–62.

53. Cazals-Hatem D, Vilgrain V, Genin P, et al. Arterial and portal circulation and parenchymal changes in Budd-Chiari syndrome: a study in 17 explanted livers. Hepatology 2003;37:510–9.

54. Casillas VJ, Amendola MA, Gascue A, et al. Imaging of nontraumatic hemorrhagic hepatic lesions. Radiographics 2000;20:367–78.

55. Perricone G. Hepatology: Fitz-Hugh-Curtis syndrome: pelvic inflammatory disease with perihepatitis. J Gastroenterol Hepatol 2014;29:1853.

56. Curtis AH. A cause of adhesions in the right upper quadrant. JAMA 1930;94:1221–2.

57. Fitz-Hugh T Jr. Acute gonococcic peritonitis of the right upper quadrant in women. JAMA 1934;102:2094–6.

58. van Dongen PW. Diagnosis of Fitz-Hugh-Curtis syndrome by ultrasound. Eur J Obstet Gynecol Reprod Biol 1993;50:159–62.

59. Kim S, Kim TU, Lee JW, et al. The perihepatic space: comprehensive anatomy and CT features of pathologic conditions. Radiographics 2007;27:129–43.

60. Nishie A, Yoshimitsu K, Irie H, et al. Fitz-Hugh-Curtis syndrome. Radiologic manifestation. J Comput Assist Tomogr 2003;27:786–91.

61. Shaffer EA. Gallstone disease: epidemiology of gallbladder stone disease. Best Pract Res Clin Gastroenterol 2006;20(6):981–96.

62. Knab LM, Boller AM, Mahvi DM. Cholecystitis. Surg Clin North Am 2014;94:455–70.

63. Lack EE. Cholecystitis, cholelithiasis and unusual infections of the gallbladder. In: Pathology of the pancreas, gallbladder, extrahepatic biliary tract, and ampullary region. Oxford (United Kingdom): Oxford, University Press; 2003. p. 414–52.

64. Tazuma S. Gallstone disease: epidemiology, pathogenesis, and classification of biliary stones (common bile duct and intrahepatic). Best Pract Res Clin Gastroenterol 2006;20:1075–83.

65. Trotman BW. Pigment gallstone disease. Gastroenterol Clin North Am 1991;20:111–26.

66. Weltman DI, Zeman RK. Acute diseases of the gallbladder and biliary ducts. Radiol Clin North Am 1994;32:933–50.

67. Cooperberg P. Imaging of the gallbladder. Radiology 1987;163:605.

68. McIntosh DM, Penney HF. Gray-scale ultrasonography as a screening procedure in the detection of gallbladder disease. Radiology 1980;136:725–7.

69. Carroll BA. Gallstones: in vitro comparison of physical, radiographic and ultrasonic characteristics. AJR Am J Roentgenol 1978;131:223.

70. Filly RA, Moss AA, Way LW. In vitro investigation of gallstone shadowing with ultrasound tomography. J Clin Ultrasound 1979;7:255–62.

71. Grossman M. Cholelithiasis and acoustic shadowing. J Clin Ultrasound 1978;6:182.

72. Desser TS, Jeffrey RB Jr, Lane MJ, et al. Tissue harmonic imaging: utility in abdominal and pelvic sonography. J Clin Ultrasound 1999;27:135–42.

73. Oktar SO, Yucel C, Ozdemer H, et al. Comparison of conventional sonography, real-time compound sonography, tissue harmonic sonography, and tissue harmonic compound sonography of abdominal and pelvic lesions. AJR Am J Roentgenol 2003; 181:1341–7.

74. Chintapalli KN, Ghiatas AA, Chopra S, et al. Sonographic findings in cases of missed gallstones. J Clin Ultrasound 1999;27:117–21.

75. MacDonald FR, Cooperberg PL, Cohen MM. The WES triad: a specific sonographic sign of gallstones in the contracted gallbladder. Gastrointest Radiol 1981;6:39–41.

76. Baron RL, Rohrmann CA, Lee SP, et al. CT evaluation of gallstones in vitro: correlation with chemical analysis. AJR Am J Roentgenol 1988;151: 1123–8.

77. Brakel K, Lameris JS, Nijs HG, et al. Predicting gallstone composition with CT: in vivo and in vitro analysis. Radiology 1990;174:337–41.

78. Paulson EK. Acute cholecystitis: CT findings. Semin Ultrasound CT MR 2000;21:56–63.

79. Barakos JA, Ralls PW, Lapin SA, et al. Cholelithiasis: evaluation with CT. Radiology 1987;162: 415–8.

80. Chan WC, Joe BN, Coakley FV, et al. Gallstone detection at CT in vitro: effect of peak voltage setting. Radiology 2006;241:546–53.

81. Tsai HM, Lin XZ, Chen CY, et al. MRI of gallstones with different compositions. AJR Am J Roentgenol 2004;182:1513–9.

82. Hartman EM, Barish MA. MR cholangiography. Magn Reson Imaging Clin North Am 2001;4: 841–55.

83. Ukayi M, Ebara M, Tsuchiya Y, et al. Diagnosis of gallstone composition in magnetic resonance imaging: in vitro analysis. Eur J Radiol 2002;41: 49–56.

84. Ko CW, Sekijima JH, Lee SP. Biliary sludge. Ann Intern Med 1999;130:301–11.

85. Lee SP. Pathogenesis of biliary sludge. Hepatology 1990;12:2005–35.

86. Friedman GD. Natural history of asymptomatic and symptomatic gallstones. Am J Surg 1993; 165:399–404.

87. Duncan CB, Riall TS. Evidence-based current surgical practice: calculous gallbladder disease. J Gastrointest Surg 2012;16:2011–25.

88. Keus F, Broeders IA, van Laarhoven CJ. Surgical aspects of symptomatic cholecystolithiasis and acute cholecystitis. Best Pract Res Clin Gastroenterol 2006;20:1031–51.

89. Laing FL, Federle MP, Jeffrey RB, et al. Ultrasonic evaluation of patients with acute right upper quadrant pain. Radiology 1981;140:449–55.

90. Yarmish GM, Smith MP, Rosen MP, et al. ACR appropriateness criteria right upper quadrant pain. J Am Coll Radiol 2014;11:316–22.

91. Kieweit JJ, Leeuwenburgh MM, Bipat S, et al. A systematic review and meta-analysis of diagnostic performance of imaging in acute cholecystitis. Radiology 2012;264:708–20.

92. Laing FC. Ultrasonography of the acute abdomen. Radiol Clin North Am 1992;30:389–404.

93. Sherman M, Ralls PW, Quinn M, et al. Intravenous cholangiography and sonography in acute cholecystitis: prospective evaluation. AJR Am J Roentgenol 1980;135:311–3.

94. Hanbidge AE, Buckler PM, O'Malley ME, et al. Imaging evaluation for acute pain in the right upper quadrant. Radiographics 2004;24:1117–35.

95. O'Connor OJ, Maher MM. Imaging of cholecystitis. AJR Am J Roentgenol 2011;196:W367–74.

96. Ralls PW, Colleti PM, Lapin SA, et al. Real-time sonography in suspected acute cholecystitis. Radiology 1985;155:767–71.

97. Paulson EK, Kliewer MA, Hertzberg BS, et al. Diagnosis of acute cholecystitis with color Doppler sonography: significance of arterial flow in

thickened gallbladder wall. AJR Am J Roentgenol 1994;162:1105–8.

98. Schiller VL, Turner RR, Sarti DA. Color Doppler imaging of the gallbladder wall in acute cholecystitis: sonographic-pathologic correlation. Abdom Imaging 1996;21:233–7.

99. Palmer EL, Scott JA, Strauss HW. Abdominal imaging. In: Practical nuclear medicine. Philadelphia: WB Saunders; 1992. p. 275–85.

100. Zeissman HA. Hepatobiliary scintigraphy in 2014. J Nucl Med 2014;55:967–75.

101. Bennett GL, Rusinek H, Lisi V, et al. CT findings of acute gangrenous cholecystitis. AJR Am J Roentgenol 2002;178:275–81.

102. Kane RA, Costello P, Duszlak E. Computed tomography in acute cholecystitis: new observations. AJR Am J Roentgenol 1983;141:697–701.

103. Fidler J, Paulson EK, Layfield L. CT evaluation of acute cholecystitis: findings and usefulness in diagnosis. AJR Am J Roentgenol 1996;166:1085–8.

104. Gore RM, Yaghmai V, Newmark GM, et al. Imaging benign and malignant disease of the gallbladder. Radiol Clin North Am 2002;40:1307–23.

105. Gore RM, Thakrar KH, Newmark GM, et al. Gallbladder imaging. Gastroenterol Clin North Am 2010;39:265–87.

106. Grand D, Horton KM, Fishman E. CT of the gallbladder: spectrum of disease. AJR Am J Roentgenol 2004;183:163–70.

107. Yamashita K, Jin MJ, Hirose Y, et al. CT findings of transient focal increased attenuation of the liver adjacent to the gallbladder in acute cholecystitis. AJR Am J Roentgenol 1995;164:343–6.

108. Ito K, Awaya H, Mitchell DG, et al. Gallbladder disease: appearance of associated transient increased attenuation in the liver at biphasic, contrast-enhanced dynamic CT. Radiology 1997;204:723–8.

109. Kim YK, Kim CS, Han YM, et al. CT findings of mild forms or early manifestations of acute cholecystitis. Clin Imaging 2009;33:274–80.

110. Cheng SM, Ng SP, Shih SL. Hyperdense gallbladder sign: an overlooked sign of acute cholecystitis on unenhanced CT examination. Clin Imaging 2004;28:128–31.

111. Soyer P, Hoeffel C, Dohan A, et al. Acute cholecystitis: quantitative and qualitative evaluation with 64-section helical CT. Acta Radiol 2013;54:477–86.

112. Adusumilli S, Siegelman ES. MR imaging of the gallbladder. Magn Reson Imaging Clin North Am 2002;10:165–84.

113. Loud PA, Semelka RC, Kettriz U, et al. MRI of acute cholecystitis: comparison with the normal gallbladder and other entities. Magn Reson Imaging 1996;14:349–55.

114. Pedrosa I, Rofsky NM. MR imaging in abdominal emergencies. Magn Reson Imaging Clin North Am 2004;12:603–35.

115. Watanabe Y, Nagayama M, Okumura A, et al. MR imaging of acute biliary disorders. Radiographics 2007;27:477–95.

116. Catalano OA, Sahani DV, Kalva SP, et al. MR imaging of the gallbladder: a pictorial essay. Radiographics 2008;28:135–55.

117. Tonolini M, Ravelli A, Villa C, et al. Urgent MRI with MR cholangiopancreatography (MRCP) of acute cholecystitis and related complications: diagnostic role and spectrum of imaging findings. Emerg Radiol 2012;19:341–8.

118. Park MS, Yu JS, Kim YH, et al. Acute cholecystitis: comparison of MR cholangiography and US. Radiology 1998;209:781–5.

119. Regan F, Schaefer DC, Smith DP, et al. The diagnostic utility of HASTE MRI in the evaluation of acute cholecystitis. Half-Fourier acquisition single-shot turbo SE. J Comput Assist Tomogr 1998;22: 638–42.

120. Altun E, Semelka RC, Elias J Jr, et al. Acute cholecystitis: MR findings and differentiation from chronic cholecystitis. Radiology 2007;244:174–83.

121. Akpinar E, Turkbeyd B, Karcaaltincaba M, et al. Initial experience on utility of gadobenate dimeglumine (GT1-weighted-BOPTA) enhanced MR cholangiography in diagnosis of acute cholecystitis. J Magn Reson Imaging 2009;30:578–85.

122. Choi Y, Cha SH, Yeom SK, et al. Diagnosis of acute cholecystitis: value of contrast agent in the gallbladder and cystic duct on Gd-EOB-DTPA enhanced MR cholangiography. Clin Imaging 2014;38:174–8.

123. Huffman JL, Schenker S. Acute acalculous cholecystitis: a review. Clin Gastroenterol Hepatol 2010;8:15–22.

124. Glenn F, Becker CG. Acute acalculous cholecystitis. An increasing entity. Ann Surg 1982;195: 131–6.

125. Barie PS, Eachempati SR. Acute acalculous cholecystitis. Gastroenterol Clin North Am 2010; 39:343–57.

126. Kang JY, Williamson RC. Cholecystitis without gallstones. HPB Surg 1990;2:83–103.

127. Parithivel VS, Gerst PH, Banerjee S, et al. Acute acalculous cholecystitis in young patients without predisposing factors. Am Surg 1999;65:366–8.

128. Savoca PE, Longo WE, Zucker KA, et al. The increasing prevalence of acalculous cholecystitis in outpatients. Ann Surg 1990;211:433–7.

129. Flancbaum L, Choban PS. Use of morphine cholescintigraphy in the diagnosis of acute cholecystitis in critically ill patients. Intensive Care Med 1995; 21:120–4.

130. Kalliafas S, Ziegler DW, Flancbaum L, et al. Acute acalculous cholecystitis: incidence, risk factors, diagnosis, and outcome. Am Surg 1998; 64:471–5.

131. Shuman WP, Rogers JV, Rudd TG, et al. Low sensitivity of sonography and cholescintigraphy in acalculous cholecystitis. AJR Am J Roentgenol 1984; 142:531–4.

132. Boland GW, Slater G, Lu DS, et al. Prevalence and significance of gallbladder abnormalities seen on sonography in intensive care unit patients. AJR Am J Roentgenol 2000;174:973–7.

133. Kalff V, Froelich JW, Lloyd R, et al. Predictive value of an abnormal hepatobiliary scan in patients with severe intercurrent illness. Radiology 1983;146: 191–4.

134. Flancbaum L, Alden SM. Morphine cholescintigraphy. Surg Gynecol Obstet 1990;171:227–32.

135. Mariat G, Mahul P, Prevot N, et al. Contribution of ultrasonography and cholescintigraphy to the diagnosis of acute acalculous cholecystitis in intensive care patients. Intensive Care Med 2000;26: 1658–63.

136. Ahvenjarvi L, Koivukangas V, Jartti A, et al. Diagnostic accuracy of computed tomography imaging of surgically treated acute acalculous cholecystitis in critically ill patients. J Trauma 2011;70:183–8.

137. McGahan JP, Lindfors KK. Percutaneous cholecystostomy: an alternative to surgical cholecystectomy for acute cholecystitis? Radiology 1989;173: 481–5.

138. Boland GW, Lee MJ, Mueller PR, et al. Gallstones in critically ill patients with acute calculous cholecystitis treated by percutaneous cholecystostomy: nonsurgical therapeutic options. AJR Am J Roentgenol 1994;162:1101–3.

139. Lo LD, Vogelzang RL, Braun MA, et al. Percutaneous cholecystostomy for the diagnosis and treatment of acute calculous and acalculous cholecystitis. J Vasc Interv Radiol 1995;6:629–34.

140. Ito K, Fujita N, Noda Y, et al. Percutaneous cholecystostomy versus gallbladder aspiration for acute cholecystitis: a prospective randomized controlled trial. AJR Am J Roentgenol 2004;183:193–6.

141. Cotran RS, Kumar V, Robbins SL. Pathologic basis of disease. 4th edition. Philadelphia: WB Saunders; 1989.

142. Morfin E, Ponka J, Brush B. Gangrenous cholecystitis. Arch Surg 1968;96:567–72.

143. Wilson AK, Kozol RA, Salwen WA, et al. Gangrenous cholecystitis in an urban VA hospital. J Surg Res 1994;56:402–4.

144. Ahmad MM, Macon WL. Gangrene of the gallbladder. Am Surg 1983;49:155–8.

145. Merriam LT, Kanaan SA, Dawes LG, et al. Gangrenous cholecystitis: analysis of risk factors and experience with laparoscopic cholecystectomy. Surgery 1999;126:680–6.

146. Jacobs M, Verdeja J, Goldstein HS. Laparoscopic cholecystectomy in acute cholecystitis. J Laparoendosc Surg 1991;1:175–7.

147. Singer JA, McKeen RV. Laparoscopic cholecystectomy for acute or gangrenous cholecystitis. Am Surg 1994;60:326–8.

148. Teefey SA, Baron RL, Radke HM, et al. Gangrenous cholecystitis: new observations on sonography. J Ultrasound Med 1991;134:191–4.

149. Jeffrey RB, Laing FC, Wong W, et al. Gangrenous cholecystitis: diagnosis by ultrasound. Radiology 1983;148:219–21.

150. Teefey SA, Dahiya N, Middleton WD, et al. Acute cholecystitis: do sonographic findings and WBC count predict gangrenous changes? AJR Am J Roentgenol 2013;200:363–9.

151. Simeone J, Brink J, Mueller P, et al. The sonographic diagnosis of acute gangrenous cholecystitis: importance of the Murphy sign. AJR Am J Roentgenol 1989;152:209–90.

152. Lamki N, Raval B, St. Ville E. Computed tomography of complicated cholecystitis. J Comput Assist Tomogr 1986;10:319–24.

153. Varma DG, Faust JM. Computed tomography of gangrenous acute postoperative acalculous cholecystitis. J Comput Tomogr 1988;12:29–31.

154. Bridges MD, Jones BC, Morgan DE, et al. Acute cholecystitis and gall-bladder necrosis: value of contrast enhanced CT [abstract]. AJR Am J Roentgenol 1999;172:34–5.

155. Wu CH, Chen CC, Wang CJ, et al. Discrimination of gangrenous from uncomplicated acute cholecystitis: accuracy of CT findings. Abdom Imaging 2011;36:174–8.

156. Liang JL, Chen MC, Huang HY, et al. Gallbladder carcinoma manifesting as acute cholecystitis: clinical and computed tomographic features. Surgery 2009;146:861–8.

157. Jenkins M, Golding RH, Cooperberg PL. Sonography and computed tomography of hemorrhagic cholecystitis. AJR Am J Roentgenol 1983;140:1197–8.

158. Shah VR, Clegg JF. Haemorrhagic cholecystitis. Br J Surg 1979;66:404–5.

159. Hudson PB, Johnson PP. Hemorrhage from the gallbladder. N Engl J Med 1946;234:438–41.

160. Moskos MM, Eschelman DJ. Hemorrhagic cholecystitis. AJR Am J Roentgenol 1991;156:1304–5.

161. Polse S, Stoney RJ, Baldwin JN. Hemorrhage from the gallbladder. Calif Med 1967;107:51–3.

162. Chinn DH, Miller EI, Piper N. Hemorrhagic cholecystitis. Sonographic appearance and clinical presentation. J Ultrasound Med 1987;6:313–7.

163. Gremmels JM, Kruskal JB, Parangi S, et al. Hemorrhagic cholecystitis simulating gallbladder carcinoma. J Ultrasound Med 2004;23:993–5.

164. Yiu-Chiu VS, Chiu LC, Wedel VJ. Current cases and concepts: acalculous hemorrhagic cholecystitis. J Comput Tomogr 1980;4:201–6.

165. Tavernaraki K, Sykara A, Tavernaraki E, et al. Massive intraperitoneal bleeding due to

hemorrhagic cholecystitis and gallbladder rupture: CT findings. Abdom Imaging 2011;36:565–8.

166. Jacob H, Appelman R, Stein HD. Emphysematous cholecystitis. Am J Gastroenterol 1979;71:325–30.

167. May RE, Strong R. Acute emphysematous cholecystitis. Br J Surg 1971;58:453–8.

168. Mentzer RM Jr, Golden GT, Chandler JG, et al. A comparative appraisal of emphysematous cholecystitis. Am J Surg 1975;129:10–5.

169. Garcio-Sancho Tellez L, Rodriguez-Montes JA, Fernandez de Lis S, et al. Acute emphysematous cholecystitis: report of twenty cases. Hepatogastroenterology 1999;46:2144–8.

170. Konno K, Ishida H, Naganuma H, et al. Emphysematous cholecystitis: sonographic findings. Abdom Imaging 2002;27:191–5.

171. Bloom RA, Libson E, Lebensart PD, et al. The ultrasound spectrum of emphysematous cholecystitis. J Clin Ultrasound 1989;17:251–6.

172. Gill KS, Chapman AH, Weston MJ. The changing face of emphysematous cholecystitis. Br J Radiol 1997;70:986–91.

173. Charalel RA, Jeffrey RB, Shin LK. Complicated cholecystitis: the complementary roles of sonography and computed tomography. Ultrasound Q 2011;27:161–70.

174. McMillin K. Computed tomography of emphysematous cholecystitis. J Comput Assist Tomogr 1985;9:330–2.

175. Chiu HH, Chen CM, Mo LR. Emphysematous cholecystitis. Am J Surg 2004;188:325–6.

176. Koenig T, Tamm EP, Kawashima A. Magnetic resonance imaging findings in emphysematous cholecystitis. Clin Radiol 2004;59:455–8.

177. Diffenbaugh WG. Gangrenous perforation of the gallbladder. Arch Surg 1949;59:743–9.

178. Strohl EL, Digffenbaugh WG, Baker JH, et al. Collective reviews: gangrene, and perforation of the gallbladder. Int Abstr Surg 1962;114:1–7.

179. Madrazo BL, Francis I, Hricak H, et al. Sonographic findings in perforation of the gallbladder. AJR Am J Roentgenol 1982;139:491–6.

180. Niemeier OW. Acute free perforation of the gallbladder. Am Surg 1934;99:922–4.

181. Fletcher AG, Ravdin IS. Perforation of the gallbladder. Am J Surg 1951;81:178–85.

182. Heuer GJ. The factors leading to death in operations upon the gallbladder and bile ducts. Ann Surg 1934;99:881–92.

183. Cowley LL, Harkins HN. Perforation of the gallbladder. Surg Gynecol Obstet 1943;77:661–8.

184. Peer A, Witz E, Manor H, et al. Intrahepatic abscess due to gallbladder perforation. Abdom Imaging 1995;20:452–5.

185. Chen JJ, Lin HH, Chiu CT, et al. Gallbladder perforation with intra-hepatic abscess formation. J Clin Ultrasound 1990;18:43–5.

186. Ikard RW. Gallstones, cholelithiasis and diabetes surgery. Gynecol Obstet 1990;171:528–32.

187. Sood BP, Kalra N, Gupta S, et al. Role of sonography in the diagnosis of gallbladder perforation. J Clin Ultrasound 2002;30:270–4.

188. Chau WK, Na WT, Feng TT, et al. Ultrasound diagnosis of perforation of the gallbladder: real time application and the demonstration of a new sonographic sign. J Clin Ultrasound 1988;16:358–60.

189. Revzin MV, Scoutt L, Smitaman E, et al. The gallbladder: uncommon gallbladder conditions and unusual presentations of common gallbladder pathological processes. Abdom Imaging 2015;40:385–99.

190. Fitoz S, Erden A, Karagulle T, et al. Interruption of gallbladder wall with pericholecystic fluid: a CT finding of perforation. Emerg Radiol 2000;7:253–5.

191. Kim PN, Lee KS, Kim IY, et al. Gallbladder perforation: comparison of US findings with CT. Abdom Imaging 1994;19:239–42.

192. Saul SH. Gallbladder and extrahepatic biliary tree. In: Steinberg SS, editor. Diagnostic surgical pathology. 3rd edition. Philadelphia: Lippincott; 1999. p. 1629–70.

193. Jagannath SB, Singh V, Cruz-Correa M, et al. A long-term cohort study of outcome after cholecystectomy for chronic acalculous cholecystitis. Am J Surg 2003;185:91–5.

194. Krishnamurthy GT, Krishnamurthy S, Brown PH. Constancy and variability of gallbladder ejection fraction: impact on diagnosis and therapy. J Nucl Med 2004;45:1872–7.

195. Poynter MT, Saba AK, Evans RA, et al. Chronic acalculous biliary tract disease: cholecystokinin cholescintigraphy is useful in formulating treatment strategy and predicting success after cholecystectomy. Am Surg 2002;68:382–4.

196. Reilly DJ, Kalogeropoulos G, Thiruchelvam D. Torsion of the gallbladder: a systematic review. HPB (Oxford) 2012;14:669–72.

197. Timpone VM, Lattin GE, Lewis RB, et al. Abdominal twists and turns: part 2, solid visceral torsion with pathologic correlation. AJR Am J Roentgenol 2011;197:97–102.

198. Quinn SF, Fazzio F, Jones E. Torsion of the gallbladder: findings on CT and sonography and role of percutaneous cholecystostomy. AJR Am J Roentgenol 1987;148:881–2.

199. Chung JC, Song OP, Kim HC. Gallbladder torsion diagnosed by MDCT and MRCP. Abdom Imaging 2010;35:462–4.

200. Liu TH, Moody FG. Pathogenesis and presentation of common bile duct stones. Semin Laparosc Surg 2000;7:224–31.

201. Lamont JT, Afdhal NH. Cholesterol gallstone disease: from pancreatitis to prevention. Curr Opin Gastroenterol 1994;10:523–5.

202. Hermann RE. The spectrum of biliary stone disease. Am J Surg 1989;158:171–3.

203. Raraty MG, Finch M, Neoptolemos JP. Acute cholangitis and pancreatitis secondary to common duct stones: management update. World J Surg 1998;22:1155–61.

204. Makary MA, Duncan MD, Harmon JW, et al. The role of magnetic resonance cholangiography in the management of patients with gallstone pancreatitis. Ann Surg 2005;241:119–24.

205. Bilbao MK, Dotter CT, Lee TG, et al. Complications of endoscopic retrograde cholangiopancreatography. A study of 10,000 cases. Gastroenterology 1976;70:314–20.

206. Lo SK, Chen J. The role of ERCP in choledocholithiasis. Abdom Imaging 1996;21:120–32.

207. Harvey RT, Miller WT Jr. Acute biliary disease: initial CT and follow-up US versus initial US and follow-up CT. Radiology 1999;213:831–6.

208. Bortoff GA, Chen MY, Ott DJ, et al. Gallbladder stones: imaging and intervention. Radiographics 2000;20:751–66.

209. Pasanen P, Partanen K, Pikkarainen P, et al. Ultrasonography, CT and ERCP in the diagnosis of choledochal stones. Acta Radiol 1992;33:53–6.

210. Stott MA, Farrands PA, Guyer PB, et al. Ultrasound of the common bile duct in patients undergoing cholecystectomy. J Clin Ultrasound 1991;19:73–6.

211. Dong B, Chen M. Improved sonographic visualization of choledocholithiasis. J Clin Ultrasound 1987;15:185–90.

212. Laing FC, Jeffrey RB, Wing VW. Improved visualization of choledocholithiasis by sonography. AJR Am J Roentgenol 1984;143:949–52.

213. Ortega D, Burns PN, Simpson DH, et al. Tissue harmonic imaging: is it a benefit for bile duct sonography? AJR Am J Roentgenol 2001;176:653–65.

214. Amouyal P, Amouyal G, Levy P, et al. Diagnosis of choledocholithiasis by endoscopic ultrasonography. Gastroenterology 1994;106:1062–7.

215. Baron RL. Common bile duct stones: reassessment of criteria for CT diagnosis. Radiology 1987;162:419–24.

216. Baron RL. Diagnosing choledocholithiasis: how far can we push helical CT? Radiology 1997;203:601–3.

217. Pickuth D. Radiologic diagnosis of common bile duct stones. Abdom Imaging 2000;25:618–21.

218. Neitlich JD, Topazian M, Smith RC, et al. Detection of choledocholithiasis: comparison of unenhanced helical CT and endoscopic retrograde cholangiopancreatography. Radiology 1997;203:753–7.

219. Soto JA, Alvarez O, Munera F, et al. Diagnosing bile duct stones: comparison of unenhanced helical CT, oral contrast-enhanced CT cholangiography, and MR cholangiography. AJR Am J Roentgenol 2000;175:1127–34.

220. Jimenez Cuenca I, del Olmo Martinez L, Perez Horns M. Helical CT without contrast in choledocholithiasis diagnosis. Eur Radiol 2001;11:197–201.

221. Van Beers BE, Pringot JH. Imaging of cholelithiasis: helical CT. Abdom Imaging 2001;26:15–20.

222. Klein HM, Wein B, Truong S, et al. Computed tomographic cholangiography using spiral scanning and 3D imaging processing. Br J Radiol 1993;66:762–7.

223. Breen DJ, Nicholson AA. The clinical utility of spiral CT cholangiography. Clin Radiol 2000;55:733–9.

224. Xu AM, Cheng HY, Jiang WB, et al. Multislice three-dimensional spiral CT cholangiography: a new technique for diagnosing biliary disease. Hepatobiliary Pancreat Dis Int 2002;1:595–603.

225. Cabada Giadas T, Sarria Octavio de Toledo L, Martinez-Berganza Asensio MT, et al. Helical CT cholangiography in the evaluation of the biliary tract: application to the diagnosis of choledocholithiasis. Abdom Imaging 2002;27:61–70.

226. Okada M, Fukada JI, Toya K, et al. The value of drip infusion cholangiography using multidetector-row helical CT in patients with choledocholithiasis. Eur Radiol 2005;15:2140–5.

227. Zandrino F, Curone P, Benzi L, et al. MR versus multislice CT cholangiography in evaluating patients with obstruction of the biliary tract. Abdom Imaging 2005;30:77–85.

228. Gibson RN, Vincent JM, Spur T, et al. Accuracy of computed tomographic intravenous cholangiography (CT-IVC) with iotrexate in the detection of choledocholithiasis. Eur Radiol 2005;15:1634–42.

229. Ahmetoglu A, Kosucu P, Kul S, et al. MDCT cholangiography with volume rendering for the assessment of patients with biliary obstruction. AJR Am J Roentgenol 2004;183:1327–32.

230. Baille J, Paulson EK, Vitellas KM. Biliary imaging: a review. Gastroenterol Clin North Am 2003;124:1686–99.

231. Fulcher AS, Turner MA. Benign disease of the biliary tract: evaluation with MR cholangiography. Semin Ultrasound CT MR 1999;20:294–303.

232. Reinhold C, Taourel P, Bret PM, et al. Choledocholithiasis: evaluation of MR cholangiography for diagnosis. Radiology 1998;209:435–42.

233. Heller SL, Lee VS. MR imaging of the gallbladder and biliary system. Magn Reson Imaging Clin North Am 2005;13:295–311.

234. Kim JH, Kim MJ, Park S, et al. MR cholangiography in symptomatic gallstones: diagnostic accuracy according to clinical risk group. Radiology 2002;224:410–6.

235. Schmidt S, Chevallier P, Novellas S, et al. Choledocholithiasis: repetitive thick-slab single-shot projection magnetic resonance cholangiopancreaticography versus endoscopic ultrasonography. Eur Radiol 2007;17:241–50.

236. Regan F, Smith D, Khazan R, et al. MR cholangiography in biliary obstruction using half-Fourier acquisition. J Comput Assist Tomogr 1996;20:627–32.

237. Kim M-J, Mitchell DG, Ito K, et al. Biliary dilatation: differentiation of benign from malignant causes–value of adding conventional MR imaging to MR cholangiography. Radiology 2000;214:173–81.

238. Eun HW, Kim JH, Hong SS. Assessment of acute cholangitis by MR imaging. Eur J Radiol 2012;81: 2476–80.

239. Wieloplski PA, Gaa J, Wielopolski DR, et al. Breath-hold MR cholangiopancreatography with three-dimensional, segmented, echo-planar imaging and volume rendering. Radiology 1999;210: 247–52.

240. Soto JA, Barish MA, Yucel E, et al. Pancreatic duct: MR cholangiopancreatography with a three-dimensional fast spin-echo technique. Radiology 1995;196:459–64.

241. Barish M, Yucel E, Soto J, et al. MR cholangiopancreatography: EFFICACY of three-dimensional turbo spin-echo technique. AJR Am J Roentgenol 1995;196:459–64.

242. McKenzie CA, Lim D, Ransil BJ, et al. Shortening MR image acquisition time for volumetric interpolated breath-hold examination with a recently developed parallel imaging reconstruction technique: clinical feasibility. Radiology 2003;230:589–94.

243. Costello JR, Kalb B, Chundru S, et al. MR Imaging of benign and malignant biliary conditions. Magn Reson Imaging Clin North Am 2014;22:467–88.

244. Watanabe Y, Dohke M, Ishimori T, et al. Pseudo-obstruction of the extrahepatic bile duct due to artifact from arterial pulsatile compression: a diagnostic pitfall of MR cholangiopancreatography. Radiology 2000;214:856–60.

245. Sugita R, Sugimura E, Itoh M, et al. Pseudolesion of the bile duct caused by flow effect: a diagnostic pitfall of MR cholangiopancreatography. AJR Am J Roentgenol 2003;180:467–71.

246. Flores C, Maguilnik I, Hadlich E, et al. Microbiology of choledochal bile in patients with choledocholithiasis admitted to a tertiary hospital. J Gastroenterol Hepatol 2003;18:333–6.

247. Patel NB, Oto A, Thomas S. Multidetector CT of emergent biliary pathologic conditions. Radiographics 2013;33:1867–88.

248. Kim SW, Shin HC, Kim HC, et al. Diagnostic performance of multidetector CT for acute cholangitis: evaluation of a CT scoring method. Br J Radiol 2012;85:770–7.

249. Menu Y, Lorphelin JM, Scherrer A, et al. Sonographic and computed tomographic evaluation of intrahepatic calculi. AJR Am J Roentgenol 1985; 145:579–83.

250. Carmona RH, Crass RA, Lim RC Jr, et al. Oriental cholangitis. Am J Surg 1984;148:117–24.

251. Sperling RM, Koch J, Sandhu JS, et al. Recurrent pyogenic cholangitis in Asian immigrants to the United States. Natural history and role of therapeutic ERCP. Dig Dis Sci 1997;42:865–71.

252. Yassa NA, Stain S, Ralls PW. Recurrent pyogenic cholangitis. Ultrasound Q 1998;14:41–7.

253. Kim M-J, Cha S-W, Mitchell DG, et al. MR imaging findings in recurrent pyogenic cholangitis. AJR Am J Roentgenol 1999;173:1545–9.

254. Chan F-L, Man S-W, Leong LL, et al. Evaluation of recurrent pyogenic cholangitis with CT: analysis of 50 patients. Radiology 1989;170:165–9.

255. Federle MP, Cello JP, Laing FC, et al. Recurrent pyogenic cholangitis in Asian immigrants. Use of ultrasonography, computed tomography and cholangiography. Radiology 1982;143:151–6.

256. Lim JH, Ko YT, Lee DH, et al. Oriental cholangiohepatitis: sonographic findings in 48 cases. AJR Am J Roentgenol 1990;155:511–4.

257. Kusano S, Okada Y, Endo T, et al. Oriental cholangiohepatitis: correlation between portal vein occlusion and hepatic atrophy. AJR Am J Roentgenol 1992;158:1011–4.

258. Sathesh-Kumar T, Saklani AP, Vinayagam R, et al. Spilled gallstones during laparoscopic cholecystectomy: a review of the literature. Postgrad Med J 2004;80:77–9.

259. Litwin DE, Girotti MJ, Poulin EC, et al. Laparoscopic cholecystectomy: Trans-Canada experience with 2201 cases. Can J Surg 1992;35:291–6.

260. Larson GM, Vitale GC, Casey J, et al. Multipractice analysis of laparoscopic cholecystectomy in 1,983 patients. Am J Surg 1992;163:221–6.

261. Cuschieri A, Dubois F, Mouiel J, et al. The European experience with laparoscopic cholecystectomy. Am J Surg 1991;161:385–7.

262. Morrin MM, Kruskal JB, Hochman MG, et al. Radiologic features of complications arising from dropped gallstones in laparoscopic cholecystectomy patients. AJR Am J Roentgenol 2000;174: 1441–5.

263. Trerotola SO, Lillemoe KD, Malloy PC, et al. Percutaneous removal of "dropped" gallstones after laparoscopic cholecystectomy. Radiology 1993; 188:419–21.

264. Campbell WB, McGarity WC. An unusual complication of laparoscopic cholecystectomy. Am Surg 1992;184:195–200.

265. Mirizzi PC. Syndrome del conducto hepatico. J Int Chir 1948;8:731–77.

266. McSherry C, Ferstenberg H, Virshup M. The Mirizzi syndrome: suggested classification and surgical therapy. Surg Gastroenterol 1982;1:219–25.

267. Abou-Saif A, Al-Kawas FH. Complications of gallstone disease: Mirizzi syndrome, cholecystocholedochal fistula and gallstone ileus. Am J Gastroenterol 2002; 97:249.

268. Sharma AK, Rangan HK, Choubey RP, et al. Pitfalls in the management of Mirizzi's syndrome. Trop Gastroenterol 1998;19:72–4.

269. Karademir S, Astarioglu H, Sokmen S, et al. Mirizzi's syndrome: diagnostic and surgical considerations in 25 patients. J Hepatobiliary Pancreat Surg 2000;7:72–7.

270. Berland LL, Lawson TL, Stanley RJ. CT appearance of Mirizzi syndrome. J Comput Assist Tomogr 1984;8:165–6.

271. Kim PN, Outwater EK, Mitchell DG. Mirizzi syndrome: evaluation by MR imaging. Am J Gastroenterol 1999;94:2546–50.

272. Wakefield EG, Vickers PM, Walters W. Intestinal obstruction caused by gallstones. Surgery 1939;5:670–3.

273. Chen MY. Gallstone ileus: CT findings. Appl Radiol 1991;20:37–8.

274. Rigler LG, Borman CN, Noble JF. Gallstone obstruction: pathogenesis and roentgen manifestations. JAMA 1941;117:1753–9.

275. Balthazar EJ, Schechter LS. Air in gallbladder: a frequent finding in gallstone ileus. AJR Am J Roentgenol 1978;131:219–22.

276. Delabrousse E, Bartholomot B, Sohm O, et al. Gallstone ileus: CT findings. Eur Radiol 2000;10:938–40.

277. Loren I, Lasson A, Nilsson A, et al. Gallstone ileus demonstrated by CT. J Comput Assist Tomogr 1994;18:262–5.

278. Swift SE, Spencer JA. Gallstone ileus: CT findings. Clin Radiol 1998;53:451–6.

Evaluating Patients with Left Upper Quadrant Pain

Jacob S. Ecanow, MD, Richard M. Gore, MD*

KEYWORDS

- Acute abdomen • Left upper quadrant (LUQ) • Splenic infarct • Splenic abscess • Gastritis
- Peptic ulcer disease (PUD) • Perforation

KEY POINTS

- Imaging plays an important role in evaluating left upper quadrant (LUQ) pain in the acute setting.
- The anatomy of the peritoneal reflections, subperitoneal space, and peritoneal spaces play an important role in clarifying the pattern and appearance of disease in the LUQ.
- Currently, the primary imaging modality for evaluating acute LUQ pain is contrast-enhanced multidetector computed tomography, although ultrasound and MR imaging play important adjunctive roles. Fluoroscopic upper gastrointestinal studies are occasionally useful.
- The most common causes of acute LUQ pain include gastritis, peptic ulcer disease, sickle cell crisis and splenic infarct, and pancreatitis; the full differential diagnosis is longer.
- Several of the causes of LUQ pain are life threatening and require rapid diagnosis and treatment.

INTRODUCTION

Acute left upper quadrant (LUQ) pain is less common than pain at other sites in the abdomen; but several of the causes of acute LUQ pain can be life threatening, and rapid accurate diagnosis is critical.[1] Frequently, the radiologist is the first person to discover that the cause of a patient's nonspecific acute abdominal pain is a disease in the LUQ.[2] In a study of patients who presented to the emergency department (ED) with abdominal pain, only 4% of patients initially complained of LUQ pain, yet the most common posttest primary diagnosis was gastritis/peptic ulcer disease (PUD) complex.[3] Imaging plays a vital role in the evaluation of patients with acute LUQ pain. Physical examination in patients with abdominal pain has low specificity and low sensitivity.[4] One study found that interrater agreement between ED attendings and residents in detecting LUQ physical examination findings was only fair and was worse than for any other area of the torso.[5] Non–imaging-based tests also provide limited benefit. Nagurney and colleagues[3] evaluated and compared the usefulness of common tests in the evaluation of patients with abdominal pain. The initial pretest diagnosis and disposition were changed in more than one-third of patients in their study, and computed tomography (CT) was identified as the most useful test in these patients. In another study evaluating 4 different models for comparing abdominal pain, Gerhardt and colleagues[4] found that noncontrast helical CT was the most accurate "clinical predictor variable" in determining the need for urgent intervention.[4] They concluded that CT is "the single most useful diagnostic adjunct to augment the clinical evaluation."[4] The problems in obtaining a meaningful history and accurate physical examination are even more difficult in elderly patients who frequently have preexisting illnesses that can alter or mask the usual manifestation of acute disease.[6] As a result, thorough familiarity with the imaging

No disclosures.
Department of Radiology, NorthShore University HealthSystem, 2650 Ridge Avenue, Suite G507, Evanston, IL 60201, USA
* Corresponding author.
E-mail address: RGore@northshore.org

Radiol Clin N Am 53 (2015) 1131–1157
http://dx.doi.org/10.1016/j.rcl.2015.06.003

manifestations of LUQ pathology and an ability to prescribe the most suitable imaging strategy for evaluation of this area are vital.

The most common causes of acute LUQ pain include gastritis, PUD, sickle cell crisis, splenic infarct, splenic abscess, and pancreatitis; a more complete differential diagnosis is given in **Box 1**.[1,7,8] This article discusses important common diseases of the spleen and stomach that cause acute LUQ pain and reviews aspects of other entities in the differential diagnosis in terms

- Left kidney
  - Renal colic
  - Pyelonephritis and renal abscess
- Left adrenal hemorrhage
- Left subphrenic abscess
- Diseases of the left hemithorax
  - Pulmonary disease (eg, left lower lobe pneumonia)
  - Diseases of the heart and pericardium (eg, coronary infarction)
- Diaphragmatic hernias

Data from Refs.[1,7,8]

Box 1
Differential diagnosis of acute LUQ pain

- Spleen
  - Infarct and sickle cell crisis
  - Splenomegaly
  - Rupture
  - Abscess and infection
  - Ruptured splenic artery aneurysm
  - Splenic torsion
  - Splenic vein thrombosis
- Gastric
  - Gastritis
  - Gastric ulcer/PUD complex
  - Volvulus and gastric outlet obstruction
  - Postoperative complication
    - Laparoscopic Roux-en-Y gastric bypass
    - Gastric banding
- LUQ complications of pancreatitis
  - Pseudocysts and fluid collections in the lesser sac, subphrenic space, and LUQ subperitoneal space
  - Intrasplenic pseudocysts, hemorrhage, infarct
  - Gastric wall
  - Colonic spasm, obstruction, and adynamic ileus
  - Pseudoaneurysm of the splenic artery
  - Splenic vein thrombosis
- Splenic flexure
  - Colitis and ischemic colitis
  - Diverticulitis
  - Carcinoma
- Jejunum
  - Jejunal obstruction and internal hernias
  - Jejunal diverticulitis

---

of their features that are unique to the LUQ. Relevant aspects of LUQ anatomy and the current role of CT, ultrasound (US), and MR imaging in evaluating this area are considered.

ANATOMY AND APPROACH TO IMAGING
Anatomy

The interpretation of imaging studies is facilitated by familiarity with the peritoneal reflections that define the spaces of the LUQ (**Table 1**) and that fix the relationship between the spleen, stomach, and splenic flexure. The loose areolar tissue that surrounds the vessels, lymphatics, and nerves running within the peritoneal reflections constitutes the subperitoneal space that serves as a pathway for the spread of disease into and out of the LUQ.[9] A systematic approach to the anatomy is useful.

The transverse mesocolon (TM) is a peritoneal fold that surrounds the transverse colon with its root running along the ventral length of the body of the pancreas.[9,10] It divides the abdomen into supramesocolic and inframesocolic compartments and, therefore, may be considered the caudal border of the LUQ. It can be appreciated in the sagittal and coronal planes in patients with ascites; in the axial plane, its position in the LUQ can be localized by following the course of the left colic vein and the veins that drain the splenic flexure as they converge on the inferior mesenteric vein (IMV) (**Fig. 1**).[11] This subperitoneal space connects the transverse colon with the pancreas and also acts as a crossroad for the spread of disease throughout the abdomen because it is contiguous with ligaments that ultimately join all of the major subperitoneal routes in the upper abdomen.[9] The classic example of an acute disease process spreading via this pathway occurs in acute

Table 1
Peritoneal spaces of the LUQ

Space	Boundaries	LUQ Imaging Landmarks	Some Potential Implications in Acute LUQ pain
Left subphrenic	Between the diaphragm and left hepatic lobe; continuous with the perisplenic space (The coronary ligament of the left hepatic lobe indents its right margin.)	Left hepatic lobe and diaphragm	Abscess after perforated gastric ulcer, ruptured splenic abscess, or postoperative Pancreatic fluid collection after pancreatitis Same as perisplenic space
Perisplenic	Surrounds spleen and contiguous with the left subphrenic space	Spleen	Hematoma after splenic rupture or laceration Abscess Same as left subphrenic space
Lesser sac	Left: SRL & GSL Ventral: GCL, stomach/duodenal bulb, & lesser omentum/(GHL, HDL) Right: caudate lobe of liver Inferior: TMC & transverse colon Dorsal: parietal peritoneum covering pancreas	Between stomach and pancreas/left kidney (retrogastric space)	Common site of pancreatic pseudocyst Abscess from perforated gastric ulcer

Abbreviations: GCL, gastrocolic ligament; GSL, gastrosplenic ligament; HDL, hepatoduodenal ligament; SRL, splenorenal ligament; TMC, transverse mesocolon.
Data from Refs.[9–11]

pancreatitis. Dissection of pancreatic fluid via the TM can cause focal pericolonic inflammation resulting in edema, spasm, or stricture of the transverse colon. Abrupt colonic narrowing that mimics an annular carcinoma called the *colon cutoff sign* can be seen on abdominal radiographs, CT, and barium lower gastrointestinal (GI) studies.[10] Although originally described at the hepatic flexure, this sign can be seen anywhere along the transverse colon and most commonly occurs

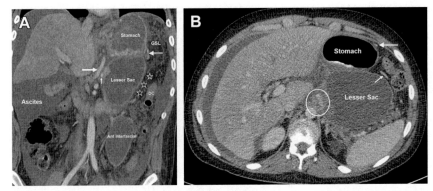

Fig. 1. Severe pancreatitis in a patient with Crohn's disease. (*A*) Coronal multidetector CT (MDCT) shows a pseudocyst with enhancing walls in the lesser sac, another in the retromesenteric anterior interfascial space (Ant Interfascial), and ascites. Note the left gastric artery (*small arrow*) and vein (*large arrow*) marking the right margin of the bursa omentalis of the lesser sac. The gastrosplenic ligament (GSL) is continuous with the base of the TM (*stars*) on the left. The short gastric vessels (*double arrow*) could be traced from the fundus to the splenic hilum and help identify the GSL. (*B*) Axial MDCT demonstrates the pseudocyst in the lesser sac. Note the left gastric artery and vein (*circle*) marking the right margin of the bursa omentalis. The TM merges with gastrocolic ligament (GCL) anteriorly on the left. A splenic flexure vein within the TM (*small arrow*) could be followed as it merged with the inferior mesenteric vein (not shown). A gastroepiploic vessel in the GCL can be seen adjacent to the greater curvature of the stomach (*double arrow*).

at the splenic flexure.[10] The same finding can be seen when pancreatic cancer invades the splenic flexure directly via the TM (**Fig. 2**).

The gastrocolic ligament (GCL) is composed of 4 layers of peritoneum and acts as a pathway between the greater curvature of the stomach and the transverse colon before continuing as the greater omentum (**Fig. 3**).[9] The gastroepiploic veins (GEVs) form an arcade in the anterior 2 layers of the greater omentum and can be used to localize the GCL on axial sections (see **Fig. 1**).[11,12] The greater omentum frequently acts to wall off or confine inflammatory processes in the abdomen and has, therefore, been referred to as "the policeman of the abdomen."[9]

The gastrosplenic ligament (GSL) is easily recognized as the fat-containing area between the stomach and spleen and is one of the suspensory ligaments of the spleen.[13] The short gastric veins run in this ligament (see **Fig. 1**). Pancreatic pseudocysts are prone to form in the GSL.[9]

The phrenicocolic ligament (PCL) is an important structure as it marks the anatomic splenic flexure, acts as a suspensory ligament for the splenic flexure as well as the spleen, and is another subperitoneal pathway in the spread of disease.[9] In some patients, the spleen and splenic flexure of the colon are displaced inferiorly by space-occupying disease in LUQ, indicating that there can be some laxity in this ligament.[11] Variations in the location of the transverse colon and splenic flexure may be encountered on normal scans. In a review of 9400 CT scans, Oldfield and Wilbur[14] described a "retrogastric colon"[14] in 21 patients in which they found the splenic flexure of the colon in the expected location of the lesser sac between

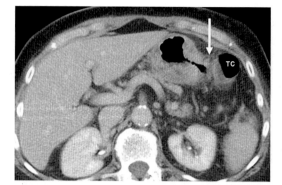

Fig. 3. Axial intravenous contrast-enhanced CT image demonstrates a mural discontinuity in the greater curvature at the site of an ulcer that has perforated into the GCL (*arrow*). TC, Transverse colon.

the stomach and pancreas (types 1 and 2) or posterior to the stomach and spleen (type 3) (**Fig. 4**).[14] Another series found 1% of patients with splenorenal, "retrogastric", or "retrosplenic colonic"[15] interpositions.[15] This anatomic variation can cause diagnostic confusion because air and fluid in the colon might be confused with an abscess or pathologic fluid collection or might also be misinterpreted as an internal hernia through the foramen of Winslow.[14,16]

The lesser sac lies between the stomach and the parietal peritoneum covering the pancreas. The margins that define the lesser sac are listed in **Table 1**. As part of the lesser omentum, the gastrohepatic ligament (GHL) is an easily recognizable structure and is a useful landmark on US and CT for the medial superior recess of the lesser sac (vestibule).[17] The lesser sac is a common site for

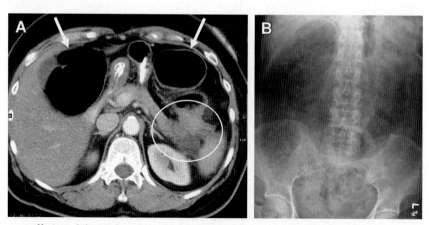

Fig. 2. Colon cutoff sign. (*A*) Axial oral and intravenous contrast-enhanced CT image demonstrates a cystic pancreatic tail mass invading directly through the TM (*circle*) into the splenic flexure causing obstruction. Dilated proximal transverse colon (*arrows*) can be seen. (*B*) Supine anteroposterior plain film radiograph of the abdomen shows the dilated colon with abrupt cutoff at the splenic flexure. This cutoff is identical to the colon cutoff sign seen in pancreatitis.

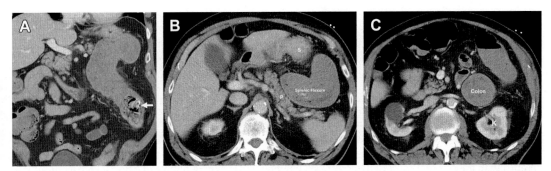

Fig. 4. Retrogastric colon. Variant anatomy in a patient with acute LUQ pain caused by descending colonic obstruction by a bezoar. The obstruction subsequently resolved spontaneously. (*A*) Coronal intravenous contrast-enhanced multidetector CT image demonstrates obstruction of the descending colon by a bezoar (*arrow*). Note the medial position of the splenic flexure. (*B*) Axial image shows the splenic flexure insinuated between the stomach (S) and the pancreas (P). (*C*) Axial image obtained more caudally shows the proximal descending colon is medial to the left kidney (K).

pancreatic pseudocysts, abscesses from perforated gastric ulcers, and splenic hemorrhage (see **Fig. 1**).

The spleen is an intraperitoneal lymphatic organ fixed by the GSL, splenorenal ligament (SRL), and PCL.[18] The tortuous splenic artery runs along the body of the pancreas in the anterior pararenal space, passes through the SRL, and then enters the spleen via the splenic hilum.[9,10,19] The splenic vein (SV) exits the spleen at the hilum and receives the short gastric veins and the left GEV.[12]

Imaging

There is no specific imaging test for evaluating LUQ pain.[8] Multidetector CT (MDCT) is currently the primary imaging examination for evaluating patients with an acute abdomen and is well suited for diagnosing and characterizing the most important causes of acute LUQ pain.[1,20,21] Patient preparation and scan protocols can be tailored to optimize the evaluation of a specific suspected diagnosis, although frequently the initial clinical diagnosis is incorrect, and the imaging protocol used should not be too narrow.[2,20] Intravenous contrast is necessary for the optimal evaluation of many of the acute LUQ diseases.[22] Contrast-enhanced dual-phase MDCT is advocated for suspected pancreatitis or left pyelonephritis and for the evaluation of splenic pathology.[1,23,24] Intravenous contrast improves the detection and characterization of LUQ abscesses, suspected diverticulitis, and suspected colonic ischemia, all of which are pertinent to the LUQ.[25–27]

The need for and optimal type of oral contrast material is also an important issue. Potential drawbacks of oral contrast agents include significant time costs, delay in surgical management, and, in the case of high-density (positive contrast) oral

agents, potentially increasing the radiation exposure of the CT scan.[22] High-density oral contrast can obscure gastric, jejunal, and splenic flexure wall enhancement; it can obscure the LUQ vasculature on CT angiography; it can make 3-dimensional (3D) postprocessing more difficult.[28] Heterogeneous mixing of high-density oral contrast with retained gastric contents can also cause diagnostic confusion or create pseudotumors in the stomach.[28] The use of high-volume low-density (neutral contrast) agents, such as water, avoids these problems and improves evaluation of the gastric wall.[28] The main specific benefit of positive oral contrast agents over neutral agents is in potentially demonstrating a site of LUQ GI perforation (**Fig. 5**). Positive oral contrast can also be helpful in identifying and characterizing LUQ abscesses, fluid collections, and inflammatory processes.[25]

Because many of the structures of the LUQ occupy multiple planes, and because the vessels are tortuous, 3D postprocessing techniques, including maximum intensity projection (MIP), multiplanar reformatting (MPR), volume rendering, and surface shading techniques, can be very useful.[23,29]

In the LUQ, US is useful in screening for renal abnormalities, determining splenic size, and detecting LUQ fluid collections; color and spectral Doppler US of the splenic vessels are occasionally helpful in confirming suspected vascular occlusion, aneurysms, pseudoaneurysms, or hemodynamic alterations. Scanning of the spleen is generally performed with a 3.5-MHz transducer using a posterolateral intercostal window along the long axis of the 10th rib.[30] One drawback of US is that it requires a cooperative patient who can follow breathing instructions, which may not be possible in the acute setting. In general, US currently provides limited benefits and is primarily an adjunct to MDCT.

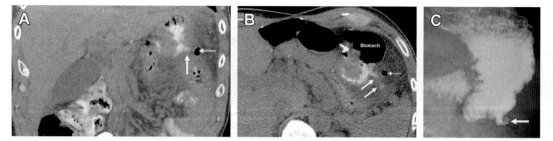

Fig. 5. Perforated greater curvature ulcer in a patient who presented with acute LUQ pain. Coronal (*A*) and axial (*B*) MDCT with positive oral contrast demonstrated pneumoperitoneum. A bubble of extraluminal air (*double arrow*) adjacent to a linear tract of oral contrast extending through the gastric wall (*arrows*) marks the site of the perforated ulcer. Barium upper GI (*C*) confirms the ulcer of the greater curvature (*arrow*).

MR imaging is commonly used for the evaluation of acute abdominal pain in the pediatric and obstetric populations.[21] In published series evaluating the performance of MR imaging in pregnant patients with acute abdominal pain, diagnoses pertinent to the LUQ, including adrenal hemorrhage, pyelonephritis, pancreatitis, colitis, diverticulitis, hydronephrosis, and urolithiasis, were facilitated by MR imaging.[31–33] False-negative rates were low in each of these series; the only reported false-negative upper abdominal disease was a case of pyelonephritis, a diagnosis for which physicians do not need imaging.[31] MR imaging has good diagnostic performance in evaluating acute pancreatitis as well as abnormalities of the spleen, including acute infections, infarcts, and hemorrhage.[18,34] A typical protocol in a cooperative patient might include a diffusion-weighted imaging sequence, T2-weighted single-shot (ss) fast spin echo (FSE) images in all 3 planes, axial ssFSE with fat saturation (fat sat), a fat-sat axial 2-dimensional coherently balanced steady-state sequence, and pre–contrast-enhanced and post–contrast-enhanced 3-phase volumetric acquisition with fat sat. Contrast is not given if patients are pregnant. The role of MR imaging in the evaluation of acute abdominal pain in general and the LUQ specifically may increase as more radiologists gain experience with interpretation and as newer pulse sequences are developed that allow for faster scan times and that have sufficient diagnostic accuracy for a wider range of abdominal diseases.

SPLENIC INFARCT

Common presenting symptoms of splenic infarction include LUQ pain, diffuse abdominal pain, nausea, vomiting, or fever.[35] Leukocytosis may be present but is not sensitive, and the physical examination is often nonspecific.[35] Infarcts in the spleen are usually caused by occlusion of small

end vessels and are most commonly seen in sickle cell disease in patients younger than 40 years and thromboembolic disease in patients older than 40 years (**Box 2**).[35–37] Occlusion of the main splenic artery resulting in global infarction is rare, usually associated with advanced pancreatic cancer, splenic torsion, or prior splenic artery interventions. Splenic infarction is usually a self-limited process that is managed conservatively. As infarcts resolve, they get progressively smaller and ultimately result in a focal scarring, calcifications, or develop into benign splenic pseudocysts.[37] Serious complications, including abscess, splenic rupture, and hemorrhage, can occur.

CT has a high sensitivity and specificity for diagnosing splenic infarcts and can demonstrate findings that suggest the cause of the infarct, such as cardiac thrombus or aortic plaque.[35,36,38] Multiple infarcts in the spleen, kidney, and liver suggests embolic disease (**Fig. 6**).[39] The appearance on CT depends on the age of the infarct. In the acute phase, noncontrast CT may show a hypoattenuating wedge-shaped peripheral lesion (**Fig. 7**).[18] The findings may be subtle or atypical, and hyperdense mottled areas can be seen because of hemorrhage (see **Fig. 6**).[39] Contrast CT is preferable because the classic wedge-shaped nonenhancing or poorly enhancing infarct can be distinguished more readily from the adjacent enhancing parenchyma.[38,39] A thin rim of enhancing capsule may overlay the infarct because the splenic capsule is supplied separately by the short gastric arteries.[18] In the subacute phase, there is progressive liquefaction with a decrease in CT attenuation and development of a more distinct margin (**Fig. 8**).[18] Infarcts can appear round, irregular, or ill defined and may be indistinguishable from other splenic lesions.[18] Follow-up imaging can help confirm the diagnosis by demonstrating changes that characterize the natural history of the infarct. CT is valuable in detecting complications of infarct and, in the case of infection, guiding percutaneous

Box 2
Causes of splenic infarction

- Hematologic
  - Hemoglobinopathies: sickle cell disease, sickle cell trait, and hemoglobin sickle cell disease
  - Hematologic malignancy: leukemias, polycythemia vera
- Infectious
  - Mononucleosis
  - AIDS
  - Malaria
  - Sepsis (especially meningococcal)
- Trauma
- Iatrogenic
  - Splenic artery interventions and therapeutic embolization
  - Intra-aortic balloon pump
  - Postoperative
  - Pharmacologic: vasopressin, erythropoietin, clofazimine
- Hypercoagulable states
- Embolic
  - Bacterial endocarditis
  - Thromboembolic
    - Atrial fibrillation
    - Patent foramen ovale
  - Atheroembolic
- Aortic dissection
- Pancreatitis and pancreatic cancer
- Splenic disorders
  - Torsion
  - Splenomegaly
- Drugs: cocaine
- Collagen vascular disease

Data from Refs.[35–37]

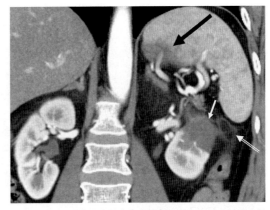

Fig. 6. Coronal MDCT image demonstrates an acute splenic infarct (*large black arrow*) with ill-defined margins and an irregular shape. A nonenhancing mature left renal infarct (*small white arrow*) is lower in density and has well-defined margins. Reactive edema in the perirenal space is seen adjacent to the upper pole of the kidney (*double arrow*). The presence of multiple infarcts suggests embolic disease.

spleen may only have a heterogeneous echotexture in the region of involvement.[40] Contrast-enhanced sonography using a spleen-specific agent may improve the sensitivity of US in these patients.[40] US is useful in following suspected infarcts with serial examinations in order to confirm the diagnosis, monitor for complications, and help guide management decisions.[37] On grayscale US, infarcts become progressively more hypoechoic over the course of several days and develop the typical wedge-shaped appearance that extends to the capsular surface.[40] If the infarct liquefies or develops into an abscess, US is very useful in demonstrating the fluid collection and for guiding percutaneous drainage. In the chronic phase, infarcts appear echogenic on US because of the development of fibrosis.

On MR imaging, infarcted splenic tissue can have low signal or high signal on T1- and T2-weighted images depending on the age of the infarct.[39,41] Nonenhancing subcapsular defects are seen on delayed postcontrast images, and associated signal changes caused by hemorrhage may also be evident.[18]

SICKLE CELL DISEASE

Splenic complications of sickle cell disease are a common cause of LUQ pain. Splenomegaly can be seen in patients with heterozygous disease and predisposes them to complications including splenic rupture, hemorrhage, and infarction.[39] The splenic parenchyma in patients with sickle cell disease typically has low signal on T1- and

drainage. The development of an enlarging fluid collection or expansion of the infarct has been described as signs of infection or impending rupture (**Fig. 9**).[18] Gas bubbles in a splenic fluid collection are diagnostic for infection.[39]

US has lower accuracy than CT in the detection of acute splenic infarcts, with sensitivity as low as 18%.[38] Acute infarcts are nearly isoechoic to normal splenic tissue on gray scale; initially, the

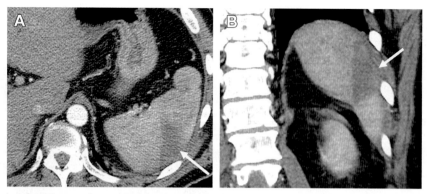

Fig. 7. Splenic infarct in a patient with thromboembolic disease. Axial (*A*) and coronal (*B*) intravenous contrast-enhanced MDCT shows the characteristic wedge-shaped nonenhancing infarct (*arrow*) extending to the capsular surface.

T2-weighted MR imaging sequences because of iron deposition from multiple blood transfusions (hemosiderosis).[42,43] Splenomegaly in a patient with sickle cell disease with acute LUQ pain and a sudden decrease in hematocrit suggests acute splenic sequestration, with the associated risk of shock and death.[39] The spleen may have a heterogeneous appearance on CT caused by interspersed areas of blood pooling, hemorrhage, and infarct.[39] MR imaging is well suited to demonstrate areas of hemorrhage in the spleen.[21]

SPLENIC INFECTIONS
Splenic Abscess

Splenic infections manifest as splenomegaly, abscess, or microabscesses.[44] The diagnosis of splenic abscess or microabscesses should be considered in patients with LUQ pain and fever especially if there is a history of infection elsewhere, malignancy, AIDS, other immune compromise states, diabetes mellitus, splenic trauma, or significant splenic infarction.[41,44,45] Abscesses are almost always caused by bacterial infection.[44,46] The pathophysiology of abscess formation follows one of 3 mechanisms: hematogenous spread from a preexisting infection (eg, endocarditis), superinfection of a splenic lesion, or direct extension from a local infection.[46] Prompt diagnosis is important because of the risk of intraperitoneal rupture and peritonitis.[39]

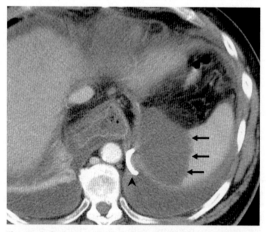

Fig. 8. Subacute splenic infarct in a postoperative patient. Axial contrast-enhanced MDCT shows an infarct with lower attenuation and well-defined margins (*arrows*). A percutaneous catheter has been placed in the left pleural space (*arrowhead*).

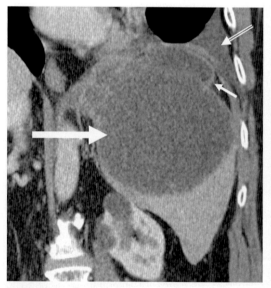

Fig. 9. LUQ pain in a patient with diffuse large B-cell lymphoma. Coronal contrast-enhanced MDCT image demonstrates a large expansile liquefied infarct (*large arrow*) and evidence for rupture into the subphrenic space (*small arrow*). A sterile left pleural effusion is also present (*double arrow*). The patient subsequently underwent splenectomy.

On CT, abscesses can have the nonspecific appearance of a low-attenuation lesion with a differential diagnosis that includes infarct, cyst, and benign or malignant tumor. The presence of gas bubbles or an air fluid level allows for a specific diagnosis of abscess.[39,47] An enhancing rim may be seen on postinfusion images but is not as conspicuous as the rim enhancement associated with abscesses elsewhere because adjacent normal splenic parenchyma usually enhances strongly (**Fig. 10**).[46] US has slightly lower sensitivity than CT and is also nonspecific.[47] Abscesses appear as hypoechoic or anechoic fluid collections with irregular walls or can appear heterogeneous with complex internal echoes (**Fig. 11**).[46] Gas in the abscess can cause internal echogenic foci (see **Fig. 11**) or "dirty shadowing."[46] Splenic abscesses frequently require follow-up imaging in order to monitor treatment; MR imaging is an appealing modality when serial examinations are needed (**Fig. 12**). On MR imaging, abscesses have low signal on T1- and intermediate or high signal on T2-weighted images.[41,46] Air is seen as a signal void, and there is frequently an enhancing rim on postcontrast images (see **Fig. 12**).[41,46]

Although the classic treatment has been antibiotics and splenectomy, percutaneous catheter drainage has gained widespread use (see **Fig. 10**).[44,48,49] The benefits of percutaneous drainage over splenectomy include external drainage of infected fluid with a low risk of intraabdominal spillage, preservation of the immune functions of the spleen, and avoidance of abdominal surgery with its potential associated morbidity.[48] The presence of multiple loculations or extensive internal septations may prevent successful drainage. Avoidance of the left pleural space is critical; therefore, accessible paths are more likely to be found for abscesses in the mid and lower pole of the spleen.[48] Reported complication rates are low and primarily involve splenic hemorrhage occasionally requiring splenectomy.[49]

Splenic Microabscesses

Splenic microabscesses are usually seen in immunocompromised patients and are most often caused by fungal or mycobacterial infection.[41,46] Splenic microabscesses appear as numerous hypodensities on CT, usually measuring less than 1 cm.[41] They are more conspicuous on postinfusion CT. Microabscesses may be very subtle on US, with detection rates of 2% or less in patients with AIDS with suspected infection.[50] The use of higher-frequency linear-array transducers increases the detection rate with US, even though only the most superficial 3 to 4 cm of the spleen can be examined.[45] Microabscesses appear as numerous small hypoechoic lesions on US and have a typical target-sign appearance caused by the differing echogenicity of the fungal elements and necrotic tissue.[45,47] MR imaging is more sensitive than CT or US for the detection of microabscesses.[42] On MR imaging, lesions are low signal on T1 and can be high signal or low signal on T2.[42,45] On gadolinium-enhanced MR imaging, the lesions show ring enhancement.[42]

SPLENOMEGALY

Splenomegaly causes LUQ pain when the splenic capsule becomes significantly stretched. The differential diagnosis is lengthy; but the more common causes include portal hypertension, lymphoproliferative disorders, complications of sickle cell disease, diffuse splenic infectious processes such as mononucleosis, and occasionally metastases. Sarcoidosis or granulomatous infections are occasionally seen, and metabolic and storage disorders are rare.[39,41] Splenomegaly increases the risk of splenic rupture, infarct, hematoma, and susceptibility to trauma.[51] Cross-sectional imaging is well suited for identifying an enlarged spleen and, in the acute setting,

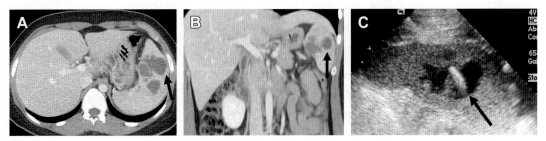

Fig. 10. LUQ pain and fever in a patient with a history of ulcerative colitis. Axial (*A*) and coronal (*B*) contrast-enhanced MDCT images demonstrate a multiloculated splenic abscess. Rim enhancement around one locule can be faintly appreciated (*arrow*) but is otherwise not conspicuous because of the adjacent splenic parenchymal enhancement. Image from the US-guided (*C*) percutaneous drainage catheter placement shows the echogenic needle entering the major locule (*arrow*).

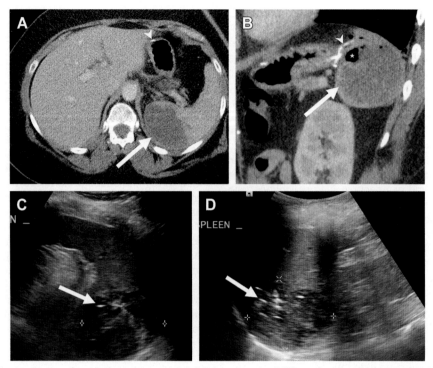

Fig. 11. Splenic abscess after cholecystectomy. Axial (*A*) and sagittal (*B*) contrast-enhanced MDCT show splenic fluid collection (*large arrow*) with bubbles of gas and an air-fluid level (*star*). Note gastric staples from prior gastric surgery (*arrowhead*). Transverse (*C*) and longitudinal (*D*) gray-scale US images show echogenic foci (*arrow*) caused by gas in the collection (*calipers*).

can occasionally narrow the differential diagnosis. Various schemes for quantitatively determining splenic size have been proposed, but in clinical practice splenomegaly is usually identified subjectively or by using a cutoff craniocaudal length of 13 to 14 cm as a rule of thumb.[41,47]

Splenic lymphoma can have several pathologic patterns that determine the imaging appearance: microscopic involvement with no specific imaging findings, splenomegaly without focal lesions, solitary focal involvement, or multifocal involvement with lesions that can be micronodular or macroscopic.[51] CT, therefore, has mediocre accuracy in demonstrating splenic involvement by lymphoma, with reported sensitivities ranging from 22% to 65%.[51] Lesions have low density compared with normal parenchyma and enhance far less than normal parenchyma after contrast

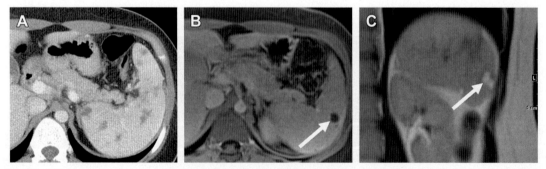

Fig. 12. Axial contrast-enhanced MDCT (*A*) shows multiple low-density bacterial abscesses in the spleen. The patient was treated with antibiotics. Three-month follow-up MR imaging (*B, C*) showed resolution of most of the abscesses. (*B*) Axial 3-minute post–contrast-enhanced T1-weighted with fat-saturated MR imaging shows low internal T1 signal with subtle wall *enhancement* in a single remaining small subcapsular abscess (*arrow*). Coronal T2 MR imaging (*C*) demonstrates high T2 signal within the same abscess (*arrow*).

administration.[51] US also has low sensitivity and may demonstrate hypoechoic lesions with scattered vascularity on color Doppler.[51,52] Lymphomatous lesions and splenic parenchyma have similar relaxation times on T1- and T2-weighted imaging sequences; therefore, the lesions are not well detected on these sequences.[41,53] Lesions are better demonstrated on gradient echo and proton density–weighted sequences.[54] In patients with splenomegaly caused by portal hypertension, MR imaging can show associated varices and can demonstrate findings in the liver that indicate the presence of cirrhosis when they are present.[42] In approximately 9% to 12% of patients with splenomegaly caused by portal hypertension, multiple low signal foci called Gamna-Gandy bodies can be seen in the splenic parenchyma on T2-weighted images because of the susceptibility artifact caused by the deposition of hemosiderin.[42,47] Splenic metastases are rare and are usually seen late in the course of the disease when other metastases are already evident (**Fig. 13**).[41] LUQ pain in these patients can be caused by splenomegaly or caused by other complications, such as hemorrhage, necrosis, or splenic rupture.[41] Lesions can appear solid, cystic, or heterogeneous with various patterns of enhancement on CT and have low or intermediate T1 and high or heterogeneous T2 signal on MR imaging.[41]

SPLENIC VEIN THROMBOSIS

SV thrombosis can present as LUQ pain and is usually the harbinger of a serious underlying disorder. Common causes include pancreatitis, pancreatic cancer, ulcerative colitis, sepsis, and hypercoagulable states.[18] Findings on CT include nonenhancement of the vein, a diminutive vessel

caliber, or a partial or complete filling defect.[12] The SV may be encased or obliterated by a malignant or inflammatory mass, usually of pancreatic origin (**Fig. 14**).[12] MPR images are very helpful in evaluating the SV, and CT venograms with curved planar reformatted images can be useful in confirming a suspected SV thrombosis when the diagnosis is uncertain because of the tortuosity of the vessel.[1,55] Varices may be seen and should be described. The main upstream tributaries of the SV are the short gastric veins that drain the gastric fundus and run in the GSL and the GEVs that run in the GCL and drain the greater omentum. SV thrombosis causes isolated gastric varices because of the elevated venous pressure in the short gastric collateral veins. Esophageal varices do not form when the portal vein is patent (see **Fig. 14**). The collateral pathway via the GEV arcade lays in the GCL and greater omentum, so that GEV varices do not lead to GI hemorrhage. They have been called the "safe varices."[56] The GEVs are often the first vessels to enlarge and may be the only dilated collaterals in the setting of acute SV occlusion.[12] MR imaging can demonstrate SV thrombus, and contrast-enhanced magnetic resonance angiography can demonstrate the anatomy of the SV and portal venous system.[42]

SPLENIC RUPTURE

Spontaneous splenic rupture is rare but may result in life-threatening hemorrhage.[57] Predisposing factors are listed in **Box 3**.[18,57–59] Hemoperitoneum is demonstrated on US as complex hypoechoic fluid with areas of hyperechoic blood, but the sensitivity for detecting the site of splenic rupture is low.[18] Hemorrhage is also well demonstrated on CT, and the hyperdense sentinel clot can help identify the site of hemorrhage.[18] Active extravasation of iodinated contrast may be seen on postinfusion CT (**Fig. 15**). Splenic rupture may require splenectomy or transcatheter embolization.[18] An unusual cause of splenic rupture without an obvious history of trauma is seen in patients with acute LUQ after optical colonoscopy.[10,60,61] Splenic laceration or rupture can occur in patients with an acutely angled colonic splenic flexure and in patients in whom the colonoscopy procedure is technically difficult (see **Fig. 15**).[60] Proposed mechanisms include direct trauma by the colonoscope, presumably as it abruptly tents the wall of the splenic flexure into the closely apposed lower pole of the spleen.[60] Another proposed mechanism is traction on the splenic capsule transmitted via the splenocolic ligament composed of the combined PCL and SRL.[9,60–62] The imaging features include subcapsular or perisplenic

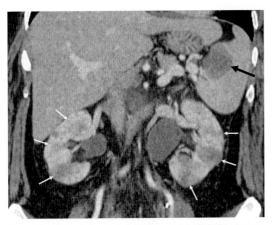

Fig. 13. Coronal contrast-enhanced MDCT image demonstrates splenic (*large black arrow*) and bilateral renal (*small white arrows*) metastases.

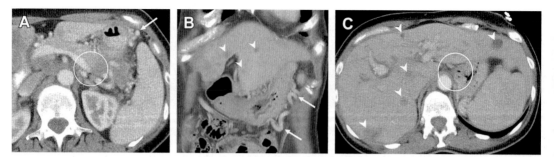

Fig. 14. Oral and intravenous contrast-enhanced MDCT images of a patient with pancreatic cancer causing SV thrombosis. Axial image (*A*) shows a small SV encased proximally by the pancreatic mass (*circle* in [*A*]). Note the distended left GEV (*arrow*) in the GCL, which could be traced to the greater omentum on serial images. Coronal image (*B*) shows the distended tortuous GEV running along the greater curvature (*arrows*). Liver metastases can be seen (*arrowheads*). Axial image at the level of the hiatus (*C*) shows absence of esophageal varices (*circle* in [*C*]), and hepatic metastases (*arrowheads*). A splenorenal shunt and varices in the GSL could be seen on other images.

hematoma, frank rupture with hemoperitoneum, and splenic artery pseudoaneurysm.[10,60,61]

SPLENIC TORSION

Splenic torsion is an uncommon cause of acute LUQ pain but is an important diagnosis because of the potential for splenic infarction, abscess, necrosis of the pancreatic tail, peritonitis, and hemoperitoneum.[18,63,64] Torsion of the vascular pedicle can occur when there is abnormal laxity of the SRL, GSL, and PCL allowing hypermobility of the spleen, referred to as a *wandering spleen*.[63] In the pediatric age group, the hypermobility is usually caused by the developmental abnormality of the dorsal mesogastrium; in the adult population, it is most commonly seen in multiparous women or in the peripartum period and is caused by hormone-induced laxity of the suspending ligaments.[13,65] Other causes include splenomegaly, trauma, and prior surgery.[18] Findings of a wandering spleen on CT or US include inferior displacement of the spleen, absence of the spleen from the left subphrenic space with a mass seen elsewhere in the abdomen or pelvis, and changing position of the spleen on serial studies.[63,65] A strategy using MR imaging has been described in which a patient was scanned in the supine, prone, and bilateral lateral decubitus positions in order to demonstrate the abnormal degree to which the spleen changed positions.[43] A balanced steady-state free precession sequence was used that allowed rapid image acquisition and demonstrated the anatomy adequately enough to appreciate the changing position of the spleen. Torsion should be considered if there is associated acute or intermittent LUQ or if there are associated imaging findings. Signs on CT include splenomegaly, abnormal ovoid or rounded splenic shape, heterogeneous or absent contrast enhancement, or the presence of infarcts.[18] US can also show the abnormal splenic size and shape, and the parenchyma may have a heterogeneous echotexture.[65] When the spleen is in its normal position in the LUQ, torsion may be more difficult to diagnose. Viewing MPR images on MDCT is helpful as inversion of the spleen may be appreciated on coronal images, which has been referred to as the "upside down spleen sign."[13] On contrast CT, a "Whirl sign"[13] consisting of the twisted vascular pedicle is seen in the splenic hilum.[18] On US, the thickened and edematous twisted pedicle may appear as a mass in the hilum.[66] Spectral Doppler shows high-resistance waveforms or absent flow in the

---

Box 3
Predisposing factors for spontaneous splenic rupture

- Infections
  - Infectious mononucleosis
  - Malaria
- Malignancy
- Amyloidosis
- Pregnancy
- Hematologic disorders and coagulopathy
  - Idiopathic thrombocytopenia purpura
  - Factor VIII deficiency
  - Sickle cell disease
- Splenomegaly
- Splenic tumors
- Splenic infarcts

Data from Refs.[18,57–59]

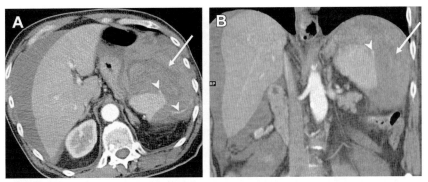

Fig. 15. Patient with LUQ pain after optical colonoscopy. Axial (*A*) and coronal (*B*) contrast-enhanced MDCT images show a deformed ruptured spleen with mixed-density fluid in the perisplenic space (*arrow*) indicating hemoperitoneum. A sentinel clot can be seen adjacent to site of rupture (*arrowhead*).

splenic vessels, and color Doppler may show absent flow in the spleen.[64,65] It is important to realize the flow may still be detected in segments of the main splenic artery or vein depending on where the twist in the pedicle occurs in relationship to arterial branches (pancreatic and short gastric) and venous tributaries (GEV and short gastric).[65] Interrogation of the vessels in the abdominal wall adjacent to the spleen and of deeper intra-abdominal vasculature is recommended to help differentiate truly diminished or absent splenic flow from lack of sufficient Doppler sensitivity or from improper Doppler settings.[65] Early diagnosis of splenic torsion is critical as it allows splenic preservation with surgical detorsion and splenopexy.[64]

RUPTURED SPLENIC ARTERY ANEURYSM

Ruptured splenic artery aneurysms (SAAs) can present with acute LUQ pain with or without hemodynamic instability.[67–69] A classic clinical presentation is that of sudden vascular collapse during the third trimester of pregnancy, a reflection of the effects of the hormones of pregnancy on the mural integrity of the splenic artery. Maternal mortality rates of 70% to 75% are reported for these cases.[68,69] Another scenario known as the double rupture phenomenon is characterized by sudden LUQ pain and hypotension with subsequent apparent hemodynamic recovery followed by sudden circulatory collapse.[70] This latter phenomenon is caused by brief tamponade of the extravasating blood in the lesser sac before generalized hemoperitoneum occurs via outflow through the foramen of Winslow.[70] SAA rupture is becoming less common as more of these lesions are being discovered as incidental findings on imaging studies performed for other indications. Current estimates are that approximately 2% to 3% of patients with SAAs present with rupture and that the overall mortality rate for these patients is 25%.[69] Unruptured SAAs can also cause LUQ pain, and surgical consultation should be obtained for symptomatic aneurysms because of the risk of sudden rupture.[70] Dual-phase MDCT with MPR imaging is the optimal method for identifying and characterizing SAAs in this setting. Tortuosity of the splenic artery can be misinterpreted as an aneurysm, and true aneurysms may be misidentified as vessel loops.

STOMACH

When acutely symptomatic, PUD and acute gastritis can have a wide range of presentations, which may include LUQ pain. There may be associated GI bleeding, nausea, vomiting, or chest pain.[71] Upper endoscopy has assumed the primary role in the evaluation of these entities; but noninvasive imaging still plays a major role, especially in the acute setting in which MDCT may be the first study that reveals an abnormality of the stomach. US and MR imaging do not play a significant role.

PEPTIC ULCER DISEASE

CT has a low diagnostic yield for the evaluation of uncomplicated PUD.[72] Shallow gastric ulcers are not well demonstrated on CT, although deep ulcers and perforated ulcers can be seen (see **Figs. 3** and **5**; **Figs. 16** and **17**).[28] The most common CT finding is nonspecific focal wall thickening.[20] In a retrospective study, Allen and colleagues[72] compared CT without oral contrast in 57 patients with endoscopically proven gastric or duodenal ulcers with 57 patients with negative endoscopies. They found that 54% of the ulcers were occult on CT, even when searched for retrospectively by 2 readers, and that sensitivity when

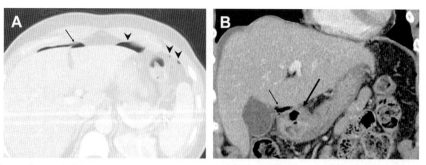

Fig. 16. Perforated antral ulcer. Axial contrast-enhanced MDCT image with lung window (*A*) shows pneumoperitoneum in the left subphrenic space (*arrowheads*). The coronary ligament is visible (*arrow*). Coronal contrast-enhanced MDCT image (*B*) shows extraluminal gas (*small arrow*) adjacent to thickened antral wall containing gas (*large arrow*).

both readers agreed was 29.6% with a specificity of 100%. The presence of 2 or more ancillary findings, including mural edema, asymmetric wall thickening, focal fat stranding, regional lymph nodes, and extraluminal gas, resulted in an odds ratio greater than 5.6 that a true ulcer was present (see **Fig. 16**). They also noted that gastric ulcers were more readily identified than duodenal or marginal ulcers. They advocated the use of multiplanar reformations to improve diagnostic performance, as have other investigators (see **Fig. 17**).[29,72]

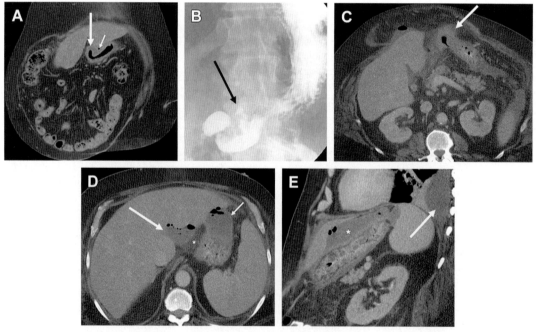

Fig. 17. Perforated antral ulcer with left subphrenic space abscess. Patient presented with acute LUQ pain. (*A*) Coronal noncontrast MDCT shows antral wall thickening and a probable antral ulcer (*large arrow*). There is free air adjacent to stomach (*small arrow*). (*B*) Subsequent barium upper GI confirmed the antral ulcer (*arrow*). Note that the configuration of the ulcer in the coronal plane is similar to the upper GI, illustrating why multiplanar reformats are very important in making the diagnosis. Subsequent MDCT scan. (*C*) Axial contrast-enhanced MDCT image at the level of the antrum demonstrates worsening mural thickening at the site of the ulcer and stranding of the adjacent fat (*arrow*). (*D*) Axial image near the fundus demonstrates 2 lobes of a left subphrenic space abscess with gas bubbles. One part of the abscess is located between the left lobe of the liver and the diaphragm (*large arrow*) and outlines fat in the GHL (*star*). The other portion is between the stomach and diaphragm (*small arrow*). (*E*) Sagittal image from the same examination demonstrates the subphrenic location of the abscess (*star*). Note the left pleural effusion (*arrow*).

In patients with epigastric pain and free intraperitoneal air, the most common diagnosis is a perforated gastric or duodenal ulcer.[73] CT viewed with lung and soft tissue windows has long been known to be the best modality for detecting small amounts of free air in the abdomen.[1,57,74,75] Extravasation of positive contrast oral agents with opacification of a tract through the wall can indicate the site of perforation (see **Fig. 5**).[1,57,76] Mortality rates for untreated perforated gastric or duodenal ulcers approaches 30%.[73] Findings that help confirm the site of perforation include visible discontinuity of the gastric wall (see **Fig. 3**) and focal gastric wall thickening with adjacent bubbles of extraluminal air or adjacent inflammatory stranding (see **Figs. 16** and **17**).[28] When the source of free air cannot be definitively established, and depending on the clinical status of patients, emergency upper GI studies with water-soluble contrast are useful.[73,77] Complications of perforated gastric ulcers include peritonitis and abscess formation. In the LUQ, abscesses can form in the left subphrenic space (see **Fig. 17**), the lesser sac, the GSL, or in the GCL (see **Fig. 3**).

GASTRITIS

MDCT with standard protocols using positive oral contrast has low sensitivity and low negative predictive value for gastritis because of poor gastric distension.[78] When the stomach is distended with air or contrast, the CT findings include diffuse, segmental, or focal wall thickening and thickened gastric folds (**Fig. 18**).[28] On arterial-phase contrast-enhanced images, the thickened gastric wall may have a layered or halo appearance caused by enhancement of the hyperemic mucosa adjacent to the hypodense edematous submucosa.[28] *Helicobacter pylori* gastritis can cause annular thickening of the antrum or focal thickening of the greater curvature that can be mistaken for malignancy.[28]

Emphysematous gastritis is a rare form of gastric mural inflammation with associated intramural pneumatosis and systemic toxicity with a mortality rate of up to 61%.[79] It is caused by infection by gas-forming organisms, such as *Clostridium perfringens*, that occurs in the setting of severe gastric mucosal injury, such as caustic ingestion, massive gastric distension, erosive gastritis, surgery, chemotherapy, alcohol, volvulus, and ischemia.[73,79,80] Emphysematous gastritis should be differentiated from the finding of gastric pneumatosis, in which gas enters the wall of the stomach directly through a breach in mucosal integrity or from extragastric sources.[80] Many of the causes of mucosal injury that

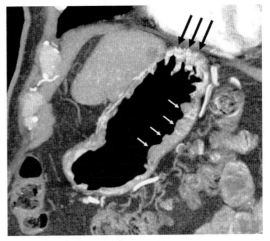

Fig. 18. Oblique coronal thick MPR contrast-enhanced MDCT image in a patient with gastritis demonstrates gastric wall and rugal fold thickening (*small white arrows*) as well as diffuse wall enhancement, which is particularly prominent adjacent to the diaphragm (*black arrows*). The findings can be appreciated because the stomach is distended with air.

predispose to emphysematous gastritis can cause simple gastric pneumatosis. Associated findings that may indicate a poor outcome include portal venous air, mural thickening and irregularity, perigastric inflammatory stranding, extragastric air, and pneumatosis elsewhere (**Fig. 19**). As is the case elsewhere in the GI tract, true intramural pneumatosis must be distinguished from peripheral intraluminal gas, especially when the stomach has retained food or secretions.[79] A search for intramural air in a nondependent portion of the stomach may be helpful in questionable cases. Depending on the clinical status of patients, upper GI endoscopy may be necessary for further evaluation and management.[81]

GASTRIC VOLVULUS

Acute gastric volvulus is a potential surgical emergency because of the risk of gastric obstruction, ischemic necrosis, and gastric perforation.[82] Mortality rates of up to 50% have been reported.[82] The stomach can rotate around the long axis from the gastroesophageal (GE) junction to the pylorus (organoaxial) (**Fig. 20**), around its mesenteric axis (mesenteroaxial) (**Fig. 21**), or rarely around both.[83] In adults, gastric volvulus is most often seen in the setting of paraesophageal hernias, but it can also occur in patients with other processes that lead to weakening of the supporting ligaments of the stomach, such as trauma, diaphragmatic eventration, and phrenic nerve palsy, as well as in patients with agenesis of the left

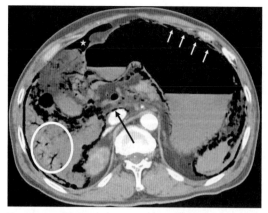

Fig. 19. Axial intravenous contrast-enhanced MDCT image demonstrates diffuse gastric pneumatosis (*small white arrows*), portal venous gas (*circle*), pneumoperitoneum (*star*), and retroperitoneal free air (*black arrow*). The constellation of findings is ominous and could have multiple causes.

hepatic lobe and patients with a wandering spleen.[82,83] Organoaxial volvulus is more common than mesenteroaxial volvulus and has a higher association with abnormalities of the diaphragm.[82] The clinical diagnosis is difficult because the instances requiring emergency surgery are rare, and the history and physical findings are nonspecific.[82,84] The clinical triad of epigastric pain, vomiting, and inability to pass a nasogastric tube (Borchardt triad) occurs in up to 70% of cases but is nonspecific.[82] A history of hiatal hernia increases the predictive value of the triad.[84]

The diagnosis has classically been made by upper gastrointestinal exam (UGI) but is currently frequently made by MDCT, especially in patients who present to the ED for abdominal pain.[85] In some cases, both are performed. US and MR imaging are not useful. Acute gastric outlet obstruction occurs when the volvulus is greater than 180°.[86] If there is less than 180° of gastric rotation, then the finding should be described as

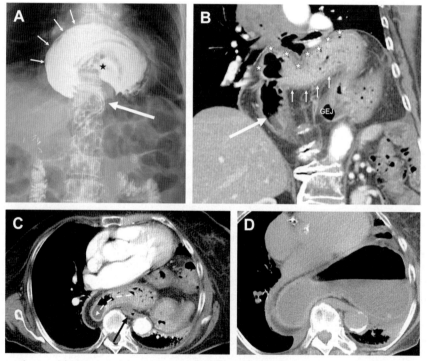

Fig. 20. Two patients with organoaxial gastric volvulus. Frontal view from a barium upper GI (*A*) demonstrates the rotated body of the stomach with the greater curve (*small arrows*) to the right and above the lesser curve, but the GE junction (GEJ) (*star*) remains above the antrum (*large arrow*). Note the counterclockwise path of the stomach. Another patient with organoaxial volvulus, which subsequently perforated (*B–D*). Initial coronal contrast-enhanced MDCT image (*B*) demonstrates the rotated body of the stomach, with the greater curve (*stars*) above and to the right of the lesser curve (*small arrows*). The antrum (*large arrow*) is to the right and slightly below the GEJ. Note the same counterclockwise path of the stomach. Axial contrast-enhanced MDCT image at the level of the hiatus (*C*) shows the GEJ (*solid black arrow*) at the same level as the antrum (*dashed white arrow* shows the direction of the antrum). Note the same counterclockwise path of the stomach. Axial image (*D*) from a subsequent noncontrast MDCT show gastric distention indicating volvulus.

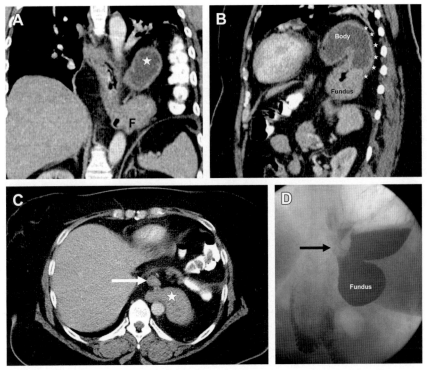

Fig. 21. Mesenteroaxial volvulus in a large hiatal hernia. Coronal (*A*) oral and intravenous contrast-enhanced MDCT image shows the fundus (F) below the body (*star*). Sagittal (*B*) oral and intravenous contrast-enhanced MDCT image demonstrates the greater curve (*stars*) posterior to the lesser curve and the fundus below the body. Axial (*C*) oral and intravenous contrast-enhanced MDCT image shows the GE junction (*arrow*) and antrum (*star*) at the same level. Frontal view from a barium upper GI (*D*) demonstrates the inverted fundus and shows how the antrum crosses over the GE junction (*arrow*). Note the counterclockwise course of the stomach.

organoaxial rotation or organoaxial position rather than volvulus.[87] However, it is important to note that, in patients with organoaxial rotation, there is a very high likelihood that the stomach will eventually go on to volvulus; therefore, surgical consultation for consideration of elective repair is warranted (see **Fig. 20**).[87] Differentiating true gastric volvulus from gastric rotation or even from a large paraesophageal hernia may be challenging. Reported CT findings are listed in **Table 2**. Millet and colleagues[83] evaluated the diagnostic performance of 9 direct CT findings of gastric volvulus, 4 associated findings, and 4 findings associated with gastric ischemia by comparing a group of 10 patients with surgically proven gastric volvulus with 20 patients who had CT scans showing gastroduodenal distension but who subsequently received diagnoses other than gastric volvulus. They found that the demonstration of the antrum at the same level or cranial to the fundus and associated with a transition point at the pylorus but with no visible abnormality of the pylorus was highly sensitive and specific for gastric volvulus. There was low interobserver agreement on whether there was reversal of the

greater and lesser curvatures; they noted that, although specific, this finding had low sensitivity (30%). CT signs of ischemia, including gastric pneumatosis, lack of mural enhancement, and pneumoperitoneum, did not correlate with pathologically proven ischemia in the 2 patients with volvulus who were subsequently proven to be ischemic. The right gastric vein has been used as a landmark to help identify the relationship of the lesser and greater curvature.[84]

LEFT UPPER QUADRANT PAIN AFTER BARIATRIC SURGERY

Gastric bypass and gastric banding procedures have become widespread, and complications are occasionally encountered in current clinical practice. Timing of the pain in relation to the surgery is important; early complications are beyond the scope of this review.

LUQ pain in patients who have undergone prior laparoscopic adjustable polymeric silicone ring gastric banding may indicate band slippage, stomal stenosis, or late perforation.[88] Late perforation is caused by erosion of the band through the

Table 2
Direct CT findings of acute gastric volvulus

Finding	Comment
Gastric dilatation	AP diameter >10 cm
Antral-pyloric transition	Evaluate antrum for visible pathology (mass or mural thickening)
Intrathoracic position of the gastric fundus	—
Intrathoracic position of the gastric body	—
Intrathoracic position of the antrum	—
Reversal of the greater and lesser curvatures	Identified by noting if the right side of the esophagus appears continuous with the greater curvature rather than the lesser curvature May be identified by following the course of the right gastric vein; if right gastric vein traverses the greater curve, suspect volvulus
Antrum at the same level or cranial to the fundus	—
Stenosis of the gastric segment passing through the esophageal hiatus	—
Perigastric intraperitoneal fluid	Attributed to venous compression

Abbreviation: AP, anteroposterior.

Data from Millet I, Orliac C, Alili C, et al. Computed tomography findings of acute gastric volvulus. Eur Radiol 2014;24:3115–22; and Larssen KS, Stimec B, Takvam JA, et al. Role of imaging in gastric volvulus: stepwise approach in three cases. Turk J Gastroenterol 2012;23(4):390–3.

gastric wall and is usually a chronic sealed perforation so that free air and contrast extravasation will not be seen.[88] On CT, part of the band may be seen in the stomach lumen and contrast may surround that portion of the band.[88] Band slippage may cause pain, stomal obstruction, band erosion, bleeding, gastric infarction, or volvulus and has been reported in up to 36% of patients.[88,89] The diagnosis can be suggested based on the anteroposterior abdominal radiograph. Signs of gastric band slippage on abdominal radiographs are listed in **Table 3**.[89] If band slippage is suspected, barium upper GI or MDCT should be obtained (**Fig. 22**).

In patients with LUQ pain who have had prior Roux-en-Y gastric bypass (RYGB), bowel obstruction should be considered. Causes of small bowel obstruction (SBO) in these patients depend on

Table 3
Signs of gastric band slippage on frontal radiographs

Sign	Definition	Sensitivity (%)	Specificity (%)
Abnormal phi angle (>58°)	Angle between a vertical line through the spinous processes of the thoracic spine and the long axis of the gastric band as seen on the frontal radiograph	91–95	52–62
O sign	Circular O appearance of the gastric band on the frontal radiograph	33–48	97
Inferior displacement of the superolateral band margin by more than 2.4 cm from the diaphragm	—	95	97–98
Presence of an air-fluid level above the band	—	95	100

Data from Swenson DW, Petryga JA, Grand DJ, et al. Gastric band slippage: a case-controlled study comparing new and old radiographic signs of this important surgical complication. AJR Am J Roentgenol 2014;203:10–6.

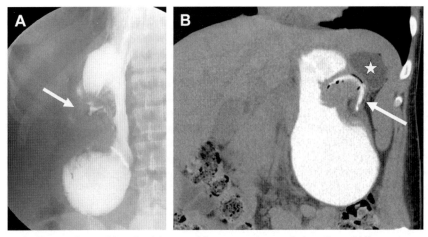

Fig. 22. LUQ pain in a patient with prior history of laparoscopic gastric banding. Oblique prone view from a barium upper GI (*A*) and coronal MPR image from an MDCT with oral contrast (*B*) demonstrate slippage of the polymeric silicone band (*arrow*) with entrapment of fluid in the fundus (*star*). The patient subsequently underwent uneventful surgical removal of the band.

whether the procedure was performed laparoscopically (LRYGB), whether the Roux limb was brought through the TM or over the TM, and on the technical details of the procedure (such as whether staples or sutures are used to close the jejunojejunostomy). Internal hernias in patients that have undergone RYGB can occur through the TM defect, through the mesentery at the jejunojejunostomy site, or between the mesentery of the Roux-limb and the TM (Petersen space).[90] The incidence is higher after laparoscopic RYGB compared with open procedures and also higher when the Roux-limb is retrogastric/retrocolic compared with ante-gastric/ante-colic.[90] The most common symptoms are intermittent postprandial pain, nausea, and vomiting, although patients may be asymptomatic or have vague complaints.[90] Identification of this entity is important because surgical repair may be necessary.[90,91] In a retrospective analysis of 1000 patients who had undergone laparoscopic RYGB, Garza and colleagues[90] reported 45 internal hernias in 43 patients, including 43 through the TM and 2 through the Petersen defect. They found that initial CT scans were diagnostic in 64% of these patients and that retrospective review of imaging studies including CT and/or upper GI showed diagnostic abnormalities in 97% of the cases.[90] CT findings include abnormal clustering of small bowel in the LUQ and congestion and crowding of the mesenteric vessels.[88] The abnormal location of the bowel loops can be a clue to the type of hernia. In a transmesenteric hernia, there may be loops adjacent to the anterior abdominal wall with no overlying omental fat.[88] If bowel loops are clustered posterior to the gastric

remnant, then a hernia through the TM should be considered. There may be mass effect on the posterior gastric remnant wall.[88] A Petersen hernia may not be recognizable on CT, or occasionally the abnormal bowel loops may be seen directly ventral to the pancreas.[88,92] Other causes of SBO in these patients should also be kept in mind. Koppman and colleagues[91] reviewed the rate of SBO in 9527 patients who had undergone LRYGB, including 615 LRYGB procedures that they had performed and 8912 LRYGB procedures reported in 16 studies in the literature. In their own 615 procedures, they found 3 obstructions caused by adhesive disease, one internal hernia into Petersen defect, one trocar site hernia, and 6 obstructions from jejunojejunostomy stenosis caused by narrowing of the afferent limb during stapled closure of the common enterotomy. When considering all 9527 patients, SBO occurred in 3.6% of the patients, with the most common causes including internal hernia, adhesive disease, jejunojejunostomy stenosis, and incisional hernia. SBO from jejunojejunostomy stenosis caused by narrowing of the afferent limb during stapled closure of the common enterotomy was the most common cause of obstruction in patients who underwent an antecolic LRYGB. SBO after retrocolic LRYGB was most often caused by transmesocolic internal hernia or caused by cicatrization at the mesocolic window.[91]

COMPLICATIONS OF PANCREATITIS SPECIFIC TO THE LEFT UPPER QUADRANT

LUQ pain can be the primary presenting symptom in patients with acute pancreatitis as inflammatory exudates containing pancreatic enzymes spread from the anterior pararenal space to the TM, SRL, GCL, and through the parietal peritoneum into the lesser sac (see **Fig. 1**).[10,19] Acute pancreatic fluid collections (APFCs) form in these areas and can extend into the adjacent LUQ structures, including the stomach, spleen, and splenic flexure.[34] Enzymes and inflammatory mediators in the APFCs cause LUQ complications: inflammation, acute necrotic collections (ANCs), pseudocysts, pseudoaneuryms, and SV thrombosis.[34] Gas bubbles indicate abscess formation.[23] MDCT with multiplanar and 3D reconstruction is invaluable in identifying the specific anatomic site of these fluid collections, helping to determine the optimal treatment, and in planning a route of percutaneous catheter drainage. MR imaging can also demonstrate fluid collections, which typically appear bright on T2-weighted images. MR imaging is useful in distinguishing between APFCs and ANCs because it is better able than CT to depict solid necrotic components when they are present.[34] Pseudocysts, abscesses, and hematomas can form in the wall of the stomach (**Fig. 23**). LUQ pain may be the first presenting symptom when colonic obstruction or adynamic ileus at the splenic flexure (associated with the colon cutoff sign discussed earlier) occurs.[10] APFCs spread to the spleen via the SRL and lesser sac. Splenic complications of pancreatitis are generally self-limited and regress with conservative treatment.[93] They include splenic infarcts, hemorrhage, intrasplenic pseudocysts, and splenic rupture.[23,94]

Careful evaluation of the splenic artery for the presence of a pseudoaneurysm is very important in all patients with pancreatitis because of the risk of spontaneous rupture or other complication.[48,69,95] There is a paucity of data indicating which pseudoaneurysms are likely to rupture; because the mortality rate after spontaneous rupture approaches 100%, multiple investigators advocate urgent treatment of pseudoaneurysms of any size, even if asymptomatic.[48,69] Classic treatment involves surgical ligation. Percutaneous treatment with coil embolization, percutaneous thrombin injection, and a combination of the two have been described and seem to have very high success rates.[48,69] Interventional management is preferred by many investigators because the operative mortality can be as high as 50% in these critically ill patients.[69]

DIVERTICULITIS OF THE SPLENIC FLEXURE

Diverticulitis of the splenic flexure and proximal descending colon can cause LUQ pain. Barium enema is rarely performed anymore because of the higher sensitivity of MDCT as well as the ability of MDCT to demonstrate complications, suggest alternative diagnoses, and guide surgical or percutaneous therapy.[20,57] CT findings related to inflammation in the pericolonic fat, including linear stranding, haziness, small fluid collections, and extraluminal gas bubbles are detected in up to 98% of cases.[20] Diverticular abscesses arising from the splenic flexure tend to form in the left subphrenic space and those from the proximal descending colon in the left paracolic gutter. Diverticulitis can be diagnosed on MR imaging with sensitivities up to 94% and specificity up to 92%.[96] Findings on MR imaging are similar to CT, including mural thickening and stranding of the pericolonic fat as well as the depiction of diverticula; abscesses can also be seen on MR imaging.[96]

COLITIS OF THE SPLENIC FLEXURE

Various forms of acute colitis may occasionally be associated with LUQ pain, although the more common presentation is either diarrhea or colicky abdominal pain.[20] The CT findings are frequently

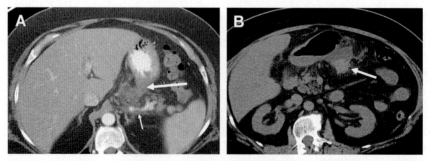

Fig. 23. MDCT scans of a patient with acute pancreatitis obtained at initial presentation (*A*) and several days later (*B*). Axial image (*A*) from an oral and intravenous contrast-enhanced MDCT demonstrates early pancreatitis with inflammatory change extending through the lesser sac to the posterior wall of the stomach (*large arrow*) and around the splenic artery (*small arrow*). Axial image from a noncontrast MDCT obtained several days later (*B*) demonstrates gastric wall hemorrhage extending into the GCL (*arrow*).

nonspecific; a differential diagnosis of infectious, inflammatory, and ischemic colitis (IC) is usually offered in the radiology report. Findings include mural thickening, mucosal enhancement, submucosal edema, and engorgement of the vasa recta. Pseudomembranous colitis caused by overgrowth of *Clostridium difficile* can cause severe mural thickening measuring up to 20 mm (**Fig. 24**).[20] When positive enteric contrast is used, it can insinuate between the markedly thickened haustra giving rise to an accordionlike appearance.[20] Pseudomembranous colitis tends to involve a long segment of the colon, although it may be predominately left sided.[97] Pericolonic inflammatory stranding or ascites may be present. Ulcerative colitis tends to predominately affect the left side of the colon and may cause nonspecific mural thickening. Rectal involvement can be a clue to the diagnosis. Complications of colitis, such as toxic megacolon, are well demonstrated with CT.

ISCHEMIC COLITIS OF THE SPLENIC FLEXURE

IC should be considered in all patients with LUQ pain, but the index of suspicion should be especially high in geriatric patients and patients with certain predisposing factors as listed in **Box 4**.[97] Patients with IC of the splenic flexure may present with mild LUQ pain and tenderness; most patients develop bloody diarrhea within 24 hours.[98] The splenic flexure is particularly sensitive to ischemia because it lies at Griffin point, the watershed between the middle colic and left colic artery blood supply.[20] Colonic ischemia (CI) is divided into 6 categories that reflect pathologic changes and clinical severity: milder forms, such as reversible ischemic colopathy and transient ulcerating IC;

Box 4
Clinical clues suggesting IC
1. Elderly
a. Coexisting cardiovascular disease
b. Low flow states and patients receiving vasoactive medications
c. Chronic renal failure with hemodialysis
d. Postsurgical patients (especially cardiac and aortic surgery)
2. Young patients
a. Trauma with shock
b. Hypercoagulable states
c. Vasculitis (systemic lupus erythematosus, polyarteritis nodosa, sickle cell disease, long distance runners, medications)
Data from Taourel P, Aufort S, Merigeaud S, et al. Imaging of ischemic colitis. Radiol Clin North Am 2008;46:909–24; and Gore RM, Yaghmai V, Thakrar KH, et al. Imaging the intestinal ischemic disorders. Radiol Clin North Am 2008;46:845–75.

severe forms, such as colonic gangrene and fulminant universal IC; and chronic forms, including colonic stricture and chronic ulcerating IC.[98] The clinical course of the disease can take 2 forms, a mild self-limited form that resolves in approximately 2 weeks in about half of patients and a fulminant form with gangrenous ischemia with a greater than 50% mortality rate.[98–100]

Plain abdominal radiographs are of limited value; the common findings, such as dilated gas-filled bowel or a gasless abdomen, are nonspecific and insensitive. Thumbprinting caused by

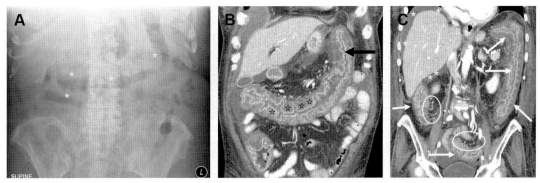

Fig. 24. *Clostridium difficile* colitis. (*A*) Supine anteroposterior radiograph of the abdomen demonstrates gaseous distension of the transverse colon with thickened haustral folds thumbprinting (*stars*). (*B*) Coronal image from an oral and intravenous contrast-enhanced MDCT demonstrates severe mural and haustral thickening of the transverse colon (*stars*). Intense mucosal enhancement is seen (*arrow*). (*C*) Coronal image obtained more posteriorly demonstrates extensive involvement of the entire colon (*arrows*). Note the engorged vasa recta (*circles*) and ascites (*stars*).

Table 4 Findings in CI		
Stage	**Pathophysiology**	**Imaging Findings**
First	Early arterial compromise	Mural thickening and submucosal edema (target sign)
	Early venous compromise	1. Mural thickening and mucosal hyperdensity (hemorrhagic areas) 2. Ascites
Second	Continued arterial compromise without reperfusion with progressive ischemia	Symmetric concentric mural thickening
	Continued venous compromise with progressive mural edema	1. Submucosal hypodensity 2. Shaggy contour with pericolonic stranding
Third	Infarction	1. Pneumatosis 2. Mesenteric and PV gas 3. Loss of parietal enhancement 4. Pneumoperitoneum

Data from Gore RM, Yaghmai V, Thakrar KH, et al. Imaging the intestinal ischemic disorders. Radiol Clin North Am 2008;46:845–75.

mucosal and submucosal edema and hemorrhage is more specific but uncommon and can also be seen with other entities, such as pseudomembranous colitis (see **Fig. 24**). Pneumatosis and portal vein (PV) gas can be seen late in the process and are better demonstrated on CT. MDCT is the preferred modality for evaluating patients with suspected IC.[97,98] Dual-phase imaging is recommended, and positive oral contrast should be avoided.[101] The imaging findings depend on the stage of the process and the underlying pathophysiology and are listed in **Table 4** (**Fig. 25**).[98,102,103] Pneumatosis is well demonstrated on CT and is an ominous sign; patients with CI who have lactic acidosis and pneumatosis have a mortality rate greater than 80%.[104]

Occlusion of the involved mesenteric vessels can be visualized at any of the stages.[98] Good-quality CT angiography (CTA) studies can demonstrate the mesenteric vessels to the level of the small distal segments.[105] US can be useful in confirming the diagnosis and differentiating IC from other forms of colitis.[97] US can demonstrate hypoechoic circumferential mural thickening; color Doppler examination of the colonic wall may reveal absent or diminished flow, which would confirm the diagnosis and might suggest necrosis.[97]

Focal segmental IC can be caused by mucosal and submucosal vascular damage because of the elevated intraluminal pressure proximal to an obstructing cancer.[106] This complication should be identified preoperatively in patients who are

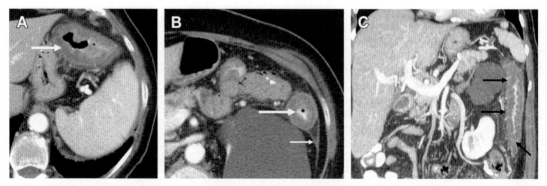

Fig. 25. IC. (*A*) Axial image from an oral and intravenous contrast-enhanced MDCT demonstrates mural thickening and submucosal edema (*arrow*) of the splenic flexure. (*B*) Axial image of the proximal descending colon shows higher-density mucosa and muscularis mucosa (*large arrow*) offsetting the edematous submucosa (*target appearance*). There is thickening of the adjacent fascial trifurcation (*small arrow*) caused by reactive edema. (*C*) Coronal image from an oral and intravenous contrast-enhanced MDCT demonstrates extensive involvement of the left side of the colon (*arrows*).

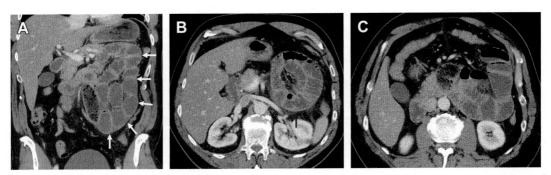

Fig. 26. Left paraduodenal hernia. Coronal (*A*) and axial (*B*) images from an intravenous contrast-enhanced MDCT demonstrate distended fluid-filled bowel loops within a hernia sac under the descending mesocolon (*arrows*). Axial image (*C*) at the level of the duodenojejunal junction shows the herniating bowel loops descending posterior to the inferior mesenteric vein (*arrow*).

undergoing resection of the tumor because it can lead to breakdown of the suture line at the site of reanastomosis. Additionally, CI adjacent to a cancer can cause diagnostic confusion regarding the extent of the cancer because ischemic congestive changes in the pericolonic fat may be interpreted as evidence of T3 invasion or because the ischemic segment may be interpreted as part of the malignancy. One helpful clue is that there is preservation of mural stratification (target sign) in IC, whereas mural thickening caused by tumor is heterogeneous.

LEFT UPPER QUADRANT SMALL BOWEL OBSTRUCTION

SBO usually presents with periumbilical or diffuse pain but can occasionally cause LUQ pain. Adhesions, inflammatory strictures, and neoplasms can involve the jejunum; several internal hernias are typically found in the LUQ. Left paraduodenal internal hernias can cause LUQ pain and can be recognized on MDCT by the characteristic saclike configuration of the involved bowel loops in the left side of the abdomen posterior to the descending mesocolon (**Fig. 26**).[92] Identification of the bowel loops entering the hernia sac posterior to the IMV helps to confirm the diagnosis (see **Fig. 26**).[92] If the obstructed bowel is seen in the lesser sac, herniation through the foramen of Winslow or a right paraduodenal hernia should be considered. Internal hernias typically cause closed-loop obstructions with an associated elevated risk of ischemia; therefore, early diagnosis and surgical referral is important.[92]

MISCELLANEOUS CAUSES

Left subphrenic abscesses can be associated with other LUQ acute pathologies described earlier, including perforated gastric ulcers, ruptured splenic abscesses, perforated splenic flexure diverticulitis, and may be seen postoperatively.[10] Left retroperitoneal diseases, such as left adrenal hemorrhage or obstructive uropathy, and infection of the left kidney can all present with LUQ pain, although left flank pain is more common. Inflammation of "jejunal pseudodiverticuli"[20] is an extremely rare cause of LUQ pain.[20] Diaphragmatic hernias are occasionally encountered, and diseases of the left hemithorax and heart should also be considered in the clinical differential diagnosis.

SUMMARY

High-quality imaging is critical in the evaluation of patients with acute LUQ pain, and imaging is frequently the key to identifying that nonspecific abdominal pain is caused by disease in the LUQ. Several acute diseases of the LUQ that rely on imaging for diagnosis, such as gastric perforation and volvulus, acute splenic sequestration or torsion, ruptured splenic artery aneurysm, internal hernia with SBO, or acute CI, may be rapidly life threatening. Contrast-enhanced MDCT is currently the primary modality for evaluating these patients, and US and MR imaging are important additional tests. MR imaging may play a greater role in the future.

REFERENCES

1. Leschka S, Alkadhi H, Wildermuth S, et al. Multi-detector computed tomography of acute abdomen. Eur Radiol 2005;15:2435–47.
2. Siewert B, Raptopoulos V, Mueller M, et al. Impact of CT on diagnosis and management of acute abdomen in patients initially treated without surgery. AJR Am J Roentgenol 1997;168:173–8.
3. Nagurney JT, Brown DFM, Chang Y, et al. Use of diagnostic testing in the emergency department

for patients presenting with non-traumatic abdominal pain. J Emerg Med 2003;25(4):363–71.

4. Gerhardt RT, Nelson BK, Keenan S, et al. Derivation of a clinical guideline for the assessment of nonspecific abdominal pain: the guideline for abdominal pain in the ED setting (GAPEDS) phase 1 study. Am J Emerg Med 2005;23:709–17.

5. Pines J, Pines LU, Hall A, et al. The interrater variation of ED abdominal examination findings in patients with acute abdominal pain. Am J Emerg Med 2005;23:483–7.

6. Ragsdale L, Southerland L. Acute abdominal pain in the older adult. Emerg Med Clin North Am 2011;29:429–48.

7. Marincek B, Heiken JP. Emergency radiology of the abdomen: the acute abdomen. In: Hodler J, Von Schulthess GK, Zollikofer CL, editors. Diseases of the abdomen and pelvis diagnostic imaging and interventional techniques. Milan (MI); New York: Springer; 2006. p. 3–9.

8. Panebianco NL, Jahnes K, Mills AM. Imaging and laboratory testing in acute abdominal pain. Emerg Med Clin North Am 2011;29:175–93.

9. Gore RM, Newmark GM, Thakrar KH, et al. Pathways of abdominal tumour spread: the role of the subperitoneal space. Cancer Imaging 2009;9: 112–20.

10. Meyers MA. Dynamic radiology of the abdomen: normal and pathologic anatomy. 4th edition. New York: Springer-Verlag; 1993.

11. van Leeuwen MS, Veldhuis WB. Dynamic approach to abdominal radiology. 1st edition. 2012. ISBN: 978-90-818819-0-6.

12. Moody AR, Poon PY. Gastroepiploic veins: CT appearance in pancreatic disease. AJR Am J Roentgenol 1992;158:779–83.

13. Cotes C, Swischuk LE. Left upper quadrant pain: upside down spleen. Pediatr Emerg Care 2013; 29(9):1009–10.

14. Oldfield AL, Wilbur AC. Retrogastric colon: CT demonstration of anatomic variations. Radiology 1993;186:557–61.

15. Bredolo F, Esposito A, Casiraghi E, et al. Intestinal interposition: the prevalence and clinical relevance of non-hepatodiaphragmatic conditions (non-Chilaiditi forms) documented by CT and review of the literature. Radiol Med 2011;116:607–19.

16. Wojtasek DA, Codner MA, Nowick EJ. CT diagnosis of cecal herniation through the foramen of Winslow. Gastrointest Radiol 1991;16:77–9.

17. Desai G, Filly RA. Sonographic anatomy of the gastrohepatic ligament. J Ultrasound Med 2010;29:87–93.

18. Alabousi A, Patlas MN, Scaglione M, et al. Cross-sectional imaging of nontraumatic emergencies of the spleen. Curr Probl Diagn Radiol 2014;43:254–67.

19. Gore RM, Balfe DM, Aizenstein RI, et al. The great escape: interfascial decompression planes of the retroperitoneum. AJR Am J Roentgenol 2000;175: 363–70.

20. Gore RM, Miller FH, Pereles FS, et al. Helical CT in the evaluation of the acute abdomen. AJR Am J Roentgenol 2000;174:901–13.

21. Singh A, Danrad R, Hahn PF, et al. MR Imaging of the acute abdomen and pelvis: acute appendicitis and beyond. Radiographics 2007;27:1419–31.

22. Anderson SW, Soto JA. Multi-detector row CT of acute non-traumatic abdominal pain: contrast and protocol considerations. Radiol Clin North Am 2012;50:137–47.

23. Urban BA, Fishman EK. Tailored helical CT evaluation of acute abdomen. Radiographics 2000;20: 725–49.

24. Katz DS, Baker ME, Rosen MP, et al. Expert Panel of Gastrointestinal Imaging: ACR appropriateness criteria® acute pancreatitis. Reston (VA): American College of Radiology; 2010 [on-line publication].

25. Grant TH, Rosen MP, Fidler JL, et al. ACR appropriateness criteria® acute abdominal pain and fever or suspected abdominal abscess. Reston (VA): American College of Radiology; 2008 [on-line publication].

26. Miller FH, Bree RL, Rosen MP, et al. ACR appropriateness criteria ® left lower quadrant pain. Reston (VA): American College of Radiology; 2008 [on-line publication].

27. Katz DS, Baker ME, Rosen MP, et al. Expert Panel of Gastrointestinal Imaging: ACR appropriateness criteria ® suspected small-bowel obstruction. Reston (VA): American College of Radiology; 2010 [on-line publication].

28. Horton KM, Fishman EK. Current role of CT in imaging of the stomach. Radiographics 2003;23: 75–87.

29. Paulson EK, Jaffe TA, Thomas J, et al. MDCT of patients with acute abdominal pain: a new perspective using coronal reformations from submillimeter isotropic voxels. AJR Am J Roentgenol 2004; 183(4):899–906.

30. Peddu P, Shah M, Sidhu PS. Splenic abnormalities: a comparative review of ultrasound, microbubble-enhanced ultrasound and computed tomography. Clin Radiol 2004;59:777–92.

31. Baron KT, Arleo EK, Robinson C, et al. Comparing the diagnostic performance of MRI versus CT in the evaluation of acute nontraumatic abdominal pain during pregnancy. Emerg Radiol 2012;19: 519–25.

32. Birchard KR, Brown MA, Hyslop WB, et al. MRI of acute abdominal and pelvic pain in pregnant patients. AJR Am J Roentgenol 2005;184:452–8.

33. Masselli G, Brunelli R, Casciani E, et al. Acute abdominal and pelvic pain in pregnancy: MR imaging as a valuable adjunct to ultrasound? Abdom Imaging 2011;36:596–603.

34. Manikkavasakar S, AlObaidy M, Busireddy KK, et al. Magnetic resonance imaging of pancreatitis: an update. World J Gastroenterol 2014;20(4): 14760–77.

35. Lawrence YR, Pokroy R, Berlowitz D, et al. Splenic infarction: an update on William Osler's observations. Isr Med Assoc J 2010;12:362–5.

36. Bitzer M, Armeanu S, Krober SM, et al. A young woman with splenic infarction. Lancet 2003; 362:1456.

37. Beeson MS. Splenic infarct presenting as acute abdominal pain in an older patient. J Emerg Med 1996;14(3):319–22.

38. Antopolsky M, Hiller N, Salameh S, et al. Splenic infarction: 10 years of experience. Am J Emerg Med 2009;27:262–5.

39. Rabushka LS, Kawashima A, Fishman EK, et al. Imaging of the spleen: CT with supplemental MR examination. Radiographics 1994;14:307–32.

40. Gorg C, Graef C, Bert T. Contrast-enhanced sonography for differential diagnosis of an inhomogeneous spleen of unknown cause in patients with pain in the left upper quadrant. J Ultrasound Med 2006;25:729–34.

41. Gaetke-Udager K, Wasnik AP, Kaza RK, et al. Multimodality imaging of splenic lesions and the role of non-vascular image-guided intervention. Abdom Imaging 2014;39(3):570–87.

42. Elsayes KM, Narra VR, Mukundan G, et al. MR Imaging of the spleen: spectrum of abnormalities. Radiographics 2005;25(4):971.

43. Clark JK, Gorman J, Lee MH, et al. Dynamic MRI in the diagnosis and post surgical evaluation of wandering spleen. J Radiol Case Rep 2014;8(10): 15–22.

44. Fotiadis C, Lavranos G, Patapis P, et al. Abscesses of the spleen: report of three cases. World J Gastroenterol 2008;14(19):3088–91.

45. Murray JG, Patel MD, Lee S, et al. Microabscesses of the liver and spleen in AIDS: detection with 5-HHz sonography. Radiology 1995;197:723–7.

46. Warshaueer DM, Hall HL. Solitary splenic lesions. Semin Ultrasound CT MR 2006;27:370–88.

47. Robertson F, Leander P, Ekberg O. Radiology of the spleen. Eur Radiol 2001;11:80–95.

48. Singh AK, Shankar S, Gervais DA, et al. Image-guided percutaneous splenic interventions. Radiographics 2012;321:523–34.

49. Lucey BC, Boland GW, Maher MM, et al. Percutaneous nonvascular splenic interventions: a 10-year review. AJR Am J Roentgenol 2002;179(6): 1591–6.

50. Smith FJ, Mathieson JR, Cooperberg PL. Abdominal abnormalities in AIDS: detection at US in a large population. Radiology 1994;192(3):691–5.

51. Bhatia K, Sahdev A, Reznek RH. Lymphoma of the spleen. Semin Ultrasound CT MR 2007;28:12–20.

52. Catalano O, Lobianco R, Sandomenico F, et al. Real-time contrast enhanced ultrasound of the spleen: examination technique and preliminary clinical experience. Radiol Med 2003;106(4): 338–56.

53. Hahn PF, Weissleder R, Stark DD, et al. MR imaging of focal splenic tumors. AJR Am J Roentgenol 1988;150(4):823–7.

54. Hess CF, Griebel J, Schmiedl U, et al. Focal lesions of the spleen: preliminary results with fast MRI imaging at 1.5 T. J Comput Assist Tomogr 1988; 12(4):569–74.

55. Gong JS, Xu JM. Role of curved planar reformations using multidetector spiral CT in diagnosis of pancreatic and peripancreatic diseases. World J Gastroenterol 2004;10(13):1943–7.

56. Bradley EL. The natural history of splenic vein thrombosis due to chronic pancreatitis: indications for surgery. Int J Pancreatol 1987;2(2):87–92.

57. Siewert B, Raptopoulos V. CT of the acute abdomen: findings and impact on diagnosis and treatment. AJR Am J Roentgenol 1994;163(3): 1317–24.

58. Farley DR, Zietlow SP, Bannon MP, et al. Spontaneous rupture of the spleen due to infectious mononucleosis. Mayo Clin Proc 1992;67:846–53.

59. Blankenship JC, Indeck M. Spontaneous splenic rupture complicating anticoagulant or thrombolytic therapy. Am J Med 1993;94(4):433–7.

60. Daly B, Lu M, Pickhardt PJ, et al. Complications of optical colonoscopy: CT findings. Radiol Clin North Am 2014;52(5):1087–99.

61. Cassar K, Munro A. Iatrogenic splenic injury. J R Coll Surg Edinb 2002;47(6):731–41.

62. Fishback SJ, Pickhardt PJ, Bhalla S, et al. Delayed presentation of splenic rupture following optical colonoscopy: clinical and CT findings. Emerg Radiol 2011;18(6):539–44.

63. Magowska A. Wandering spleen: a medical enigma, its natural history and rationalization. World J Surg 2013;37:545–50.

64. Lubner MG, Simard ML, Peterson CM, et al. Emergent and nonemergent nonbowel torsion: spectrum of imaging and clinical findings. Radiographics 2013;33:155–73.

65. Nemcek AA, Miller FH, Fizgerald SW. Acute torsion of a wandering spleen: diagnosis by CT and duplex Doppler and color flow sonography. AJR Am J Roentgenol 1991;157:307–9.

66. Kessler A, Miller E, Keider S, et al. Mass at the splenic hilum: a clue to torsion of a wandering spleen located in a normal left upper quadrant position. J Ultrasound Med 2003;22:527–30.

67. Agrawal GA, Johnson PT, Fishman EK. Splenic artery aneurysms and pseudoaneurysms: clinical distinctions and CT appearances. AJR Am J Roentgenol 2007;188(4):992–9.

68. Abbas MA, Stone WM, Fowl RJ, et al. Splenic artery aneurysms: two decades experience at Mayo Clinic. Ann Vasc Surg 2002;16(4):442–9.

69. Al-Habbal Y, Christophi C, Muralidharan V. Aneurysms of the splenic artery – a review. Surgeon 2010;8(4):223–31.

70. Mattar SG, Lumsden AB. The management of splenic artery aneurysms: experience with 23 cases. Am J Surg 1995;169:580–4.

71. Gore RM, Levine MS. High yield imaging: gastrointestinal. Philadelphia: Saunders; 2010. p. 162.

72. Allen BC, Tirman P, Tobben JP, et al. Gastroduodenal ulcers on CT: forgotten, but not gone. Abdom Imaging 2015;40(1):19–25.

73. Gore RM, Levine MS. High yield imaging: gastrointestinal. Philadelphia: Saunders; 2010.

74. Jeffrey R, Federle M, Wall S. Value of computed tomography in detecting occult gastrointestinal perforation. J Comput Assist Tomogr 1983;7:825–7.

75. Earls JP, Dachman AH, Colon E, et al. Prevalence and duration of postoperative pneumoperitoneum: sensitivity of CT vs left lateral decubitus radiography. AJR Am J Roentgenol 1993;161:781–5.

76. Maniatis V, Chryssikopoulos H, Roussakis A, et al. Perforation of the alimentary tract: evaluation with computed tomography. Abdom Imaging 2000; 25(4):373–9.

77. Rice RP, Thompson WM, Gedgaudas RK. The diagnosis and significance of extraluminal gas in the abdomen. Radiol Clin North Am 1982;20:819–37.

78. Ham M, McInnes MD, Woo M, et al. Negative predictive value of intravenous contrast-enhanced CT of the abdomen for patients presenting to the emergency department with undifferentiated upper abdominal pain. Emerg Radiol 2012;19:19–26.

79. Moosvi AR, Saravolatz LD, Wong DH, et al. Emphysematous gastritis: case report and review. Rev Infect Dis 1990;12(5):848–55.

80. Johnson PT, Horton KM, Edil BH, et al. Gastric pneumatosis: the role of CT in diagnosis and patient management. Emerg Radiol 2011;18:65–73.

81. Cordum NR, Dixon A, Campbell DR. Gastroduodenal pneumatosis: endoscopic and histological findings. Am J Gastroenterol 1997;92:692–5.

82. Rashid F, Thangarajah T, Mulvey D, et al. A review article on gastric volvulus: a challenge to diagnosis and management. Int J Surg 2010;8:18–24.

83. Millet I, Orliac C, Alili C, et al. Computed tomography findings of acute gastric volvulus. Eur Radiol 2014;24:3115–22.

84. Larssen KS, Stimec B, Takvam JA, et al. Role of imaging in gastric volvulus: stepwise approach in three cases. Turk J Gastroenterol 2012;23(4): 390–3.

85. Shivanand G, Seema S, Srivastava DN, et al. Gastric volvulus acute and chronic presentation. Clin Imaging 2003;27:265–8.

86. Carter R, Brewer LA, Hinshaw DB. Acute gastric volvulus. Am J Surg 1980;140(1):99–106.

87. Peterson CM, Anderson JS, Hara AK, et al. Volvulus of the gastrointestinal tract: appearances at multimodality imaging. Radiographics 2009; 29(5):1281–93.

88. Blachar A, Federle MP, Pealer KM, et al. Radiographic manifestations of normal postoperative anatomy and gastrointestinal complications of bariatric surgery, with emphasis on CT imaging findings. Semin Ultrasound CT MR 2004;25(3):239–51.

89. Swenson DW, Petryga JA, Grand DJ, et al. Gastric band slippage: a case-controlled study comparing new and old radiographic signs of this important surgical complication. AJR Am J Roentgenol 2014;203:10–6.

90. Garza E, Kuhn J, Arnold D, et al. Internal hernias after laparoscopic Roux-en-Y gastric bypass. Am J Surg 2004;188:796–800.

91. Koppman JS, Li C, Gandsas A. Small bowel obstruction after laparoscopic Roux-En-Y gastric bypass: a review of 9,527 patients. J Am Coll Surg 2008;206(3):571–84.

92. Santillan CS. Computed tomography of small bowel obstruction. Radiol Clin North Am 2013;51: 17–27.

93. Rypens F, Deviere J, Zalcman M, et al. Splenic parenchymal complications of pancreatitis: CT findings and natural history. J Comput Assist Tomogr 1997;21(1):89–93.

94. Fishman EK, Soyer P, Bliss DF, et al. Splenic Involvement in pancreatitis: spectrum of CT findings. AJR Am J Roentgenol 1995;164:631–5.

95. Tessier DJ, Stone WM, Fowl RJ, et al. Clinical features and management of splenic artery pseudoaneurysm: case series and cumulative review of literature. J Vasc Surg 2003;38:969–74.

96. Liu B, Ramalho M, AlObaidy M, et al. Gastrointestinal imaging – practical magnetic resonance imaging approach. World J Radiol 2014;6(8): 544–66.

97. Taourel P, Aufort S, Merigeaud S, et al. Imaging of ischemic colitis. Radiol Clin North Am 2008;46: 909–24.

98. Gore RM, Yaghmai V, Thakrar KH, et al. Imaging the intestinal ischemic disorders. Radiol Clin North Am 2008;46:845–75.

99. Rosai J. Gastrointestinal tract. In: Rosai J, editor. Surgical pathology. 9th edition. Edinburgh (United Kingdom): Mosby; 2004. p. 615–872.

100. Goldin SB, Rosemurgy A. Anatomy and physiology of the mesenteric circulation. In: Yeo CJ, Dempsey DT, Klein AS, et al, editors. Surgery of the alimentary tract. 6th edition. Philadelphia: Saunders; 2005. p. 1235–46.

101. Lee SS, Park SH. Computed tomography evaluation of gastrointestinal bleeding and acute

mesenteric ischemia. Radiol Clin North Am 2013;51:29–43.

102. Romano S, Lassandro F, Scaglione M, et al. Ischemia and infarction of the small bowel and colon: spectrum of imaging findings. Abdom Imaging 2006;31:277–92.

103. Romano S, Romano L, Grassi R. Multidetector row computed tomography findings from ischemia to infarction of the large bowel. Eur J Radiol 2007; 61:433–41.

104. Hawn MT, Canon CL, Lockhart ME, et al. Serum lactic acid determines outcomes of CT diagnosis of pneumatosis of the gastrointestinal tract. Am Surg 2004;70:19–23.

105. Horton KM, Fishman EK. Multidetector CT angiography in the diagnosis of mesenteric ischemia. Radiol Clin North Am 2007;45:275–88.

106. Ko GY, Ha HK, Lee HJ, et al. Usefulness of CT in patients with ischemic colitis proximal to colonic cancer. AJR Am J Roentgenol 1997;168:951–6.

Evaluating the Patient with Right Lower Quadrant Pain

Neel B. Patel, MD[a],*, Daniel R. Wenzke, MD[b]

KEYWORDS

- Abdominal pain • Appendicitis • Diverticulitis • Epiploic appendagitis • Meckel's diverticulum
- Omental infarct • Neutropenic colitis • Inflammatory bowel disease

KEY POINTS

- Right lower quadrant pain may be caused by a variety of conditions and clinical diagnosis is often challenging due to nonspecific clinical symptoms.
- Computed tomography (CT) is the primary imaging modality for the evaluation of right lower quadrant pain in most patients because it provides a rapid general survey of anatomy and potential pathology.
- CT protocol for the evaluation of suspected appendicitis or right lower quadrant pain will depend on the needs of referring clinicians, usually the emergency department, and individual work flow considerations of each radiology department.

INTRODUCTION

Right lower quadrant abdominal pain is a common presenting symptom in the emergency department and can result from a wide spectrum of conditions, ranging from benign and self-limiting to those require urgent surgical or percutaneous intervention.[1] Optimal evaluation necessitates integration of patient history, clinical examination, laboratory tests, and imaging studies. The initial consideration in most patients is acute appendicitis; however, several other conditions may present with similar clinical, physical, and laboratory features. Other causes of right lower quadrant pain include mesenteric adenitis, Meckel diverticulum, neutropenic colitis, right-sided diverticulitis, epiploic appendagitis, omental infarct, and inflammatory bowel disease.

IMAGING OF RIGHT LOWER QUADRANT PAIN

Computed tomography (CT) is the primary imaging modality for the evaluation of acute abdominal pain in most patients because it provides a general survey of anatomy and potential pathology. The vast majority of imaging studies for evaluating right lower quadrant pain center on the diagnosis of acute appendicitis, the most frequent cause of abdominal pain requiring surgery. Delayed diagnosis can result in substantial morbidity.

CT imaging has proven to be a highly effective and accurate means of diagnosing acute appendicitis, with reported sensitivities of 90% to 100%, specificities of 91% to 99%, accuracies of 94% to 98%, positive predictive values of 92% to 98%, and negative predictive values of 95% to 100%.[2–7] The optimal CT technique for acute appendicitis remains controversial and most commonly consists of oral enteric and intravenous contrast-enhanced examinations. Many studies have focused on modifying CT protocols in an attempt to reduce patient radiation dose, eliminate adverse reaction and nephrotoxicity risk with intravenous contrast, and enable earlier scanning rather than waiting for bowel transit of oral contrast

[a] Jupiter Imaging Associates, Sheridan Healthcorp, Jupiter, FL, USA; [b] NorthShore University HealthSystem, University of Chicago, Pritzker School of Medicine, 2650 Ridge Avenue, Evanston, IL 60201, USA
* Corresponding author.
E-mail address: neelbpatel@hotmail.com

Radiol Clin N Am 53 (2015) 1159–1170
http://dx.doi.org/10.1016/j.rcl.2015.06.004

material. Investigated strategies include scanning without intravenous and/or oral contrast, addition of rectal contrast, targeted imaging of the right lower quadrant, and reduced radiation dose scanning techniques.[7–15]

CT scans performed without oral, rectal, or intravenous contrast allow immediate scanning of symptomatic patients at a lower cost and without the risk of a contrast reaction. Lack of oral contrast may be a disadvantage in patients with a paucity of intra-abdominal fat, limiting detection of the appendix and subtle inflammatory changes in the right lower quadrant.[2,16] Identification of bowel wall thickening and luminal narrowing is also limited without enteric contrast.[17] Lack of intravenous contrast limits assessment of appendiceal wall thickening, differentiation of the appendix from surrounding vasculature, and reduces the ability to make an alternative diagnosis.[9,18]

Ultimately, the CT protocol for the evaluation of suspected appendicitis or right lower quadrant pain will depend on the needs of referring clinicians, usually the emergency department, and individual work flow considerations of each radiology department. For example, emergency departments are under increasing pressure to reduce average length of stay. Intravenous contrast-only protocol for select patients with abdominal pain reduced length of stay by 2 hours compared with oral contrast–prepped examinations.[19]

ACUTE APPENDICITIS

Appendicitis is the most frequent cause of acute abdominal pain requiring surgical intervention and is the most common emergent abdominal operation performed in the United States.[18,20] The annual incidence of acute appendicitis across all ages is approximately 9.4 cases per 10,000, with the highest incidence of 15.3 cases per 10,000 occurring in the 10-year-old to 19-year-old age group.[21]

The appendix is a true diverticulum located at the base of the cecum near the ileocecal valve. Although the base of the appendix is relatively constant in position, the tip may migrate into a variety of positions, most commonly retrocecal, pelvic, and less commonly retroileal, preileal, subileal, postileal, and subcecal.[22] The appendix typically measures 6 to 9 cm in length, but can vary considerably, with longest reported appendix measuring 55 cm.[23]

Clinical examination remains an essential component of evaluating a patient with suspected acute appendicitis; however, overall diagnostic accuracy is approximately 80% with a range of 78% to 92% in male patients and 58% to 85% in female patients.[18] The lower diagnostic accuracy in females is likely due to gynecologic and obstetric pathologies presenting with right lower quadrant pain. Most patients with acute appendicitis present with abdominal pain, although the classic presentation sequence of poorly localized periumbilical pain, followed by nausea and vomiting, and later migration of the pain to the right lower quadrant occurs in only one-half to two-thirds of all patients.[24] Diagnosis is complicated by variable clinical symptoms based on anatomic position of the appendix. In patients with a retrocecal appendix, the pain may be referred to the right flank, costovertebral angle, or, in males, the right testis. Patients with a pelvic or retroileal appendix may experience pain in the pelvis, rectum, adnexa, or, less commonly, left lower quadrant.[24]

CT findings of acute appendicitis generally reflect the severity of inflammation. Mild cases may have subtle imaging findings with a minimally distended, fluid-filled appendix measuring 5 to 6 mm in diameter and without appreciable periappendiceal fat stranding (Fig. 1).[18] Typically, acute appendicitis presents with luminal distension of 7 to 15 mm in diameter, circumferential wall thickening, appendiceal wall enhancement (homogeneous or stratified in a so-called "target sign"), and periappendiceal inflammatory change, occasionally with an appendicolith (Figs. 2–4).[12,18] Reactive inflammation may spread to the adjacent cecum. Triangular-shaped thickening of the cecum surrounding the appendiceal orifice is known as the "arrowhead sign" (Fig. 5), whereas linear inflammatory change separating the base

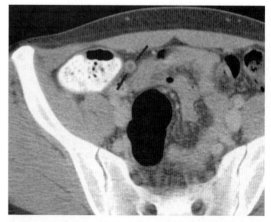

Fig. 1. Acute appendicitis. Contrast-enhanced axial CT image shows an abnormal appendix (*arrows*) with mild luminal distension and abnormal mural enhancement and thickening. No significant periappendiceal inflammatory stranding is present. (*From* Wenzke DR, Jacobs JE, Balthazar EJ, et al. Diseases of the appendix. In: Gore RM, Levine MS, editors. Textbook of gastrointestinal radiology. 4th edition. Philadelphia: Elsevier/Saunders; 2014. p. 964; with permission.)

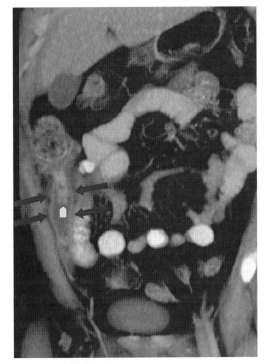

Fig. 2. Acute appendicitis. Contrast-enhanced coronal multiplanar reconstruction CT image shows a fluid-distended appendix (*arrows*) with mural wall enhancement and periappendiceal inflammatory changes. Multiple obstructing appendicoliths are present (yellow *arrowhead*). (*From* Wenzke DR, Jacobs JE, Balthazar EJ, et al. Diseases of the appendix. In: Gore RM, Levine MS, editors. Textbook of gastrointestinal radiology. 4th edition. Philadelphia: Elsevier/Saunders; 2014. p. 963; with permission.)

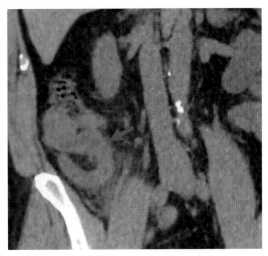

Fig. 4. Acute appendicitis. Unenhanced coronal multiplanar reconstruction CT image shows a fluid-filled dilated appendix (*circled*) with periappendiceal inflammatory changes.

of the appendix from a contrast-filled cecum is known as the "cecal bar" sign.[12]

CT signs of appendiceal perforation include abscess, phlegmon, extraluminal air, extraluminal appendicolith, and focal defect in the enhancing appendiceal wall. When used collectively, these 5 findings yield a sensitivity and specificity of approximately 95% for differentiating perforated from nonperforated appendicitis (**Fig. 6**).[25]

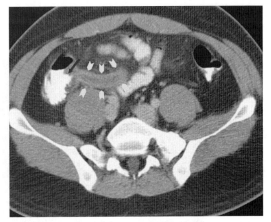

Fig. 5. Acute appendicitis. Contrast-enhanced axial CT image shows a dilated appendix (*arrowheads*) with enhancing mural wall thickening and periappendiceal inflammatory changes. Triangular-shaped thickening of the cecal base at the appendiceal orifice (*arrow*) denotes the "arrowhead sign." (*From* Wenzke DR, Jacobs JE, Balthazar EJ, et al. Diseases of the appendix. In: Gore RM, Levine MS, editors. Textbook of gastrointestinal radiology. 4th edition. Philadelphia: Elsevier/Saunders; 2014. p. 964; with permission.)

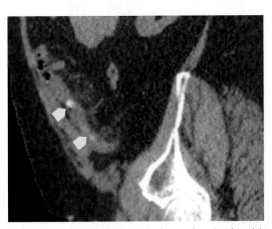

Fig. 3. Acute appendicitis. Unenhanced sagittal multiplanar reconstruction CT image shows a fluid-filled dilated appendix (*arrow*) with multiple appendicoliths (*arrowheads*) and periappendiceal inflammatory changes.

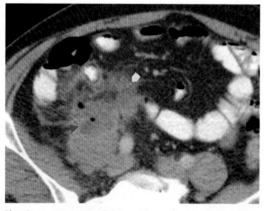

Fig. 6. Acute appendicitis with perforation. Contrast-enhanced axial CT image shows a rim-enhancing fluid collection (*arrow*) containing foci of gas with extension into the right psoas muscle. Extensive inflammatory changes in the right lower quadrant mesentery are present (*arrowhead*).

Localized lymphadenopathy, peritonitis, and small bowel obstruction also may be present (**Fig. 7**).

It is essential to evaluate the entire length of the appendix because inflammatory changes may be confined to the distal appendix, also known as tip appendicitis.[26] Patients with previous appendectomies may uncommonly present with inflammatory changes surrounding residual appendiceal tissue, also known as stump appendicitis.[27]

MESENTERIC ADENITIS

Mesenteric adenitis is inflammation affecting mesenteric lymph nodes that can lead to acute and chronic abdominal pain. The clinical presentation is nonspecific and often leads to a broad differential diagnosis for right lower quadrant abdominal pain. It is the second most common cause of right lower quadrant pain after acute appendicitis, accounting for 2% to 14% of patients suspected of having appendicitis.[28–31]

Mesenteric adenitis is primarily an imaging diagnosis and can be classified into 2 groups: primary and secondary. Primary mesenteric adenitis is defined as a cluster of 3 or more right lower quadrant lymph nodes measuring 5 mm or larger without an identifiable acute inflammatory process or with mild terminal ileal wall thickening (<5 mm) (**Fig. 8**).[29] Underlying infectious terminal ileitis is postulated as the cause of most cases of primary mesenteric adenitis.[28,29,31] Secondary mesenteric adenitis is related to an identifiable underlying condition and possibilities include appendicitis, Crohn disease, infectious colitis, ulcerative colitis, systemic lupus erythematosus, and ascending colon diverticulitis (**Fig. 9**).[29]

MECKEL DIVERTICULUM

Meckel diverticulum is the most common congenital gastrointestinal tract anomaly.[32] It is a true diverticulum arising from the antimesenteric border of the middle to distal ileum due to a remnant proximal omphalomesenteric duct, which normally obliterates during the fifth to seventh week of fetal development. Meckel diverticulum is classically referred to by the rule of "2's": affecting 2% of the population, located within 2 feet of the ileocecal valve, approximately 2 inches

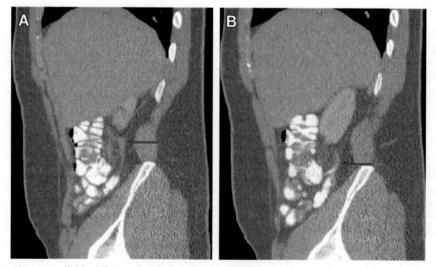

Fig. 7. Acute tip appendicitis. (*A*) Unenhanced sagittal multiplanar reconstruction CT image shows a thickened appendiceal tip (*arrow*) with periappendiceal stranding. (*B*) Unenhanced sagittal multiplanar reconstruction CT image shows normal diameter proximal and mid appendix (*arrow*).

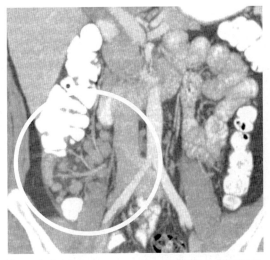

Fig. 8. Primary mesenteric adenitis. Contrast-enhanced coronal maximal intensity projection CT image shows several enlarged mesenteric lymph nodes (*circled*) in the right lower quadrant.

in length, and often clinically symptomatic before 2 years of age.[32,33]

Meckel diverticulum is usually lined by normal ileal mucosa; however, approximately 12% to 19% of Meckel diverticula contain ectopic tissue.[34–36] Ectopic tissue is most commonly gastric in origin, but also may be pancreatic, carcinoid, duodenal, or lipomatous in histology.[35] Although usually clinical silent, Meckel diverticulum may present with a variety of symptoms; 43% of symptomatic patients compared with 12% of

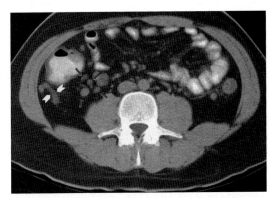

Fig. 9. Secondary mesenteric adenitis with Crohn disease. Contrast-enhanced axial CT image shows multiple enlarged mesenteric lymph nodes (*arrows*) in the right lower quadrant. The appendix is normal (*arrowheads*). (*From* Wenzke DR, Jacobs JE, Balthazar EJ, et al. Diseases of the appendix. In: Gore RM, Levine MS, editors. Textbook of gastrointestinal radiology. 4th edition. Philadelphia: Elsevier/Saunders; 2014. p. 955–83; with permission.)

asymptomatic patients had heterotopic tissue in the Meckel diverticulum.[35] Among adults in a case series at the Mayo Clinic, the most common presentations were bleeding (38%), obstruction (34%), and diverticulitis (28%).[35]

Gastrointestinal bleeding due to Meckel diverticulum is typically caused by ectopic gastric tissue. ^{99m}Tc-Na-pertechnetate scintigraphy is helpful in identifying ectopic gastric mucosa, as pertechnetate is taken up by gastric mucin-secreting cells; a Meckel diverticulum without gastric mucosa will not be detected by this scintigraphy. The sensitivity of ^{99m}Tc-Na-pertechnetate scintigraphy in adults is approximately 60% in adults and 60% to 94% in children.[37–39] Pretreatment with pentagastrin, histamine H2 blockers, and/or glucagon can increase sensitivity of ^{99m}Tc-Na-pertechnetate scintigraphy.[40]

A normal Meckel diverticulum is difficult to differentiate from normal small bowel, although in some cases a blind-ending structure in continuity with the ileum may be identified (**Fig. 10**). Similar to other etiologies of right lower quadrant pain, CT is particularly helpful in identify complications of Meckel diverticulum, including obstruction, inflammation, perforation, and neoplasm. An inflamed diverticulum appears as a blind-ending pouch that usually contains fluid, air, and/or particulate material (**Fig. 11**).[41] Mural enhancement also is present, unless the diverticulum is complicated by gangrenous or severe ischemia. A residual fibrous band connecting the diverticulum to the mesentery or anterior abdominal wall increases the risk of small bowel obstruction.[41]

NEUTROPENIC ENTEROCOLITIS (TYPHLITIS)

Neutropenic enterocolitis, or typhlitis, is a necrotizing enterocolitis occurring in neutropenic patients and characterized by edema and inflammation of the cecum, ascending colon, and occasionally the small bowel. Pathogenesis is likely multifactorial, including chemotherapy-induced mucosal injury facilitating aerobic and anaerobic infection, impaired host immune response allowing propagation of infection, and direct cytotoxic injury from chemotherapy.[42,43] Although originally described in children with acute leukemia, neutropenic enterocolitis may occur during therapy for a variety of hematological and solid malignancies in both children and adults.[44,45]

Neutropenic enterocolitis should be a diagnostic consideration in any neutropenic patient (absolute neutrophil count <500 cells/mm^3) who presents with fever, abdominal pain,

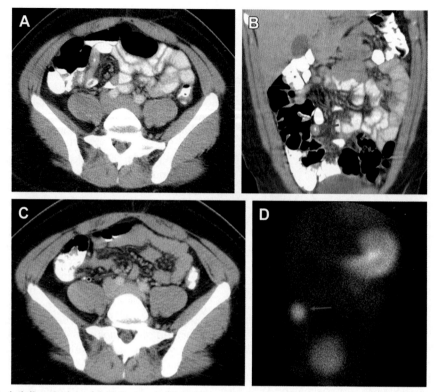

Fig. 10. Meckel diverticulum. (*A, B*) Contrast-enhanced axial (*A*) and coronal multiplanar reconstruction (*B*) CT images show a tubular blind-ending structure (*arrow*) in the right lower quadrant in continuity with the ileum. (*C*) Contrast-enhanced axial CT image at a more caudal level shows a normal appendix (*arrow*). (*D*) Tc-99m pertechnetate scan shows a focus of radiotracer accumulation in the right lower quadrant (*arrow*) corresponding to Meckel diverticulum seen in (*A, B*). (*Courtesy of* Dr Seth J. Crapp, Jupiter Imaging Associates, Sheridan Healthcorp, Jupiter, FL.)

gastrointestinal bleeding, and/or diarrhea. In a large systematic review, neutropenic enterocolitis occurs in approximately 5% of patients hospitalized for treatment.[46]

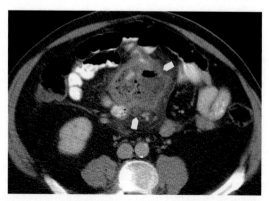

Fig. 11. Meckel diverticulitis with perforation. Contrast-enhanced axial CT image shows a blind-ending tubular structure (*star*) contiguous with the ileum with adjacent extraluminal fluid and gas (*arrowheads*), representing perforation and abscess.

CT is the preferred imaging modality for the diagnosis of neutropenic enterocolitis. CT most commonly shows circumferential thickening of the cecum and ascending colon. It may show low-attenuation edema and inflammatory changes in the adjacent mesentery (**Fig. 12**).[47] Although classically reported to affect the right colon, neutropenic enterocolitis may affect the small bowel in up to 66% of cases.[48] Pneumatosis intestinalis may affect up to 21% of cases, and prompt diagnosis is essential to prevent subsequent transmural necrosis and perforation.

RIGHT-SIDED DIVERTICULITIS

Right-sided diverticulitis is caused by inflammation of a colonic diverticulum in the cecum or ascending colon. Right-sided diverticula tend to be congenital and true diverticula, having all 3 layers of the colonic wall. Left-sided diverticula tend to be acquired and false diverticula. The epidemiology of right-sided diverticulosis is significantly different between Western and Asian countries, likely due to a combination of

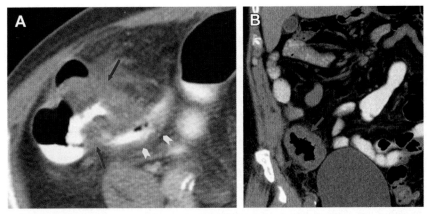

Fig. 12. Neutropenic colitis. (*A*) Contrast-enhanced axial CT image in a patient with acute myelogenous leukemia shows marked mural wall thickening of the cecum (*arrows*) and terminal ileum (*arrowheads*) with surrounding inflammatory changes. (*B*) Unenhanced coronal multiplanar reconstruction CT image shows mural wall thickening of the cecum (*arrows*) in a patient with lung cancer. (*From* [*A*] Wenzke DR, Jacobs JE, Balthazar EJ, et al. Diseases of the appendix. In: Gore RM, Levine MS, editors. Textbook of gastrointestinal radiology. 4th edition. Philadelphia: Elsevier/Saunders; 2014. p. 972; with permission.)

dietary and genetic factors. In Western countries, right-sided diverticulitis accounts for 1.5% of diverticulitis cases, whereas in Asian countries, right-sided diverticulitis accounts for up to 75% of diverticulitis cases.[49] Compared with left-sided diverticular disease, right-sided diverticular disease presents at a younger mean age of 35 to 45.[49]

As right-sided diverticulitis is uncommon, it is often misdiagnosed, usually for the more common pathology, acute appendicitis.[50] CT is the preferred modality for evaluation, as accurate diagnosis guides management. The treatment for acute appendicitis is generally surgical,

whereas the treatment for uncomplicated right-sided diverticulitis is typically antibiotic therapy. CT findings of right-sided diverticulitis are similar to those of left-sided diverticulitis. CT shows an inflamed diverticulum, peridiverticular inflammation, and localized thickening of the colonic wall that may be eccentric or circumferential (**Fig. 13**).[50,51]

EPIPLOIC APPENDAGITIS

Primary epiploic appendagitis is a generally benign, self-limiting condition that is the result of ischemia, torsion, or infarction of an epiploic

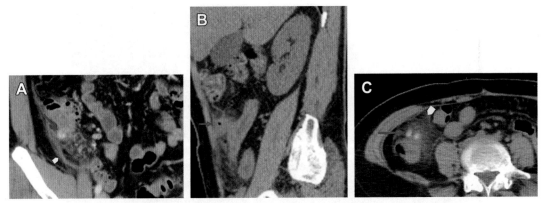

Fig. 13. Right-sided diverticulitis. (*A*) Contrast-enhanced coronal multiplanar reconstruction CT image shows a high-attenuation inflamed cecal diverticulum and cecal wall thickening (*arrow*) with pericecal fascial thickening and inflammatory changes (*arrowhead*). (*B*) Unenhanced sagittal multiplanar reconstruction CT image shows a pericecal inflammatory mass containing a focus of air (*arrow*), representing a locally ruptured cecal diverticulum. (*C*) Unenhanced axial CT image shows 2 high-attenuation cecal diverticula (*arrow*) with surrounding per-cecal inflammatory change (*arrowhead*).

appendage. Epiploic appendages are lobulated masses of subserosal fat oriented in 2 parallel rows adjacent to the anterior (tenia libera) and posterolateral (tenia omentalis) tenia coli between the cecum and rectosigmoid junction.[52] Approximately 50 to 100 epiploic appendages are supplied by a vascular stalk consisting of 2 endarteries and a single vein.[52] The limited blood supply and lobulated shape of an epiploic appendage predispose to increased mobility and risk of torsion.

Clinical symptoms of epiploic appendagitis include acute and subacute localized, nonmigratory abdominal pain. In a case series of 58 patients in the radiology literature, 48% of epiploic appendagitis cases occurred in the sigmoid colon, 28% in the descending colon, 7% in the transverse colon, and 17% in the ascending colon.[25] When epiploic appendagitis occurs in the right lower quadrant, it can simulate appendicitis and accounts for right lower quadrant pain in 1% of patients suspected of having appendicitis.[53] Due to a lack of pathognomonic clinical features and rarity of the condition, imaging diagnosis is typically made by CT examination.

CT most commonly shows a 1.5-cm to 3.5-cm fat-attenuation lesion with a hyperattenuating rim abutting the serosal surface of the colon (**Fig. 14**).[54] Occasionally a focus of central high attenuation within the fatty mass is present and may represent the thrombosed vein. Focal wall thickening of the adjacent colon and infiltration of the adjacent mesenteric fat also may be present. Long-segment colonic wall thickening should raise suspicion for right-sided diverticulitis. Additional differential considerations for a benign inflammatory fatty mass include omental infarction and mesenteric panniculitis.

Epiploic appendagitis can be managed conservatively with oral anti-inflammatory medications and does not typically require hospitalization or antibiotics. Rarely, adhesions or bands from epiploic appendagitis can cause small bowel obstruction and necessitate surgery.[55] Once the clinical symptoms subside, the infarcted epiploic appendage may undergo aseptic fat necrosis, calcify, and become a loose body within the peritoneal cavity.[52]

OMENTAL INFARCTION

Omental infarction is a rare cause of abdominal pain in children and adults. Primary omental torsion has a predilection for the right abdomen due to greater length and mobility of the omentum in the right lower quadrant.[56] Preexisting abdominal pathology, such as adhesions, hernias, and masses, can predispose to secondary omental torsion. Omental infarction without torsion may be associated with obesity, trauma, overeating, overexertion, previous surgery, vasculitis, and congestive heart failure.[56,57] Nevertheless, omental infarction is rare because of copious collateral circulation in the omentum and has a reported incidence of 0.37% in a series of 2135 patients with clinically suspected acute appendicitis.[58]

Omental infarction may present with a variety of symptoms, including abdominal pain, right lower quadrant tenderness, nausea, vomiting, and diarrhea. Clinical overlap with several other right lower quadrant pathologies often precludes a definitive

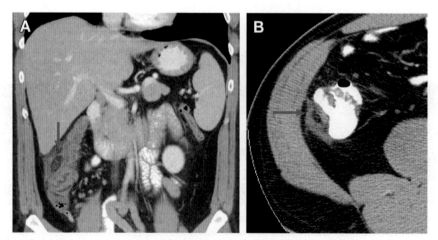

Fig. 14. Right-sided epiploic appendagitis. (*A*) Contrast-enhanced coronal multiplanar reconstruction CT image shows an inflamed epiploic appendage as a low-attenuation oval structure surrounded by thickened rim contiguous with the ascending colon. (*B*) Unenhanced axial CT image shows a low-attenuation epiploic appendage (*arrow*) with surrounding peritoneal thickening contiguous with the ascending colon.

diagnosis. Diagnosis of omental infarction is primarily based on CT examination and is rarely suspected clinically given its very low incidence.

CT findings include a triangular or oval heterogeneous fat-attenuation mass located between the abdominal wall and colon and usually measuring larger than 5 cm.[56] Presence of a whirled pattern of concentric vessels and/or stranding can be associated with omental torsion.[56,59] Unlike epiploic appendagitis, omental infarcts are not surrounded by a continuous hyperattenuating rim abutting the adjacent colon and do not contain a focus of central high attenuation (**Fig. 15**).[56] Rarely, extension of omental inflammation may cause thickening of the adjacent bowel. However, if bowel wall thickening is present, alternative etiologies, such as diverticulitis, generally should be considered first. Omental infarction may be seen with other modalities. Sonography, for example, may show a focal area of noncompressible avascular echogenic fat corresponding to a site of tenderness. PET/CT shows mild uptake of fluorine 18 (18F) fluorodeoxyglucose (FDG) corresponding to the encapsulated fat-attenuation mass.[59]

Omental infarction may be managed conservatively with oral analgesics, nonsteroidal anti-inflammatory drugs, and/or prophylactic antibiotics.[60] However, if conservative management fails because of intractable pain, peritoneal signs, or complication, such as abscess or bowel obstruction due to persistence of infarct omental tissue, laparoscopy may be performed to provide prompt symptomatic relief.[60]

INFLAMMATORY BOWEL DISEASE

Crohn disease and ulcerative colitis represent the 2 major types of inflammatory bowel disease. Inflammatory bowel disease affects approximately

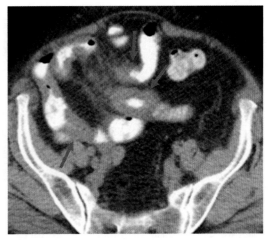

Fig. 16. Crohn disease. Unenhanced axial CT image shows multifocal short segment small bowel mural wall thickening (*arrows*) with intervening normal segments of small bowel ("skip lesions").

1.0 to 1.4 million people in the United States, with a peak onset between 15 and 30 years of age.[61,62] Crohn disease is slightly more common in females, whereas ulcerative colitis is slightly more frequent in males.

Crohn disease is characterized by transmural inflammation and skip lesions throughout the gastrointestinal tract, most commonly affecting the ileum and right colon. Ulcerative colitis is characterized by inflammation confined to the mucosal layer of the colon and almost invariably involves the rectum with proximal extension in a continuous fashion.

Crohn disease is more likely to present with right lower quadrant pain because of its predilection to affect the ileocecal region. Additional symptoms include fatigue, weight loss, fever, and diarrhea

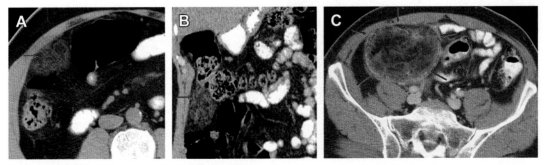

Fig. 15. Right-sided omental infarct. (*A, B*) Unenhanced axial (*A*) and coronal (*B*) multiplanar reconstruction CT images show a low-attenuation fatty mass (*arrow*) adjacent to the ascending colon without a continuous hyperattenuating rim. (*C*) Contrast-enhanced axial CT images show a heterogeneous fatty and soft tissue component mass (*arrows*) in the right lower quadrant that exerts mass effect on the adjacent small bowel. (*From* Wenzke DR, Jacobs JE, Balthazar EJ, et al. Diseases of the appendix. In: Gore RM, Levine MS, editors. Textbook of gastrointestinal radiology. 4th edition. Philadelphia: Elsevier/Saunders; 2014. p. 971; with permission.)

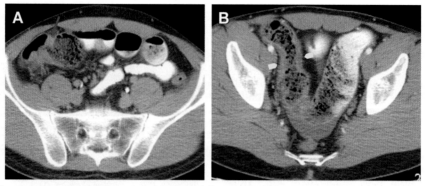

Fig. 17. Crohn disease with small bowel obstruction. (*A*) Unenhanced axial CT image shows a fibro-stenotic terminal ileum (*arrows*) with prestenotic dilated terminal ileum with feceslike material. (*B*) Unenhanced axial CT image caudal to (*A*) shows mural wall thickening of the ileum (*arrowheads*) with feceslike material ("small bowel feces sign") and a small amount of pelvic ascites (*arrow*).

with or without gastrointestinal bleeding. Although Crohn disease generally manifests with chronic, intermittent symptoms, acute exacerbations can mimic other causes of right lower quadrant pain.

In a patient with known or suspected Crohn disease, optimal evaluation is with CT or magnetic resonance (MR) enterography, with a preference toward MR examinations in the pediatric and adolescent population due to the exposure to ionizing radiation.[63] In cases of known Crohn disease with acute exacerbation, CT may be performed with standard oral and intravenous contrast if the patient is unable to tolerate the large volume of contrast typically required for enterography protocols.[63]

Common CT findings of Crohn disease include mucosal hyperenhancement and bowel wall thickening, with an average mural thickness of approximately 11 mm (**Fig. 16**).[64] Intramural edema and engorgement of the vasa recta ("comb sign") correlate with active disease.[65] CT is particularly helpful in identifying complications, such as bowel obstruction, strictures, fistulas/sinus tracts, and interloop abscesses (**Figs. 17 and 18**). CT signs of chronic inflammation include intramural fat deposition and fibrofatty proliferation along the mesenteric border of afflicted bowel.[66] Nongastrointestinal manifestations of Crohn disease that also may be present on CT include renal calculi, biliary calculi, and sacroiliitis.

SUMMARY

Acute causes of right lower quadrant pain encompass a variety of conditions that may be self-limiting or require emergent surgical intervention. Imaging plays a critical role in diagnosis because the clinical presentation of right quadrant pain is often nonspecific. Recognition of CT imaging features of various causes of right lower quadrant pain is essential for proper diagnosis and treatment referral.

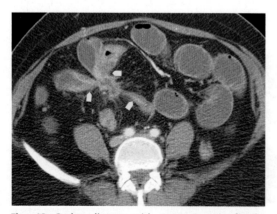

Fig. 18. Crohn disease with enteroenteric fistula. Contrast-enhanced axial CT images shows convergence of multiple tracts (*arrowheads*) in the right lower quadrant mesentery representing enteroenteric (interloop) fistulas. Multiple dilated loops of small bowel indicate obstruction.

REFERENCES

1. Martin RF, Rossi RL. The acute abdomen. An overview and algorithms. Surg Clin North Am 1997; 77(6):1227–43.
2. Lane MJ, Liu DM, Huynh MD, et al. Suspected acute appendicitis: nonenhanced helical CT in 300 consecutive patients. Radiology 1999;213(2):341–6.
3. Lane MJ, Katz DS, Ross BA, et al. Unenhanced helical CT for suspected acute appendicitis. AJR Am J Roentgenol 1997;168(2):405–9.
4. Schuler JG, Shortsleeve MJ, Goldenson RS, et al. Is there a role for abdominal computed tomographic

scans in appendicitis? Arch Surg 1998;133(4):373–6 [discussion: 377].

5. Rao PM, Rhea JT, Novelline RA, et al. Helical CT combined with contrast material administered only through the colon for imaging of suspected appendicitis. AJR Am J Roentgenol 1997;169(5):1275–80.

6. Rao PM, Rhea JT, Novelline RA. Helical CT of appendicitis and diverticulitis. Radiol Clin North Am 1999; 37(5):895–910.

7. Rao PM, Rhea JT, Novelline RA, et al. Helical CT technique for the diagnosis of appendicitis: prospective evaluation of a focused appendix CT examination. Radiology 1997;202(1):139–44.

8. Litz C, Danielson PD, Gould J, et al. Financial impact of surgical technique in the treatment of acute appendicitis in children. Am Surg 2013; 79(9):857–60.

9. Jacobs JE, Birnbaum BA, Macari M, et al. Acute appendicitis: comparison of helical CT diagnosis focused technique with oral contrast material versus nonfocused technique with oral and intravenous contrast material. Radiology 2001;220(3):683–90.

10. Kim SY, Lee KH, Kim K, et al. Acute appendicitis in young adults: low- versus standard-radiation-dose contrast-enhanced abdominal CT for diagnosis. Radiology 2011;260(2):437–45.

11. Johnson PT, Horton KM, Mahesh M, et al. Multidetector computed tomography for suspected appendicitis: multi-institutional survey of 16-MDCT data acquisition protocols and review of pertinent literature. J Comput Assist Tomogr 2006;30(5):758–64.

12. Pinto Leite N, Pereira JM, Cunha R, et al. CT evaluation of appendicitis and its complications: imaging techniques and key diagnostic findings. AJR Am J Roentgenol 2005;185(2):406–17.

13. Anderson BA, Salem L, Flum DR. A systematic review of whether oral contrast is necessary for the computed tomography diagnosis of appendicitis in adults. Am J Surg 2005;190(3):474–8.

14. O'Malley ME, Halpern E, Mueller PR, et al. Helical CT protocols for the abdomen and pelvis: a survey. AJR Am J Roentgenol 2000;175(1):109–13.

15. Rhea JT, Rao PM, Novelline RA, et al. A focused appendiceal CT technique to reduce the cost of caring for patients with clinically suspected appendicitis. AJR Am J Roentgenol 1997;169(1):113–8.

16. Malone AJ, Wolf CR, Malmed AS, et al. Diagnosis of acute appendicitis: value of unenhanced CT. AJR Am J Roentgenol 1993;160(4):763–6.

17. Federle MP. Focused appendix CT technique: a commentary. Radiology 1997;202(1):20–1.

18. Birnbaum BA, Wilson SR. Appendicitis at the millennium. Radiology 2000;215(2):337–48.

19. Hopkins CL, Madsen T, Foy Z, et al. Does limiting oral contrast decrease emergency department length of stay? West J Emerg Med 2012;13(5): 383–7.

20. Owings MF, Kozak LJ. Ambulatory and inpatient procedures in the United States, 1996. Vital Health Stat 13 1998;139:1–119.

21. Buckius MT, McGrath B, Monk J, et al. Changing epidemiology of acute appendicitis in the United States: study period 1993–2008. J Surg Res 2012; 175(2):185–90.

22. Wakeley CP. The position of the vermiform appendix as ascertained by an analysis of 10,000 cases. J Anat 1933;67(Pt 2):277–83.

23. Samaha AH, Tawfik AS, Abbas TO, et al. Megaloappendix: a case report. Case Rep Surg 2011;2011: 729304.

24. Graffeo CS, Counselman FL. Appendicitis. Emerg Med Clin North Am 1996;14(4):653–71.

25. Horrow MM, White DS, Horrow JC. Differentiation of perforated from nonperforated appendicitis at CT. Radiology 2003;227(1):46–51.

26. Rao PM, Rhea JT, Novelline RA. Distal appendicitis: CT appearance and diagnosis. Radiology 1997; 204(3):709–12.

27. Kanona H, Al Samaraee A, Nice C, et al. Stump appendicitis: a review. Int J Surg 2012;10(9):425–8.

28. Rao PM, Rhea JT, Novelline RA. CT diagnosis of mesenteric adenitis. Radiology 1997;202(1):145–9.

29. Macari M, Hines J, Balthazar E, et al. Mesenteric adenitis: CT diagnosis of primary versus secondary causes, incidence, and clinical significance in pediatric and adult patients. AJR Am J Roentgenol 2002; 178(4):853–8.

30. Puylaert JB. Mesenteric adenitis and acute terminal ileitis: US evaluation using graded compression. Radiology 1986;161(3):691–5.

31. Puylaert JB, van der Zant FM. Mesenteric lymphadenitis or appendicitis? AJR Am J Roentgenol 1995; 165(2):490.

32. Sagar J, Kumar V, Shah DK. Meckel's diverticulum: a systematic review. J R Soc Med 2006;99(10):501–5.

33. Pollack ES. Pediatric abdominal surgical emergencies. Pediatr Ann 1996;25(8):448–57.

34. Ueberrueck T, Meyer L, Koch A, et al. The significance of Meckel's diverticulum in appendicitis–a retrospective analysis of 233 cases. World J Surg 2005;29(4):455–8.

35. Park JJ, Wolff BG, Tollefson MK, et al. Meckel diverticulum: the Mayo Clinic experience with 1476 patients (1950–2002). Ann Surg 2005;241(3):529–33.

36. Cserni G. Gastric pathology in Meckel's diverticulum. Review of cases resected between 1965 and 1995. Am J Clin Pathol 1996;106(6):782–5.

37. Sinha CK, Pallewatte A, Easty M, et al. Meckel's scan in children: a review of 183 cases referred to two paediatric surgery specialist centres over 18 years. Pediatr Surg Int 2013;29(5):511–7.

38. Poulsen KA, Qvist N. Sodium pertechnetate scintigraphy in detection of Meckel's diverticulum: is it usable? Eur J Pediatr Surg 2000;10(4):228–31.

39. Lin S, Suhocki PV, Ludwig KA, et al. Gastrointestinal bleeding in adult patients with Meckel's diverticulum: the role of technetium 99m pertechnetate scan. South Med J 2002;95(11):1338–41.

40. Ford PV, Bartold SP, Fink-Bennett DM, et al. Procedure guideline for gastrointestinal bleeding and Meckel's diverticulum scintigraphy. Society of Nuclear Medicine. J Nucl Med 1999;40(7):1226–32.

41. Bennett GL, Birnbaum BA, Balthazar EJ. CT of Meckel's diverticulitis in 11 patients. AJR Am J Roentgenol 2004;182(3):625–9.

42. Rolston KV, Bodey GP, Safdar A. Polymicrobial infection in patients with cancer: an underappreciated and underreported entity. Clin Infect Dis 2007;45(2):228–33.

43. Urbach DR, Rotstein OD. Typhlitis. Can J Surg 1999;42(6):415–9.

44. Wagner ML, Rosenberg HS, Fernbach DJ, et al. Typhlitis: a complication of leukemia in childhood. Am J Roentgenol Radium Ther Nucl Med 1970;109(2):341–50.

45. Davila ML. Neutropenic enterocolitis. Curr Opin Gastroenterol 2006;22(1):44–7.

46. Gorschlüter M, Mey U, Strehl J, et al. Neutropenic enterocolitis in adults: systematic analysis of evidence quality. Eur J Haematol 2005;75(1):1–13.

47. Frick MP, Maile CW, Crass JR, et al. Computed tomography of neutropenic colitis. AJR Am J Roentgenol 1984;143(4):763–5.

48. Kirkpatrick ID, Greenberg HM. Gastrointestinal complications in the neutropenic patient: characterization and differentiation with abdominal CT. Radiology 2003;226(3):668–74.

49. Telem DA, Buch KE, Nguyen SQ, et al. Current recommendations on diagnosis and management of right-sided diverticulitis. Gastroenterol Res Pract 2009;2009:359485.

50. Scatarige JC, Fishman EK, Crist DW, et al. Diverticulitis of the right colon: CT observations. AJR Am J Roentgenol 1987;148(4):737–9.

51. Jang HJ, Lim HK, Lee SJ, et al. Acute diverticulitis of the cecum and ascending colon: the value of thin-section helical CT findings in excluding colonic carcinoma. AJR Am J Roentgenol 2000;174(5):1397–402.

52. Ghahremani GG, White EM, Hoff FL, et al. Appendices epiploicae of the colon: radiologic and pathologic features. Radiographics 1992;12(1):59–77.

53. Van Breda Vriesman AC, de Mol van Otterloo AJ, Puylaert JB. Epiploic appendagitis and omental infarction. Eur J Surg 2001;167(10):723–7.

54. Singh AK, Gervais DA, Hahn PF, et al. CT appearance of acute appendagitis. AJR Am J Roentgenol 2004;183(5):1303–7.

55. Puppala AR, Mustafa SG, Moorman RH, et al. Small bowel obstruction due to disease of epiploic appendage. Am J Gastroenterol 1981;75(5):382–3.

56. Singh AK, Gervais DA, Lee P, et al. Omental infarct: CT imaging features. Abdom Imaging 2006;31(5):549–54.

57. Wiesner W, Kaplan V, Bongartz G. Omental infarction associated with right-sided heart failure. Eur Radiol 2000;10(7):1130–2.

58. Pinedo-Onofre JA, Guevara-Torres L. Omental torsion. An acute abdomen etiology. Gac Méd Méx 2007;143(1):17–20 [in Spanish].

59. Kamaya A, Federle MP, Desser TS. Imaging manifestations of abdominal fat necrosis and its mimics. Radiographics 2011;31(7):2021–34.

60. Itenberg E, Mariadason J, Khersonsky J, et al. Modern management of omental torsion and omental infarction: a surgeon's perspective. J Surg Educ 2010;67(1):44–7.

61. Loftus EV. Clinical epidemiology of inflammatory bowel disease: incidence, prevalence, and environmental influences. Gastroenterology 2004;126(6):1504–17.

62. Kappelman MD, Rifas-Shiman SL, Kleinman K, et al. The prevalence and geographic distribution of Crohn's disease and ulcerative colitis in the United States. Clin Gastroenterol Hepatol 2007;5(12):1424–9.

63. Huprich JE, Rosen MP, Fidler JL, et al. ACR appropriateness criteria on Crohn's disease. J Am Coll Radiol 2010;7(2):94–102.

64. Philpotts LE, Heiken JP, Westcott MA, et al. Colitis: use of CT findings in differential diagnosis. Radiology 1994;190(2):445–9.

65. Lee S, Ha HK, Yang SK, et al. CT of prominent pericolic or perienteric vasculature in patients with Crohn's disease: correlation with clinical disease activity and findings on barium studies. AJR Am J Roentgenol 2002;179(4):1029–36.

66. Hara AK, Swartz PG. CT enterography of Crohn's disease. Abdom Imaging 2009;34(3):289–95.

Evaluating the Patient with Left Lower Quadrant Abdominal Pain

Nicholas A. Bodmer, MD[a],*, Kiran H. Thakrar, MD[b]

KEYWORDS

- Diverticulitis • Epiploic appendagitis • Urolithiasis • Colitis • Stercoral perforation
- Retroperitoneal hematoma • Rectus sheath hematoma

KEY POINTS

- Diverticulitis management is determined by computed tomography findings, including the presence and size of abscesses and free peritoneal air.
- Urinary tract stone size and location predict passage. Density and skin-to-stone distance predict treatment success.
- Stercoral perforation occurs in the setting of fecal impaction and is a surgical emergency.
- Epiploic appendagitis is an imaging diagnosis. The management is nonsurgical.
- Spontaneous retroperitoneal and rectus sheath hemorrhage typically occur in patients on anticoagulant medication but without supratherapeutic international normalized ratio or activated partial thromboplastin time.

INTRODUCTION

Abdominal pain is the most common reason to visit the emergency department (ED) in the United States, accounting for 11% of all adult noninjury visits from 2007 to 2008 in a Centers for Disease Control and Prevention and National Hospital Ambulatory Medical Care Survey. In this database, 17% of patients were eventually found to have a serious diagnosis and 20% were admitted, transferred, or died.[1] No published study has teased out the epidemiology of abdominal pain by quadrant. Therefore, the incidence of left lower quadrant pain compared with right lower quadrant pain, for example, is unknown.

Advanced imaging for abdominal pain in the ED increased from 20% of cases in 1999 to 2000 to 44% in 2007 to 2008 in the United States.[1] However, a more recent study found decreased growth of computed tomography (CT) and MR imaging,

and a significant decline in overall imaging ordered per ED visit between 2004 and 2012.[2] Given the cost and prevalence of imaging, there is controversy about overutilization. A study examining the yield of CT for abdominal pain found that it detected a cause of abdominal pain in 48% of patients. An unsuspected diagnosis was found in 27%. Predictors of a positive CT included being a pediatric patient, having leukocytosis, and having a specified pre-CT diagnosis.[3]

Left lower quadrant pain may be caused by gastrointestinal, urinary, mesenteric, vascular, and musculoskeletal disease processes. The type of imaging evaluation is dictated by the clinical differential diagnosis. CT is indicated for left lower quadrant pain when diverticulitis is suspected to confirm the diagnosis, evaluate the severity, or identify other causes of pain. Ultrasound is indicated for suspected gynecologic causes of pain. MR imaging may be used in special situations

Author disclosures: none.
[a] Department of Radiology, Advocate Good Samaritan Hospital, 3815 Highland Avenue, Downers Grove, IL 60515, USA; [b] Department of Radiology, Evanston NorthShore University, 2650 Ridge Avenue, Evanston, IL 60201, USA
* Corresponding author.
E-mail address: nbodmer@gmail.com

Radiol Clin N Am 53 (2015) 1171–1188
http://dx.doi.org/10.1016/j.rcl.2015.06.005

when radiation exposure is of high concern, such as in pregnant patients, pediatric patients, or those with multiple prior CT examinations.

ACUTE DIVERTICULITIS
Epidemiology

Acute diverticulitis is a common cause of left lower quadrant pain (**Box 1**). In Western countries, colonic diverticula are seen in 5% of the population by 40 years of age, 33% to 50% after 50 years of age, and in more than 50% of the population after 80 years of age.[4,5] The sigmoid colon is estimated to be involved in up to 95% of patients.[6]

It is estimated that 10% to 25% of patients with diverticulosis will develop diverticulitis.[7,8] The true incidence is probably less, with one study demonstrating an incidence closer to 4% in Department of Veterans of Affairs patients.[9] In 2012, diverticulosis and diverticulitis are listed as the discharge diagnosis of 305,700 patients in the US, accumulating $10.7 billion in charges.

Pathophysiology

Diverticulitis occurs when a diverticulum becomes inflamed or perforated. The exact mechanism is unclear but may be secondary to inflammation of the mucosal lining of the diverticular wall by inspissated fecal material leading to erosion and subsequent perforation.[4,5] It is important to realize that the inflammatory change begins at the apex of the diverticulum and that it spreads into the adjacent pericolonic fat.[4,5]

Clinical Presentation

The classic clinical triad of acute diverticulitis is left lower quadrant pain, fever, and leukocytosis. These 3 findings are not always present. Abdominal pain, sometimes vague, is the most likely to be present.[10] The severity of the clinical presentation can help to determine whether patients can be treated as outpatients, need to be hospitalized, or in more severe cases require emergent radiologic and surgical intervention.

Imaging

Methods and techniques
CT is the gold standard in the evaluation of acute diverticulitis. It evaluates the extent of colonic and extracolonic findings and guides management when combined with the clinical picture. CT has a reported accuracy of up to 99%.[11,12] The American College of Radiology's (ACR) appropriateness criteria recommend CT with intravenous (IV) contrast as the first-line imaging in patients with suspected acute diverticulitis.[13] Oral or rectal contrast is not necessary in the acute setting but may identify fistulae in the chronic setting. Although diverticulitis can be seen without IV contrast, evaluating for abscess is made clear with the use of IV contrast.

Although CT is the primary modality in suspected diverticulitis, ultrasound may be ordered for patients with ambiguous abdominal pain and for pregnant patients. Although ultrasound does well in uncomplicated diverticulitis, there is significant discordance with CT in more complicated cases and, hence, may adversely affect clinical decision making.[14]

MR imaging is sensitive and specific in diagnosing diverticulitis. One study demonstrated sensitivity of 94% and specificity of 88%.[15] Currently, MR imaging has a limited role in patients with suspected diverticulitis, given long scan times, susceptibility artifact from bowel gas, and the high cost. MR imaging may be considered in special situations, such as the evaluation of a pregnant woman.

Box 1
Diverticulitis key points

Pearls	Bowel wall thickening, pericolonic inflammation, and diverticulosis are the most sensitive findings.
	Inflamed diverticula may be hyperdense on noncontrast CT.
	Hinchey classification system guides treatment of diverticulitis.
Pitfalls	Perforated colon cancer can mimic perforated diverticulitis.
	Avoid search satisfaction and evaluate for complications, such as portal vein thrombosis and small bowel obstruction.
	Colovesical fistulae may be suggested by soft tissue stranding extending from the colon to a thickened bladder wall, sometimes with gas in an uncatheterized bladder.
Controversies	Antibiotics may not be necessary for uncomplicated diverticulitis. Antiinflammatory medication alone may be adequate.
	Follow-up colonoscopy to exclude colon cancer is not necessary in all cases.

Findings

Computed tomography Highly-sensitive (>90%) findings of diverticulitis include bowel wall thickening (>3 mm), pericolonic inflammation, and diverticulosis.[12] Pericolonic fascial thickening, free fluid, and identification of the inflamed diverticulum are additional, less sensitive signs.[12] On noncontrast studies, the inflamed diverticulum can be identified as hyperdense (**Fig. 1A**).

A modified Hinchey classification has been developed to stratify the findings in acute diverticulitis and direct clinical, radiologic, and surgical management (**Box 2**).[16,17] CT has been shown to be 42% sensitive and 95% specific in identifying Hinchey 3 diverticulitis, increasing to 100% sensitivity and 91% specificity in Hinchey 4 diverticulitis.[18] Abscess, free air, and free fluid are commonly encountered and guide the clinical or surgical management. Abscesses may be filled with fluid or a combination of fluid and gas. When an abscess is identified, the size and location should be reported. Extraluminal fecal material may be seen in Hinchey stage 4 diverticulitis.

CT can also assess pertinent sequelae of diverticulitis. Large bowel obstruction, or less commonly small bowel obstruction, may be encountered because of the inflammatory change. Diverticulitis is the cause in approximately 10% of large bowel obstructions.[19] Pylephlebitis or portal vein thrombosis may result from acute diverticulitis and carries a high morbidity/mortality.

Fistulae are associated with diverticulitis but occur most commonly in the subacute or chronic setting.[20,21]

Perforated colon cancer can mimic perforated diverticulitis. These two entities can be indistinguishable. Significant inflammation and an inflamed diverticulum favor acute diverticulitis, whereas lymphadenopathy or a discrete intraluminal mass with shouldering suggests an underlying neoplasm.[22–24] Typically, the segment of involved colon in a colonic neoplasm will not demonstrate diverticulosis.[25]

Ultrasound Ultrasound demonstrates a hypoechoic segment of colon, reflecting underlying colonic wall thickening. The adjacent pericolonic fat is noncompressible with inflamed diverticula demonstrating bright echogenic reflectors. There may be adjacent free fluid or organized fluid collections representing abscesses.[26,27]

MR imaging MR imaging findings of acute diverticulitis are mural thickening of the colon with inflammation in the adjacent fat and are seen on

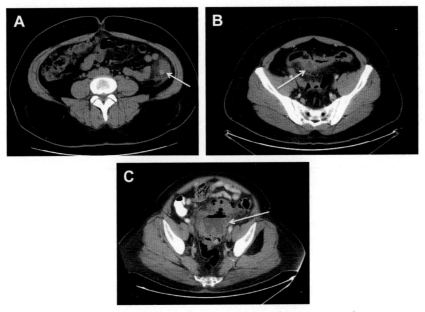

Fig. 1. (*A*) Acute diverticulitis, Hinchey 1a. Axial noncontrast CT without contrast demonstrates a hyperdense diverticulum (*arrow*) in the descending colon with surrounding fat stranding. This condition would likely be treated with antibiotics. (*B*) Acute diverticulitis, Hinchey 1b. Axial postcontrast CT without contrast demonstrates diverticulosis, pericolonic fat stranding, fascial thickening, and small pericolonic abscess (*arrow*). This condition would likely be treated conservatively with antibiotics. (*C*) Acute diverticulitis, Hinchey 2. Axial postcontrast CT without contrast demonstrates diverticulosis, pericolonic fat stranding, and large pelvic abscess distant from the colon (*arrow*). This condition would likely be treated with a percutaneous drain.

Box 2
Diverticulitis staging

Stage	Modified Hinchey Classification	CT Staging
0	Mild clinical diverticulitis	Diverticula with or without wall thickening
Ia	Confined pericolic inflammation/phlegmon	Colonic wall thickening with pericolic soft tissue changes
Ib	Pericolic/mesocolic abscess	Ia changes with pericolic/mesocolic abscess
II	Pelvic, distant intra-abdominal, retroperitoneal abscess	Ia changes with distant abscess
III	Generalized purulent peritonitis	Free air with localized or generalized ascites
IV	Generalized feculent peritonitis	Same findings as III

---

both fat-suppressed and non–fat-suppressed images. Abscesses and sinus tracts can be seen on T2-weighted and postgadolinium sequences.[28]

Clinical Management and Prognosis

Simple or uncomplicated diverticulitis will occur in 75% of initial presentations.[29] In one study of 465 patients, 17% demonstrated an associated abscess.[30] In-hospital deaths are listed at 1895 patients (0.62%).[31]

Mild or uncomplicated diverticulitis is traditionally treated with antibiotics. A Danish study demonstrated that antiinflammatory medications alone may also be successful.[32] Small pericolonic abscesses (3 cm or less) can be treated medically with antibiotics (**Fig. 1**B). Abscesses greater than 3 to 4 cm can be considered for percutaneous drainage with or without subsequent surgery (**Fig. 1**C).[33] Laparoscopic lavage for Hinchey 3 diverticulitis has been successful in select patients.[34] Colonic resection with or without anastomosis is reserved for Hinchey 4 diverticulitis.

Follow-up imaging is not routinely indicated for diverticulitis. The question of whether to perform a colonoscopy after an episode is evolving. Although colonoscopy was routinely recommended after a bout of diverticulitis previously, in the absence of suspicious feature, such as a colonic mass, lymphadenopathy, abscess, or fistula, colonoscopy should only be performed as part of routine screening guidelines.[35]

UROLITHIASIS
Epidemiology

An estimated 10% to 15% of people living in the United States will be diagnosed with a kidney stone during their lifetime (**Box 3**).[36] Urolithiasis accounts for 1.0% to 1.7% of ED visits per year and more than $5 billion in hospital charges.[37,38] Obesity, diabetes, increasing age, male sex, Caucasian race, lower socioeconomic status, diuretic use, and residence in a warmer climate increase the odds of developing urolithiasis.[36,39]

Clinical Presentation

Ureteral stones typically present with severe flank pain. Nausea, vomiting, hematuria, and pain radiating the groin may also be present.

Box 3
Urolithiasis key points

Pearls	Stone size and location are most predictive of spontaneous passage.
	Most stones less than 5 mm pass spontaneously.
	Stone density and skin-to-stone distance help predict ESWL success.
	Denser stones and larger skin-to-stone distance predict less successful ESWL.
Pitfalls	Stones must be visible with fluoroscopy or ultrasound to treat with ESWL, which is inferred by visibility on radiographs or CT scout images.
	Obstruction with superimposed infection requires emergent decompression with nephrostomy or stent.
	Calcium and uric acid stones overlap in density, and routine CT in isolation cannot predict composition.
Controversies	Stone measurement on CT is not standardized and affects the reported size (whether to measure size in axial or coronal plane and whether to measure size on soft tissue or bone algorithm).[119]
	Ultrasound may approach CT for the initial diagnosis in the ED on clinical outcomes.[120]

Pathophysiology

Calcium oxalate (CaOx) and calcium phosphate are by far the most common stone composition.[40] Randall plaques are present in all idiopathic CaOx stone formers. CaOx stones form when organic matrix and CaOx from the urine attach to the plaques.[41] Medullary pyramid density of 34 Hounsfield units (HU) or greater is thought to represent the presence of Randall plaques and identifies idiopathic stone formers with a sensitivity and specificity of 90% compared with controls.[42]

Uric acid and cystine stones form because of supersaturation of uric acid or cystine in the urine. Infection stones are caused by infection with urease-producing organisms and are more common in women.[40,41,43]

Imaging

Methods and techniques

The ACR's appropriateness criteria recommend noncontrast CT (NCCT) for suspected stone disease. NCCT consistently approaches a sensitivity and specificity near 100% for detection of urolithiasis.[44] Postcontrast CT is nearly equivalent to NCCT in detecting stones 3 mm or greater.[45] Low-radiation-dose CT has been shown to be comparable with standard-dose CT, with some studies reporting no difference and others reporting slightly decreased sensitivity for stones 3 mm or less.[46–48]

Radiographs are not adequate for initial diagnosis but are often used to track passage of the stone with treatment. A baseline radiograph performed before patients leave the ED improves the assessment of subsequent serial radiographs and may prevent follow-up CT.[49,50] The ability to visualize the stone on the CT scout image should also be reported and can obviate a baseline radiograph.[50] Radiographs detect approximately 15% to 25% more stones than scout images.[49,50]

Ultrasound is recommended by the ACR for acute onset of suspected stone disease in pregnancy but receives an equal recommendation to NCCT for recurrent stone disease in all patients. MR imaging of the abdomen and pelvis may be appropriate is situations when radiation is of higher concern.[44]

Findings

Computed tomography Identifying a calcification in the ureter makes the diagnosis of ureterolithiasis (**Fig. 2**A). The stone location, size, density, internal structure, and whether it is visible on the scout image should be reported.

Secondary findings Secondary findings of urinary obstruction help make the diagnosis but do not correlate with treatment outcomes.[51] Dilation of the urinary collecting system or adjacent stranding are secondary signs that support urinary obstruction (**Fig. 2**B). Phleboliths are venous calcifications that are common in the pelvis and may be confused with urinary stones. The tissue rim sign is defined as a circumferential rind of soft tissue attenuation surrounding a calcification that is specific for distinguishing a ureteral stone from a phlebolith.[52]

Size and location Stone size and location are the most important factors to predict spontaneous passage. The most common locations for stones to impact are the ureterovesical junction (UVJ), pelvic brim, and ureteropelvic junction.[53] The smaller the stone and the more distal in the ureter, the more likely it will pass spontaneously. Stone size compared with the rate of spontaneous passage has traditionally been based on radiograph measurements. Only one study has directly compared CT-measured stone size to spontaneous passage. Stones 4 mm or smaller passed spontaneously from the UVJ in 92% of cases

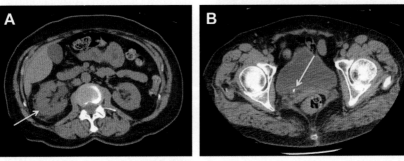

Fig. 2. (*A*) Renal obstruction with secondary signs on CT. Axial noncontrast CT image demonstrates enlargement, hypodensity, perinephric stranding, and hydronephrosis of the right kidney (*arrow*). (*B*) Renal obstruction with secondary signs on CT. Axial noncontrast CT image in the pelvis demonstrates a small obstructing ureterovesical junction stone (*arrow*). This condition would likely be treated with medical expulsive therapy and expected to pass spontaneously.

and from the upper ureter in 47% of cases. Stones greater than 7 mm passed spontaneously from the UVJ in 33% and from the upper ureter in 25%.[54]

Composition Stones of all compositions are radiodense on CT except for the rare protease inhibitor stones, such as from indinavir. The attenuation value can be accurately measured for stones 5 mm or larger. Attenuation values in stones less than 5 mm are unreliable.[55] The likelihood of extracorporeal shock-wave lithotripsy (ESWL) success decreases as the stone density increases.[56–58] There is a large range of overlap between calcium and uric acid stone density. Combining other markers with CT improves accuracy. Using a CT density of 500 HU or less and urine pH of 5.5 or less provides a positive predictive value of 90% for uric acid stones.[55,57,59–62]

Ultrasound Ultrasound shows urinary stones as hyperechoic foci that may have posterior acoustic shadowing. Hydronephrosis may indicate an obstructing ureteral stone. The twinkle artifact is a multicolor signal generated deep to a stone when interrogated with color Doppler and has been shown to increase sensitivity.[63]

MR imaging MR imaging demonstrates the secondary signs of urinary obstruction, including collecting system dilation, perinephric edema, and urothelial thickening, but is less sensitive than NCCT for the direct detection of stones (**Fig. 3**).[64]

Clinical Management and Prognosis

Nonobstructing renal stones detected incidentally on CT do not require active removal unless associated with pain, infection, or documented growth.[38]

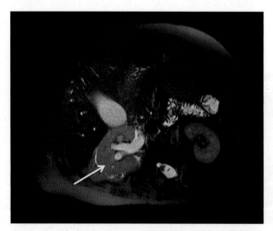

Fig. 3. Renal obstruction on MR imaging. T2-weighted, fat-suppressed axial images demonstrate secondary signs of renal obstruction with asymmetric T2 hyperintensity of the right kidney compared with the left, hydronephrosis, and perinephric fat stranding (*arrow*).

Medical expulsive therapy (primarily alphablockers) and observation can be offered for ureteral stones less than 10 mm. Most stones less than 5 mm will pass spontaneously. If there is persistent pain, infection, poor renal function, or failure of the stone to pass within 6 weeks, ESWL or ureteroscopy (URS) are indicated.[53]

ESWL or URS are generally required for ureteral stones greater than 10 mm. Both are acceptable first-line treatments. URS has a higher success rate with a single procedure but has more complications, such as ureteral perforation and stricture. URS is favored for mid and upper ureteral stones with a low probability of spontaneous passage.[53]

In ESWL, an external source of energy generates and focuses shock waves at the stone. Fluoroscopy or ultrasound is used to localize the stone during ESWL; hence, the targeted stone must be visible at one of these modalities. Imaging may also be used to measure the skin-to-stone distance on CT, with a distance of less than 9 cm predictive of ESWL success.[65]

Open or laparoscopic surgery is considered when ESWL, URS, and percutaneous treatments fail or are likely to fail, such as very large, impacted stones or multiple ureteral stones.

Uric acid stones are difficult to treat with ESWL because they are radiolucent on fluoroscopy. The first-line treatment is alkalization of the urine to dissolve the stone and prevent future stone formation.[53]

FECAL IMPACTION AND STERCORAL PERFORATION
Epidemiology

Fecal impaction and stercoral perforation are disorders associated with fecal retention (**Box 4**).

Constipation is defined by symptoms of infrequent stools or difficulty passing stool and should not be diagnosed on imaging. By definition, irritable bowel syndrome is associated with abdominal pain or discomfort, but constipation is not.[66] Suggesting constipation as the cause of abdominal pain on an otherwise negative CT is, therefore, incorrect and misleading.

Fecal impaction is most common in pediatric and geriatric patients. Studies of elderly or nursing home patients have found a prevalence of 5% to 10%, though one study estimated up to 42%.[67,68] Paradoxic diarrhea with fecal incontinence is the most common complication, potentially leading to decubitus ulcers and urinary tract infection.[68,69]

The term *stercoral* is synonymous with fecal. *Stercoral colitis*, *necrotic stercoral colitis*, *stercoral ulcer*, and *stercoral perforation* are terms used in the literature to describe the continuum of

---

Box 4
Fecal impaction and stercoral perforation key points

Pearls	Fecal impaction is diagnosed when the bowel is distended by stool, but the wall remains thin.
	Stercoral colitis is diagnosed with bowel wall thickening and fat stranding at a site of fecal impaction.
	Free air, feces bulging through the bowel wall, or a defect in the bowel wall indicate stercoral perforation.
Pitfalls	Bowel wall thickening in stercoral colitis may be subtle and focal.
	Stercoral perforation is a surgical emergency.
	Distal colon and rectum should be evaluated to exclude an obstructing mass as an underlying cause of fecal impaction or stercoral colitis.
	Constipation is defined by clinical symptoms that do not include abdominal pain and should not be suggested as a cause of pain on an otherwise negative CT.
Controversies	No published criteria exist to quantify fecal loading on CT.

---

pressure-induced ischemia, erosion, and perforation of the bowel in the setting of fecal impaction. Risk factors include chronic constipation, advanced age, nursing home residence, neurologic impairment, and medications associated with constipation, such as opiates and tricyclic antidepressants.[70,71] Stercoral perforation involves the sigmoid colon in 50%, the rectosigmoid junction in 24%, and the rectum in 7%, most commonly occurring on the antimesenteric side.[71]

Clinical Presentation

Immobilized elderly patients may present with nonspecific symptoms, such as general health deterioration or agitation. More specific symptoms include abdominal pain, distention, nausea and vomiting, overflow incontinence with diarrhea, and changes in bowel habits.[68] Stercoral colitis presents with similar symptoms, sometimes with the addition of leukocytosis, hemodynamic instability, or sepsis.[72]

Pathophysiology

Fecal impaction does not have a standard definition. A recent article in the gastroenterology literature defines it as constipation with a hard fecal mass obstructing the rectum or colon, with or without dilation of the proximal bowel, based on digital rectal examination or imaging.[68] Fecal impaction develops in the setting of chronic constipation. A hard fecal mass develops as salt and water is absorbed from a site of retained stool, subsequently leading to decreased peristalsis and further stool retention.[68]

The sigmoid is the narrowest segment of colon, and the rectosigmoid is a site of vascular watershed between sigmoid and superior rectal branches of the inferior mesenteric artery (Sudeck point), making this site susceptible to both fecal impaction and ischemia. As the colon becomes distended at a site of fecal impaction, the luminal pressure becomes greater than the bowel wall perfusion pressure, causing ischemia. The ischemia progresses to ulceration and perforation, often at multiple sites over a segment of involved bowel.[69] This finding is in contrast to diverticular perforations that are at a single site.

Imaging

Methods and techniques

There are no published studies that provide objective criteria to quantify fecal loading on CT. Abdominal radiographs are generally not useful either. Multiple objective scales have been studied to quantify fecal loading on abdominal radiographs, mostly in pediatrics, and none are reliable.[73-79] Stercoral colitis is often not suspected before imaging and first suggested on CT.[80] There is no publication describing the MR imaging or ultrasound appearance of stercoral colitis.

Findings

Fecal impaction is diagnosed on CT when the colon is distended by stool, but the bowel wall remains thin.[70] A fecaloma is a hard mass of inspissated or calcified stool that is typically equal to or larger than the diameter of the colon (Fig. 4).[69] Fecal impaction is differentiated from stercoral colitis by the lack of signs of ischemia or perforation. Fecal impaction may be complicated by obstruction, volvulus, or rectal prolapse.[68,69] The distal colon and rectum should be evaluated to exclude a stricture or neoplasm as the cause of fecal impaction and obstruction. Water-soluble contrast enema may evaluate for stricture or neoplasm and can be used to attempt disimpaction, assuming there is no evidence of perforation or obstructing colon lesion.[69]

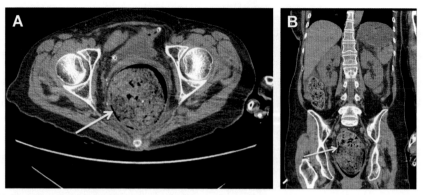

Fig. 4. Fecal impaction. Axial (*A*) and coronal (*B*) noncontrast CT images demonstrate a fecaloma distending the rectum with thin bowel wall (*arrow*).

The most common findings of stercoral colitis are bowel wall thickening and pericolonic fat stranding at a site of fecal impaction. The bowel wall thickening may be focal and subtle.[70] A retrospective study of fatal stercoral colitis compared with nonfatal stercoral colitis found that dense mucosa, perfusion defect, ascites, and extraluminal gas were significantly more common in fatal cases. In this study, colon dilation was uncommon.[80] Diagnostic features of stercoral perforation are present on CT in 90% of cases. Fecal impaction, free air, pericolonic stranding, and extraluminal feces are the most common findings, in decreasing order of frequency.[71] Discontinuity of the bowel wall and feces protruding through the bowel wall may also be seen (**Fig. 5**).[69] Colonic neoplasm may lead to fecal impaction and subsequent stercoral colitis. In these cases, perforation may be stercoral rather than caused directly by ulceration of the neoplasm.[69]

Clinical Management and Prognosis

Fecal impaction is treated with disimpaction and colon evacuation, followed by prophylactic measures to prevent recurrence. Disimpaction is performed manually or endoscopically and should not be performed in the presence of perforation. Surgery may be necessary if there is severe abdominal pain.[68]

Stercoral perforation accounts for 3.2% of all colonic perforations, with a mortality of 32% to 57%. The diagnosis is often missed preoperatively.[80] Stercoral perforations are often multiple and tend to be gaping round defects that do not resolve with conservative management like a contained diverticular perforation.[69] Therefore, the management is generally emergent laparotomy and Hartmann procedure with resection of the involved segment.[71]

PRIMARY EPIPLOIC APPENDAGITIS

Primary epiploic appendagitis is a rare cause of left lower quadrant pain (**Box 5**). Normal noninflamed epiploic appendages are not seen on CT unless there is ascites present. Approximately 100 epiploic appendages are present throughout the colon, with a preponderance (56%) in the sigmoid

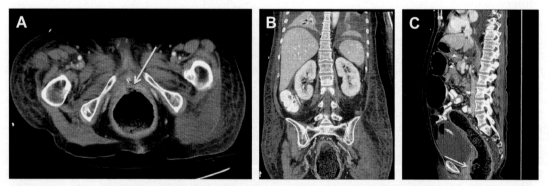

Fig. 5. Stercoral colitis and stercoral perforation. Axial (*A*), coronal (*B*), and sagittal (*C*) postcontrast CT images of the same patient 2 weeks later demonstrate rectal and sigmoid bowel wall thickening, increased pericolonic fat stranding, and discontinuity of the anterior rectal wall at a site of stercoral ulceration and perforation (*arrow*). Notice that the colon has partially decompressed compared with **Fig. 1**. Decreased dilation or lack of dilation should not exclude the diagnosis of stercoral perforation.

Box 5
Primary epiploic appendagitis key points

Pearls	Normal epiploic appendages are not visualized on CT unless outlined by ascites.
	Epiploic appendagitis occurs in the left abdomen and presents as an oval fat-density mass with a central dot and an inflamed peripheral hyperdense rim.
	Chronic epiploic appendagitis is a common cause of calcified peritoneal loose body.
Pitfalls	Treatment is conservative, not surgical.
	Omental infarction occurs in the right abdomen, lacks peripheral hyperdense rim, and is larger than an inflamed epiploic appendage.

---

colon.[81] One study of epiploic appendagitis demonstrated 82% (41 out of 50) of cases involved the sigmoid or descending colon.[82]

Clinical Presentation

Patients usually present with focal left lower quadrant pain, without fever, nausea, or vomiting.[83,84] Typically, patients can pinpoint the location of the pain. A mild leukocytosis may be seen.[83,84]

Pathophysiology

Primary epiploic appendagitis occurs where there is torsion or spontaneous venous thrombosis of the involved appendage.[81,85]

Imaging

Methods and techniques
Primary epiploic appendagitis may be detected on postcontrast or noncontrast CT. It may also be detected on MR imaging or ultrasound.

Findings
Computed tomography The inflamed appendage manifests as a 2- to 3-cm fat-density lesion along the anterior margin of the colon with peripheral rim of hyperdensity, representing inflamed peritoneum **(Fig. 6)**.[82,86] A central dot within the fat is usually

seen and represents a thrombosed vessel.[86] There is usually no wall thickening of the adjacent colon.[82] If there is wall thickening, it is asymmetric to the anterior side. Lack of wall thickening, as well as nonvisualization of an inflamed diverticulum, can help differentiate from diverticulitis. Although often mentioned in the same breath, an omental infarction has a differing location and appearance and should not be misinterpreted as epiploic appendagitis. An omental infarction is usually on the right side, lacks a hyperdense rim on CT, and is usually greater than 5 cm.[87,88]

In the chronic state, the inflamed appendage can calcify and detach. It is a common cause of an intra-abdominal loose body.[89]

Ultrasound Although CT is used more commonly for acute left lower quadrant pain, ultrasound can identify an inflamed appendage as a noncompressible echogenic mass at the specific site of pain.[90] A hypoechoic rim may be present representing the inflamed peritoneum.[90]

Magnetic resonance Magnetic resonance findings of epiploic appendagitis include a T1, hyperintense structure anterior to the colon with a T1, hypointense rim. The rim shows enhancement on postcontrast fat-saturated images, representing the inflamed peritoneum.[91]

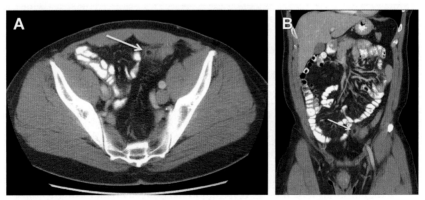

Fig. 6. Epiploic appendagitis. Axial (*A*) and coronal (*B*) CT images demonstrate a 2- to 3-cm fat-density mass at the anterior margin of the colon with hyperdense rim and mesenteric fat stranding.

Clinical Management

Treatment of epiploic appendagitis is conservative with the use of antiinflammatory medication. Before the routine use of CT, these were treated surgically with simple excision. Follow-up imaging is not necessary.

COLITIS
Epidemiology

Ischemic, ulcerative, pseudomembranous, and some types of infectious colitis favor the left colon over the right (**Box 6**).

Epidemiology differs based on the cause of colitis. Ischemic colitis is most common in older patients, with an incidence of up to 44 per 100,000 person-years; however, it is probably underdiagnosed.[92,93] Ulcerative colitis is more common than Crohn disease in adults, with an annual incidence of 1.2 to 20.3 cases per year.[94] Lower gastrointestinal infection is the primary diagnosis in 61 per 100,000 hospital discharges in the United States.[95,96] The number of patients not requiring hospitalization as well as the incidence and mortality in developing countries are much higher.[95,97] Pseudomembranous colitis specifically accounts for $1.5 billion in annual health care costs in the United States.[98,99]

Pathophysiology

Ischemic colitis is most commonly caused by a low-flow state. Mucosal ulceration and submucosal edema or hemorrhage are caused by the combination of ischemia and reperfusion injury. The distal transverse and distal left colon are watershed areas and, therefore, most susceptible.[93]

Ulcerative colitis is associated with genetics, alteration of intestinal flora, prior infectious colitis, and diet. Cigarette smoking is associated with a lower incidence and milder form of disease. Prior appendectomy is associated with a lower incidence of ulcerative colitis but higher incidence of Crohn disease.[100,101]

Schistosomiasis, shigella, herpes, gonorrhea, syphilis, and lymphogranuloma venereum more commonly involve the left colon compared with the right.[102] The infectious agent may directly invade the colonic mucosa or incite an inflammatory response and disrupt the epithelium of the colon without invasion.[95,103]

Pseudomembranous colitis is caused by *Clostridium difficile* infection in the presence of disturbed intestinal flora, most commonly by antibiotic medication.[104]

Clinical Presentation

Ischemic and ulcerative colitis present with bloody diarrhea and abdominal pain. Infectious colitis presents with diarrhea, which may be accompanied by abdominal pain, fever, or bloody stool.[95] Pseudomembranous colitis presents with watery diarrhea, abdominal pain, and severe leukocytosis.[105]

Imaging

Methods and techniques
In the emergent setting, CT is the imaging modality of choice to evaluate the colon. Ultrasound has a role in pediatric bowel diagnoses such as intussusception and pyloric stenosis. MR imaging is more commonly used in the follow-up of inflammatory bowel disease in the nonemergent setting.

Findings
Bowel wall thickening, fat stranding, and ascites are found in most types of colitis. The normal

---

Box 6
Colitis key points

Pearls	Bowel wall thickening, pericolonic fat stranding, and ascites are the most common features of colitis.
	Crohn and pseudomembranous colitis tend to have more severe wall thickening compared with ischemic and ulcerative colitis.
	An empty colon sign favors infectious colitis over ischemic or inflammatory.
Pitfalls	Ischemic colitis imaging findings usually reflect reperfusion injury rather than ongoing ischemia.
	Ischemic colitis may present with luminal dilation and a thin bowel wall if the cause of ischemia is unresolved at the time of imaging.
	Pseudomembranous colitis may have skip areas, causing confusion with Crohn colitis.
Controversies	Total colectomy has been the standard procedure for pseudomembranous colitis requiring surgery, though diverting loop ileostomy with colonic irrigation is being investigated as a colon-sparing alternative.[104]

bowel wall measures 1 to 2 mm when the lumen is distended and 3 to 4 mm when the lumen is collapsed. Bowel wall thickening is typically stratified, with enhancing mucosa, hypodense submucosal edema, and enhancing muscularis and serosa, also referred to as a target appearance or double halo.[102] Imaging findings overlap, but there are features that favor specific causes.

Ischemic colitis findings are usually related to the reperfusion of injured, leaky capillaries, with bowel wall thickening as the predominant finding (Fig. 7). Rarely, patients are imaged before reperfusion. In these cases, the bowel lumen is dilated with a thin, nonenhancing wall or homogenous, nonenhancing, mild wall thickening. Pneumatosis or venous gas in the setting of ischemia suggests bowel infarction.[93,102]

Bowel wall thickening in ulcerative colitis is continuous, symmetric, and nearly always left sided or diffuse. The wall thickening tends to be less than Crohn disease and pseudomembranous colitis, averaging 8 mm. A stratified attenuation pattern with submucosal edema implies active disease.

An empty colon sign, defined as lack of gas, fluid, or feces, was found to be an independent predictor of infectious colitis compared with inflammatory or ischemic with a PPV of 80%.[106] Pericolonic fat stranding and a "comb sign" are less common in infectious colitis compared with ischemic and inflammatory colitis.[102,106]

Pseudomembranous colitis invariably involves the rectosigmoid colon and may present with pancolitis or segmental involvement with skip areas. Bowel wall thickening is severe, with an average thickness of 15 mm.[102]

Clinical Management and Prognosis

Treatment and prognosis depend on the cause and severity of the colitis.

Ischemic colitis is treated with medical management in most cases. Indications for surgery are clinical deterioration, peritonitis, deep necrotic ulcerations on colonoscopy, or stricture.[92]

Medication regimens are used for induction and maintenance of remission of ulcerative colitis. Indications for surgery include toxic megacolon, perforation, uncontrollable bleeding, failure of medical management, and cancer.[101]

Antibiotics are prescribed based on the causative organism in infectious colitis. Fluid resuscitation and electrolyte replenishment are added if needed.[103]

Pseudomembranous colitis is initially treated with antibiotics. Monoclonal antibodies and immunoglobulins are newer therapies with encouraging early data. Stool transplant via a nasogastric tube or enema has also been effective. Surgery is indicated for worsening clinical condition, peritonitis, and shock.[104]

SPONTANEOUS RETROPERITONEAL AND RECTUS SHEATH HEMORRHAGE
Epidemiology

Retroperitoneal hemorrhage may be spontaneous, traumatic, or iatrogenic (Box 7). Spontaneous retroperitoneal hemorrhage indicates the lack of a traumatic or iatrogenic cause and has a reported incidence of 0.6% to 6.6% in patients on therapeutic anticoagulation.[107–110] In a series of 89 patients with spontaneous retroperitoneal hemorrhage, 66% were on anticoagulant medication, but only one-third had a supratherapeutic

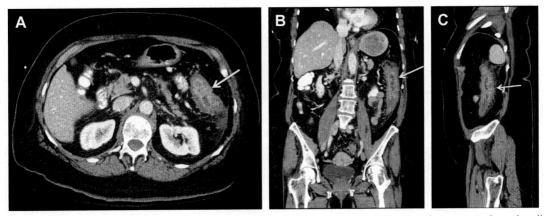

Fig. 7. Ischemic colitis. Axial (A), coronal (B), and sagittal (C) postcontrast CT images demonstrate bowel wall thickening with mucosal enhancement and submucosal edema, pericolonic fat stranding, and engorgement of the vasa recta in the distal transverse and descending colon. This pattern reflects reperfusion injury rather than ongoing ischemia.

international normalized ratio (INR) or activated partial thromboplastin time.[111]

Rectus sheath hematoma also typically occurs in patients on systemic anticoagulation without a supratherapeutic INR.[112]

Clinical Presentation

Abdominal pain is the most common presenting symptom in spontaneous retroperitoneal hematoma, followed by leg and back pain.[111]

The most common presentations of a rectus sheath hematoma are abdominal pain and abdominal wall mass.[112]

Pathophysiology

Both spontaneous retroperitoneal and rectus sheath hemorrhage occur most commonly in the setting of anticoagulation medication. Genetic bleeding diatheses and chronic hemodialysis, particularly in combination with anticoagulation, also predispose to hemorrhage.[110] The most common source of hemorrhage is vascular. Rectus sheath hemorrhage is caused by tearing of the epigastric vessels, which are fixed in position, and subject to shearing forces.

Spontaneous retroperitoneal hemorrhage may also arise from the kidneys, adrenal glands, or pancreas. Spontaneous perirenal hemorrhage should prompt a diligent evaluation and follow-up for occult neoplasm.[113]

Although technically nontraumatic, there is speculation that spontaneous retroperitoneal and rectus sheath hemorrhages are initiated by unrecognized minor trauma, such as vomiting or coughing fits, which then progresses to a large hemorrhage in susceptible patients.[110]

The arcuate line is an important demarcation of the rectus sheath. Above the arcuate line there is an anterior and posterior aponeurosis, formed by contributions from the external oblique, internal oblique, and transverse abdominis muscles. Below the arcuate line, only an anterior aponeurosis is present, with the posterior margin of the rectus muscle adjacent to the transversalis fascia. This explains why hematomas above the arcuate line are spindle shaped, and those below are spherical in shape.

Imaging

Methods and techniques

CT is the definitive imaging modality to evaluate for retroperitoneal or rectus hemorrhage. Ideally, multiphase CT with arterial and delayed IV contrast phases is performed to detect the hemorrhage and to distinguish arterial from venous bleeding, which alters management.[113] Ultrasound is not sensitive or specific for the diagnosis of retroperitoneal hemorrhage.[113] Ultrasound may perform better in rectus sheath hemorrhage. In one small study, ultrasound was 71% sensitive using CT as the gold standard.[114] MR imaging is generally not ordered for suspected retroperitoneal hemorrhage but may detect it incidentally, for example, on a lumbar spine examination.

Findings

Computed tomography Retroperitoneal hemorrhage presents with enlargement of musculature or hyperdense fluid surrounding retroperitoneal organs, depending on the location (**Fig. 8**). Rectus sheath hemorrhage presents with a muscle enlargement or a hyperdense mass along the posterior margin of the rectus (**Fig. 9**). The shape of the hematoma is affected by its location relative to the arcuate line. Above the arcuate line, there is an anterior and posterior aponeurosis. Below the arcuate line, only an anterior aponeurosis is present, with the posterior margin of the rectus muscle adjacent to the transversalis fascia. As a result, hematomas above the arcuate line are spindle shaped and those below are spherical.[115]

Acute hemorrhage measures 30 to 50 HU. As blood clots, the density increases greater than 60

Box 7
Spontaneous retroperitoneal and rectus sheath hemorrhage key points

Pearls	Fluid-fluid level or hematocrit sign occurs in patients with coagulopathy.
	Active extravasation may be arterial or venous and may be differentiated on multiphase contrast CT.
	Arcuate line divides the rectus sheath and affects the imaging appearance of rectus sheath hematomas.
Pitfalls	Occult renal neoplasm may cause spontaneous perirenal retroperitoneal hemorrhage.
	Most occur in patients on anticoagulant medication, though most do not have supratherapeutic international normalized ratio or activated partial thromboplastin time.
Controversies	Although nontraumatic by definition, spontaneous hemorrhage is likely caused by unrecognized minor trauma in susceptible patients

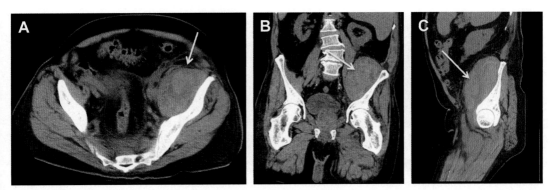

Fig. 8. Retroperitoneal hematoma. Axial (*A*), coronal (*B*), and sagittal (*C*) noncontrast CT images demonstrate a left iliacus intramuscular hematoma with enlargement and heterogeneous density of the muscle (*arrow*). There is fascial thickening adjacent to the hemorrhage.

HU, often with a hyperdense sentinel clot near the source of hemorrhage, surrounded by hypodense serum. A fluid-fluid level or hematocrit sign caused by the separation of cellular elements and serum is highly sensitive and specific for a coagulopathic hemorrhage.[116] If active hemorrhage is present, contrast extravasates into the hematoma between the cellular and serum layers.[113]

Active extravasation may be arterial or venous. Arterial bleeding appears on the arterial phase of contrast imaging in a multiphase CT. Venous bleeding is more common and does not appear

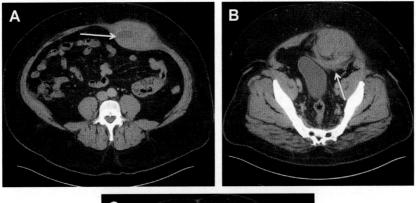

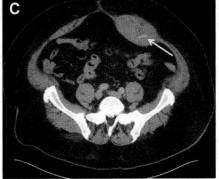

Fig. 9. (*A*) Rectus sheath hematoma. Axial noncontrast CT image demonstrates hyperdensity and enlargement of the left recuts abdominis muscle with a fluid level (*arrow*). (*B*) Rectus sheath hematoma. Axial noncontrast CT image more inferiorly shows extension of the hemorrhage into the adjacent extraperitoneal space (*arrow*). (*C*) Rectus sheath hematoma. Axial delayed-phase noncontrast CT image in a different patient shows active extravasation into the hematoma (*arrow*). The patient was treated with embolization.

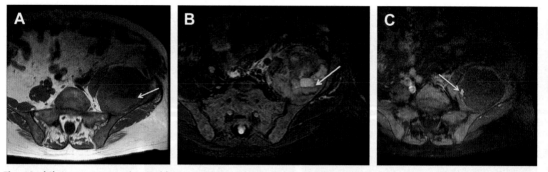

Fig. 10. (A) Acute retroperitoneal hematoma. Axial T1-weighted MR image in the same patient as Fig. 8 demonstrate the iliacus hematoma. Fluid-fluid level indicates coagulopathy (arrow). The dependent portion containing proteinaceous hematocrit is intrinsically T1 hyperintense. (B) Acute retroperitoneal hematoma. T2-weighted fat-suppressed MR image better demonstrates the fluid-fluid levels indicating coagulopathy (arrow). (C) Acute retroperitoneal hematoma. T1-weighted fat-suppressed postcontrast MR image in the venous phase shows active extravasation (arrow).

on the arterial phase. Active hemorrhage and pseudoaneurysm are distinguished on the delayed contrast phase. An area of uncontained hemorrhage continues to accumulate contrast and enlarge, whereas a pseudoaneurysm washes out on the delayed phase.[113]

Ultrasound Sonographic findings are typical of a hematoma with a mixed echogenicity mass without definite color Doppler flow.[115]

MR imaging MR imaging is able to detect fluid levels and active extravasation (Fig. 10). Signal characteristics of the hemorrhage depend on its age.[117]

Clinical Management and Prognosis

Retroperitoneal hemorrhage without active bleeding may be treated conservatively with fluid resuscitation, blood transfusion, and correction of coagulopathy. Active extravasation is more commonly venous, which can also be managed conservatively if patients are clinically stable. Endovascular embolization is recommended in the presence of arterial bleeding or contained vascular injury (pseudoaneurysm). Surgery is performed for patients who are unstable despite volume resuscitation, arterial active hemorrhage, or complications, such as abdominal compartment syndrome.[110,113,116]

Treatment of rectus hematoma is usually supportive and may include blood transfusion and reversal of anticoagulation. In select cases, percutaneous arterial embolization may be performed.[118] Surgical evacuation can also be considered in severe cases.

Mortality of spontaneous retroperitoneal hemorrhage was 6% within a week, 10% within a month, and 19% within 6 months in the series of 89 patients referenced earlier.[111]

SUMMARY

Abdominal pain is the most common cause of ED visits in the United States. CT is the current imaging modality of choice for nongynecologic causes of pain. The epidemiology, clinical presentation, pathophysiology, imaging features, and treatment of nongynecologic causes of left lower quadrant pain are reviewed.

REFERENCES

1. Bhuiya FA, Pitts SR, McCaig LF. Emergency department visits for chest pain and abdominal pain: United States, 1999–2008. NCHS Data Brief 2010;43:1–8.
2. Arasu VA, Abujudeh HH, Biddinger PD, et al. Diagnostic emergency imaging utilization at an academic trauma center from 1996 to 2012. J Am Coll Radiol 2015;12(5):467–74.
3. Modahl L, Digumarthy SR, Rhea JT, et al. Emergency department abdominal computed tomography for nontraumatic abdominal pain: optimizing utilization. J Am Coll Radiol 2006;3(11):860–6.
4. Papaconstantinou HT, Simmang CL. Diverticular Disease. In: Weinstein WM, Hawkey CJ, Bosch J, editors. Clinical Gastroenterology and Hepatology. New York: Elsevier; 2005. p. 463–72.
5. Fox JM, Stollman NH. Diverticular Disease of the Colon. In: Feldman M, Friedman LS, Brandt LJ, editors. Sleisenger and Fordtran's Gastrointestinal and Liver Disease: Pathophysiology, Diagnosis, Management. Philadelphia: Elsevier; 2010. p. 2073–89.
6. Parks TG. Natural history of diverticular disease of the colon. A review of 521 cases. Br Med J 1969; 4(5684):639–42.
7. Parks TG. Natural history of diverticular disease of the colon. Clin Gastroenterol 1975;4(1):53–69.

8. Rafferty J, Shellito P, Hyman NH, et al. Practice parameters for sigmoid diverticulitis. Dis Colon Rectum 2006;49(7):939–44.

9. Shahedi K, Fuller G, Bolus R, et al. Long-term risk of acute diverticulitis among patients with incidental diverticulosis found during colonoscopy. Clin Gastroenterol Hepatol 2013;11(12):1609–13.

10. Iyer R, Longstreth GF, Chu LH, et al. Acute colonic diverticulitis: diagnostic evidence, demographic and clinical features in three practice settings. J Gastrointestin Liver Dis 2014;23(4):379–86.

11. Rotert H, Nöldge G, Encke J, et al. The value of CT for the diagnosis of acute diverticulitis. Radiologe 2003;43(1):51–8 [in German].

12. Kircher MF, Rhea JT, Kihiczak D, et al. Frequency, sensitivity, and specificity of individual signs of diverticulitis on thin-section helical CT with colonic contrast material: experience with 312 cases. AJR Am J Roentgenol 2002;178(6):1313–8.

13. McNamara MM, L T, Camacho MA, et al. ACR appropriateness criteria: left lower quadrant pain – suspected diverticulitis [online publication]. Reston (VA): American College of Radiology (ACR); p. 7.

14. Nielsen K, Richir MC, Stolk TT, et al. The limited role of ultrasound in the diagnostic process of colonic diverticulitis. World J Surg 2014;38(7):1814–8.

15. Heverhagen JT, Sitter H, Zielke A, et al. Prospective evaluation of the value of magnetic resonance imaging in suspected acute sigmoid diverticulitis. Dis Colon Rectum 2008;51(12):1810–5.

16. Wasvary H, Turfah F, Kadro O, et al. Same hospitalization resection for acute diverticulitis. Am Surg 1999;65(7):632–5.

17. Kaiser AM, Jiang JK, Lake JP, et al. The management of complicated diverticulitis and the role of computed tomography. Am J Gastroenterol 2005;100(4):910–7.

18. Gielens MP, Mulder IM, van der Harst E, et al. Preoperative staging of perforated diverticulitis by computed tomography scanning. Tech Coloproctol 2012;16(5):363–8.

19. Taourel P, Kessler N, Lesnik A, et al. Helical CT of large bowel obstruction. Abdom Imaging 2003;28(2):267–75.

20. Woods RJ, Lavery IC, Fazio VW, et al. Internal fistulas in diverticular disease. Dis Colon Rectum 1988;31(8):591–6.

21. Goldman SM, Fishman EK, Gatewood OM, et al. CT in the diagnosis of enterovesical fistulae. AJR Am J Roentgenol 1985;144(6):1229–33.

22. Chintapalli KN, Chopra S, Ghiatas AA, et al. Diverticulitis versus colon cancer: differentiation with helical CT findings. Radiology 1999;210(2):429–35.

23. Chintapalli KN, Esola CC, Chopra S, et al. Pericolic mesenteric lymph nodes: an aid in distinguishing diverticulitis from cancer of the colon. AJR Am J Roentgenol 1997;169(5):1253–5.

24. Goh V, Halligan S, Taylor SA, et al. Differentiation between diverticulitis and colorectal cancer: quantitative CT perfusion measurements versus morphologic criteria–initial experience. Radiology 2007;242(2):456–62.

25. Lips LM, Cremers PT, Pickhardt PJ, et al. Sigmoid cancer versus chronic diverticular disease: differentiating features at CT colonography. Radiology 2015;275(1):127–35.

26. Baker JB, Mandavia D, Swadron SP. Diagnosis of diverticulitis by bedside ultrasound in the emergency department. J Emerg Med 2006;30(3):327–9.

27. Vijayaraghavan SB. High-resolution sonographic spectrum of diverticulosis, diverticulitis, and their complications. J Ultrasound Med 2006;25(1):75–85.

28. Buckley O, Geoghegan T, McAuley G, et al. Pictorial review: magnetic resonance imaging of colonic diverticulitis. Eur Radiol 2007;17(1):221–7.

29. Young-Fadok TM, Sarr MG. Diverticular disease of the colon. In: Yamada K, editor. Textbook of Gastroenterology. Hoboken, NJ: Wiley-Blackwell; 2009. p. 1574–97.

30. Ambrosetti P, Becker C, Terrier F. Colonic diverticulitis: impact of imaging on surgical management – a prospective study of 542 patients. Eur Radiol 2002;12(5):1145–9.

31. HCUPnet Agency for Healthcare Research and Quality. Available at: http://hcupnet.ahrq.gov/HCUPnet.jsp. Accessed January 15, 2015.

32. Chabok A, Påhlman L, Hjern F, et al. Randomized clinical trial of antibiotics in acute uncomplicated diverticulitis. Br J Surg 2012;99(4):532–9.

33. Kumar RR, Kim JT, Haukoos JS, et al. Factors affecting the successful management of intra-abdominal abscesses with antibiotics and the need for percutaneous drainage. Dis Colon Rectum 2006;49(2):183–9.

34. Alamili M, Gogenur I, Rosenberg J. Acute complicated diverticulitis managed by laparoscopic lavage. Dis Colon Rectum 2009;52(7):1345–9.

35. Elmi A, Hedgire SS, Pargaonkar V, et al. Is early colonoscopy beneficial in patients with CT-diagnosed diverticulitis? AJR Am J Roentgenol 2013;200(6):1269–74.

36. Stamatelou KK, Francis ME, Jones CA, et al. Time trends in reported prevalence of kidney stones in the United States: 1976–1994. Kidney Int 2003;63(5):1817–23.

37. Ghani KR, Roghmann F, Sammon JD, et al. Emergency department visits in the United States for upper urinary tract stones: trends in hospitalization and charges. J Urol 2014;191(1):90–6.

38. Pearle MS. Shock-wave lithotripsy for renal calculi. N Engl J Med 2012;367(1):50–7.

39. Scales CD Jr, Smith AC, Hanley JM, et al. Prevalence of kidney stones in the United States. Eur Urol 2012;62(1):160–5.

40. Knoll T, Schubert AB, Fahlenkamp D, et al. Urolithiasis through the ages: data on more than 200,000 urinary stone analyses. J Urol 2011; 185(4):1304–11.

41. Knoll T. Epidemiology, pathogenesis, and pathophysiology of urolithiasis. Eur Urol Suppl 2010; 9(12):802–6.

42. Bhuskute NM, Yap WW, Wah TM. A retrospective evaluation of Randall's plaque theory of nephrolithiasis with CT attenuation values. Eur J Radiol 2009;72(3):470–2.

43. Flannigan R, Choy WH, Chew B, et al. Renal struvite stones–pathogenesis, microbiology, and management strategies. Nat Rev Urol 2014;11(6): 333–41.

44. Coursey CA, Casalino DD, Remer EM, et al. ACR appropriateness criteria (R) acute onset flank pain–suspicion of stone disease. Ultrasound Q 2012;28(3):227–33.

45. Dym RJ, Duncan DR, Spektor M, et al. Renal stones on portal venous phase contrast-enhanced CT: does intravenous contrast interfere with detection? Abdom Imaging 2014;39(3):526–32.

46. Kim BS, Hwang IK, Choi YW, et al. Low-dose and standard-dose unenhanced helical computed tomography for the assessment of acute renal colic: prospective comparative study. Acta Radiol 2005; 46(7):756–63.

47. Poletti PA, Platon A, Rutschmann OT, et al. Low-dose versus standard-dose CT protocol in patients with clinically suspected renal colic. AJR Am J Roentgenol 2007;188(4):927–33.

48. Sohn W, Clayman RV, Lee JY, et al. Low-dose and standard computed tomography scans yield equivalent stone measurements. Urology 2013;81(2): 231–4.

49. Foell K, Ordon M, Ghiculete D, et al. Does baseline radiography of the kidneys, ureters, and bladder help facilitate stone management in patients presenting to the emergency department with renal colic? J Endourol 2013;27(12):1425–30.

50. Yap WW, Belfield JC, Bhatnagar P, et al. Evaluation of the sensitivity of scout radiographs on unenhanced helical CT in identifying ureteric calculi: a large UK tertiary referral centre experience. Br J Radiol 2012;85(1014):800–6.

51. Seitz C, Memarsadeghi M, Fajkovic H, et al. Secondary signs of non-enhanced CT prior to laser ureterolithotripsy: is treatment outcome predictable? J Endourol 2008;22(3):415–8.

52. Kawashima A, Sandler CM, Boridy IC, et al. Unenhanced helical CT of ureterolithiasis: value of the tissue rim sign. AJR Am J Roentgenol 1997; 168(4):997–1000.

53. Preminger GM, Tiselius HG, Assimos DG, et al. 2007 guideline for the management of ureteral calculi. Eur Urol 2007;52(6):1610–31.

54. Coll DM, Varanelli MJ, Smith RC. Relationship of spontaneous passage of ureteral calculi to stone size and location as revealed by unenhanced helical CT. AJR Am J Roentgenol 2002;178(1):101–3.

55. Stewart G, Johnson L, Ganesh H, et al. Stone size limits the use of Hounsfield units for prediction of calcium oxalate stone composition. Urology 2015; 85(2):292–5.

56. Shah K, Kurien A, Mishra S, et al. Predicting effectiveness of extracorporeal shockwave lithotripsy by stone attenuation value. J Endourol 2010;24(7): 1169–73.

57. Gucuk A, Uyeturk U. Usefulness of Hounsfield unit and density in the assessment and treatment of urinary stones. World J Nephrol 2014;3(4):282–6.

58. Ouzaid I, Al-qahtani S, Dominique S, et al. A 970 Hounsfield units (HU) threshold of kidney stone density on non-contrast computed tomography (NCCT) improves patients' selection for extracorporeal shockwave lithotripsy (ESWL): evidence from a prospective study. BJU Int 2012;110(11 Pt B):E438–42.

59. Leng S, Shiung M, Ai S, et al. Feasibility of discriminating uric acid from non-uric acid renal stones using consecutive spatially registered low- and high-energy scans obtained on a conventional CT scanner. AJR Am J Roentgenol 2015;204(1):92–7.

60. Marchini GS, Remer EM, Gebreselassie S, et al. Stone characteristics on noncontrast computed tomography: establishing definitive patterns to discriminate calcium and uric acid compositions. Urology 2013;82(3):539–46.

61. Torricelli FC, Marchini GS, De S, et al. Predicting urinary stone composition based on single-energy noncontrast computed tomography: the challenge of cystine. Urology 2014;83(6):1258–63.

62. Wisenbaugh ES, Paden RG, Silva AC, et al. Dual-energy vs conventional computed tomography in determining stone composition. Urology 2014; 83(6):1243–7.

63. Ripolles T, Martínez-Pérez MJ, Vizuete J, et al. Sonographic diagnosis of symptomatic ureteral calculi: usefulness of the twinkling artifact. Abdom Imaging 2013;38(4):863–9.

64. Kalb B, Sharma P, Salman K, et al. Acute abdominal pain: is there a potential role for MRI in the setting of the emergency department in a patient with renal calculi? J Magn Reson Imaging 2010; 32(5):1012–23.

65. Perks AE, Schuler TD, Lee J, et al. Stone attenuation and skin-to-stone distance on computed tomography predicts for stone fragmentation by shock wave lithotripsy. Urology 2008;72(4):765–9.

66. Ford AC, Moayyedi P, Lacy BE, et al. American College of Gastroenterology monograph on the management of irritable bowel syndrome and chronic idiopathic constipation. Am J Gastroenterol 2014; 109(Suppl 1):S2–26 [quiz: S27].

67. Read NW, Abouzekry L, Read MG, et al. Anorectal function in elderly patients with fecal impaction. Gastroenterology 1985;89(5):959–66.

68. Hussain ZH, Whitehead DA, Lacy BE. Fecal impaction. Curr Gastroenterol Rep 2014;16(9):404.

69. Kumar P, Pearce O, Higginson A. Imaging manifestations of faecal impaction and stercoral perforation. Clin Radiol 2011;66(1):83–8.

70. Heffernan C, Pachter HL, Megibow AJ, et al. Stercoral colitis leading to fatal peritonitis: CT findings. AJR Am J Roentgenol 2005;184(4):1189–93.

71. Chakravartty S, Chang A, Nunoo-Mensah J. A systematic review of stercoral perforation. Colorectal Dis 2013;15(8):930–5.

72. Saksonov M, Bachar GN, Morgenstern S, et al. Stercoral colitis: a lethal disease-computed tomographic findings and clinical characteristic. J Comput Assist Tomogr 2014;38(5):721–6.

73. Rao SS, Meduri K. What is necessary to diagnose constipation? Best Pract Res Clin Gastroenterol 2011;25(1):127–40.

74. Koh H, Lee MJ, Kim MJ, et al. Simple diagnostic approach to childhood fecal retention using the Leech score and Bristol stool form scale in medical practice. J Gastroenterol Hepatol 2010; 25(2):334–8.

75. Jackson CR, Lee RE, Wylie AB, et al. Diagnostic accuracy of the Barr and Blethyn radiological scoring systems for childhood constipation assessed using colonic transit time as the gold standard. Pediatr Radiol 2009;39(7):664–7.

76. de Lorijn F, van Rijn RR, Heijmans J, et al. The Leech method for diagnosing constipation: intra- and interobserver variability and accuracy. Pediatr Radiol 2006;36(1):43–9.

77. Rao SS, Ozturk R, Laine L. Clinical utility of diagnostic tests for constipation in adults: a systematic review. Am J Gastroenterol 2005;100(7):1605–15.

78. Bongers ME, Voskuijl WP, van Rijn RR, et al. The value of the abdominal radiograph in children with functional gastrointestinal disorders. Eur J Radiol 2006;59(1):8–13.

79. Moylan S, Armstrong J, Diaz-Saldano D, et al. Are abdominal x-rays a reliable way to assess for constipation? J Urol 2010;184(4 Suppl):1692–8.

80. Wu CH, Huang CC, Wang LJ, et al. Value of CT in the discrimination of fatal from non-fatal stercoral colitis. Korean J Radiol 2012;13(3):283–9.

81. Fieber SS, Forman J. Appendices epiploicae: clinical and pathological considerations; report of three cases and statistical analysis on one hundred five cases. AMA Arch Surg 1953;66(3):329–38.

82. Singh AK, Gervais DA, Hahn PF, et al. CT appearance of acute appendagitis. AJR Am J Roentgenol 2004;183(5):1303–7.

83. Chen JH, Wu CC, Wu PH. Epiploic appendagitis: an uncommon and easily misdiagnosed disease. J Dig Dis 2011;12(6):448–52.

84. Ozdemir S, Gulpinar K, Leventoglu S, et al. Torsion of the primary epiploic appendagitis: a case series and review of the literature. Am J Surg 2010;199(4): 453–8.

85. Boardman J, Kaplan KJ, Hollcraft C, et al. Radiologic-pathologic conference of Keller Army Community Hospital at West Point, the United States Military Academy: torsion of the epiploic appendage. AJR Am J Roentgenol 2003;180(3):748.

86. Ozkurt H, Karatag O, Karaarslan E, et al. CT findings in epiploic appendagitis. Surgery 2007; 141(4):530–2.

87. Singh AK, Gervais DA, Hahn PF, et al. Acute epiploic appendagitis and its mimics. Radiographics 2005;25(6):1521–34.

88. Puylaert JB. Right-sided segmental infarction of the omentum: clinical, US, and CT findings. Radiology 1992;185(1):169–72.

89. Ghahremani GG, White EM, Hoff FL, et al. Appendices epiploicae of the colon: radiologic and pathologic features. Radiographics 1992;12(1):59–77.

90. Rioux M, Langis P. Primary epiploic appendagitis: clinical, US, and CT findings in 14 cases. Radiology 1994;191(2):523–6.

91. Sirvanci M, Balci NC, Karaman K, et al. Primary epiploic appendagitis: MRI findings. Magn Reson Imaging 2002;20(1):137–9.

92. O'Neill S, Yalamarthi S. Systematic review of the management of ischaemic colitis. Colorectal Dis 2012;14(11):e751–63.

93. Taourel P, Aufort S, Merigeaud S, et al. Imaging of ischemic colitis. Radiol Clin North Am 2008;46(5): 909–24, vi.

94. Loftus EV Jr. Clinical epidemiology of inflammatory bowel disease: incidence, prevalence, and environmental influences. Gastroenterology 2004; 126(6):1504–17.

95. Navaneethan U, Giannella RA. Infectious colitis. Curr Opin Gastroenterol 2011;27(1):66–71.

96. Everhart JE, Ruhl CE. Burden of digestive diseases in the United States part II: lower gastrointestinal diseases. Gastroenterology 2009;136(3):741–54.

97. Kosek M, Bern C, Guerrant RL. The global burden of diarrhoeal disease, as estimated from studies published between 1992 and 2000. Bull World Health Organ 2003;81(3):197–204.

98. Bagdasarian N, Rao K, Malani PN. Diagnosis and treatment of Clostridium difficile in adults: a systematic review. JAMA 2015;313(4):398–408.

99. Zimlichman E, Henderson D, Tamir O, et al. Health care-associated infections: a meta-analysis of

costs and financial impact on the US health care system. JAMA Intern Med 2013;173(22):2039–46.

100. Adams SM, Bornemann PH. Ulcerative colitis. Am Fam Physician 2013;87(10):699–705.

101. Danese S, Fiocchi C. Ulcerative colitis. N Engl J Med 2011;365(18):1713–25.

102. Thoeni RF, Cello JP. CT imaging of colitis. Radiology 2006;240(3):623–38.

103. DuPont HL. Approach to the patient with infectious colitis. Curr Opin Gastroenterol 2012;28(1):39–46.

104. To KB, Napolitano LM. Clostridium difficile infection: update on diagnosis, epidemiology, and treatment strategies. Surg Infect (Larchmt) 2014;15(5):490–502.

105. Goudarzi M, Seyedjavadi SS, Goudarzi H, et al. Clostridium difficile infection: epidemiology, pathogenesis, risk factors, and therapeutic options. Scientifica (Cairo) 2014;2014:916826.

106. Plastaras L, Vuitton L, Badet N, et al. Acute colitis: differential diagnosis using multidetector CT. Clin Radiol 2015;70(3):262–9.

107. Forfar JC. A 7-year analysis of haemorrhage in patients on long-term anticoagulant treatment. Br Heart J 1979;42(2):128–32.

108. Mant MJ, O'Brien BD, Thong KL, et al. Haemorrhagic complications of heparin therapy. Lancet 1977;1(8022):1133–5.

109. Estivill Palleja X, Domingo P, Fontcuberta J, et al. Spontaneous retroperitoneal hemorrhage during oral anticoagulant therapy. Arch Intern Med 1985;145(8):1531–4.

110. Chan YC, Morales JP, Reidy JF, et al. Management of spontaneous and iatrogenic retroperitoneal haemorrhage: conservative management, endovascular intervention or open surgery? Int J Clin Pract 2008;62(10):1604–13.

111. Sunga KL, Bellolio MF, Gilmore RM, et al. Spontaneous retroperitoneal hematoma: etiology, characteristics, management, and outcome. J Emerg Med 2012;43(2):e157–61.

112. Cherry WB, Mueller PS. Rectus sheath hematoma: review of 126 cases at a single institution. Medicine (Baltimore) 2006;85(2):105–10.

113. Caleo O, Bocchini G, Paoletta S, et al. Spontaneous non-aortic retroperitoneal hemorrhage: etiology, imaging characterization and impact of MDCT on management. A multicentric study. Radiol Med 2015;120(1):133–48.

114. Moreno Gallego A, Aguayo JL, Flores B, et al. Ultrasonography and computed tomography reduce unnecessary surgery in abdominal rectus sheath haematoma. Br J Surg 1997;84(9):1295–7.

115. Berna JD, Garcia-Medina V, Guirao J, et al. Rectus sheath hematoma: diagnostic classification by CT. Abdom Imaging 1996;21(1):62–4.

116. Furlan A, Fakhran S, Federle MP. Spontaneous abdominal hemorrhage: causes, CT findings, and clinical implications. AJR Am J Roentgenol 2009;193(4):1077–87.

117. Balci NC, Sirvanci M, Tüfek I, et al. Spontaneous retroperitoneal hemorrhage secondary to subcapsular renal hematoma: MRI findings. Magn Reson Imaging 2001;19(8):1145–8.

118. Rimola J, Perendreu J, Falcó J, et al. Percutaneous arterial embolization in the management of rectus sheath hematoma. AJR Am J Roentgenol 2007;188(6):W497–502.

119. Liden M, Andersson T, Geijer H. Making renal stones change size-impact of CT image post processing and reader variability. Eur Radiol 2011;21(10):2218–25.

120. Smith-Bindman R, Aubin C, Bailitz J, et al. Ultrasonography versus computed tomography for suspected nephrolithiasis. N Engl J Med 2014;371(12):1100–10.

Imaging of Acute Pancreatitis

Ruedi F. Thoeni, MD

KEYWORDS

- Acute pancreatitis • Interstitial edematous pancreatitis • Necrotizing pancreatitis
- Acute peripancreatic fluid collections • Acute necrotic collection • Pseudocyst
- Walled-off pancreatic necrosis • Systemic inflammatory response syndrome

KEY POINTS

- The revised Atlanta classification of acute pancreatitis provides a consistent and universally adaptable system for defining acute pancreatitis in its various stages.
- The revised Atlanta classification of acute pancreatitis distinguishes interstitial edematous pancreatitis from necrotizing pancreatitis and defines early and late phases.
- The revised Atlanta classification of acute pancreatitis divides severity into mild, moderately severe, and severe form and describes transient (≤48 hours) and persistent (>48 hours) organ failure, the presence or absence of which defines these stages.
- The revised Atlanta classification of acute pancreatitis provides a new and clear definition for pancreatic fluid collections (local complications) based on the absence or presence of necrosis: acute peripancreatic fluid collection, acute necrotic collection, pseudocyst, walled-off necrosis, and postnecrosectomy pseudocyst. All fluid collections may be sterile or infected.
- In the first week, only clinical parameters are important for treatment planning, but after the first week, morphologic criteria defined by computed tomography combine with clinical parameters to determine care.

INTRODUCTION

Acute pancreatitis represents an acute inflammatory disorder of the pancreas that is initiated by premature activation of digestive enzymes in the pancreatic acinar cells, leading to autodigestion of the pancreas. The process consists of local inflammation of the pancreas and an exaggerated systemic inflammatory response syndrome (SIRS) to the pancreatic injuries, which may result in multisystem organ failure.[1] Its incidence is increasing worldwide related to well-established risk factors, such as obesity, increased aging of the general population, and rising incidence of gallstone disease.[2] In the United States, alcohol abuse and gallstone disease are the most common causes of acute pancreatitis.[2,3] About 80% to 85% of patients suffer only from the mild form of pancreatitis, whereas approximately 15% to 20% develop a severe course with complications that can include organ failure, local complications, and even death.[4]

In 1992, the original Atlanta classification system was introduced as a method for defining terminology of acute pancreatitis, its severity, organ failure, and complications.[5] However, over the years, many researchers and clinicians found this classification system insufficient and at times confusing. The need for revision also was prompted by new insights into the pathophysiology of the disease, markedly improved imaging, and new treatment options. These new treatment options included minimally invasive radiologic, endoscopic, and operative procedures for local complications that

Department of Radiology and Biomedical Imaging, University of California, San Francisco, Medical School, PO Box 2829, San Francisco, CA 94126-2829, USA
E-mail address: remo148@yahoo.com

Radiol Clin N Am 53 (2015) 1189–1208
http://dx.doi.org/10.1016/j.rcl.2015.06.006
0033-8389/15/$ – see front matter © 2015 Elsevier Inc. All rights reserved.

changed the management of patients. Therefore, an international working group on acute pancreatitis was formed to revise the Atlanta classification and published its revision in 2013.[6] The important topics that were included in this revision were a clear assessment and definition of clinical and morphologic severity of disease and clear definition of the various pancreatic and peripancreatic fluid collections that develop over the course of this disease. It also outlined what radiologists should look for when evaluating a patient with acute pancreatitis who undergoes imaging. Importantly, it stressed that in the early phase of the disease, there is no correlation between the severity of clinical disease and morphologic manifestations as seen by imaging, which limits the role of imaging in the early phase.

Because computed tomography (CT) is widely available and considered the standard in evaluating patients with acute pancreatitis, the emphasis of this revision is on CT. Magnetic resonance (MR) was recommended in selected cases to define the nature of a fluid collection or when CT is contraindicated. Both ultrasound and MR are considered superior to CT in diagnosing the heterogeneity of pancreatic collections and visualizing the presence of nonliquefied necrotic material, which is important for management. It remains to be seen if dual-energy CT might improve results in this area.[7] This article addresses the clinical definition of acute pancreatitis, defines the various pancreatic fluid collections and complications as demonstrated by CT and MR, and assesses the role of imaging in these patients.

REVISED TERMINOLOGY AND CLASSIFICATION
Diagnosis of Acute Pancreatitis

The clinical diagnosis of acute pancreatitis is based on 2 of 3 features[6]:

1. Abdominal pain highly suggestive of acute pancreatitis (acute onset of severe epigastric pain, often radiating to the back).
2. Serum lipase or amylase activity at least 3 times the upper limits of normal.
3. Characteristic features of acute pancreatitis on CT and less commonly on MR imaging or ultrasound.

If serum lipase and amylase are not sufficiently elevated but symptoms strongly suggest acute pancreatitis, imaging needs to be used to confirm the diagnosis. Imaging is usually not required in the emergency department or on the first day of admission if acute pancreatitis can be diagnosed based on typical symptoms and elevated lipase/amylase activity. However, imaging may be needed in patients with inconclusive presentations.

Onset of acute pancreatitis is defined by the beginning of acute abdominal pain and not by the time of arrival in the hospital or emergency room.

Phases of Pancreatitis

The revised Atlanta classification distinguishes between an early (within the first week) and a late phase (after the first week).[6]

Early phase
This phase usually takes place in the first week only but occasionally extends into the second week. The early phase is characterized by a systemic response to the pancreatic injury. As a result of a cytokine cascade caused by the inflammatory injury to the pancreas, a SIRS develops. If SIRS persists, organ failure may develop. During the early phase of acute pancreatitis, the severity of the attack is determined by the presence and duration of organ failure. The Atlanta classification defines organ failure as transient if it lasts for 48 hours or less, and as persistent if it lasts for greater than 48 hours. It may affect a single organ or multiple organs (multiorgan failure). In the early stage, possible pancreatic necrosis cannot by diagnosed with certainty. Local complications do not determine severity, because there is no direct correlation between the degree of morphologic changes and the severity of organ failure. In the early phase, the categorization of acute pancreatitis as moderately severe or severe is defined by the presence and duration of organ failure, which is determined based entirely on clinical criteria.

Late phase
The late phase occurs only in patients with moderately severe or severe pancreatitis because it is characterized by persistence of systemic signs of inflammation or by development of local or systemic complications. Local complications evolve over time and CT plays an important role in defining the type and extent of complications for best management. Nevertheless, persistent organ failure is an important factor in determining severity, and this phase is categorized based on both clinical data and morphologic findings.

Types of Pancreatitis

According to the revised Atlanta classification, acute pancreatitis is split into interstitial edematous pancreatitis and necrotizing pancreatitis.[6]

Interstitial edematous pancreatitis
In interstitial, edematous pancreatitis, the pancreas shows diffuse and sometimes localized

enlargement of the parenchyma with heterogeneous and occasionally homogeneous enhancement and peripancreatic fat stranding or fluid collections (see discussion under fluid collections). Usually the symptoms in patients with interstitial edematous pancreatitis resolve within 1 week.[8]

Necrotizing pancreatitis

Necrotizing pancreatitis may involve the pancreatic parenchyma and peripancreatic tissue, the peripancreatic tissue alone, or the pancreas parenchyma alone. The combination of pancreas parenchyma and peripancreatic tissue necrosis is most common, and necrosis of the pancreatic parenchyma alone is the least common.[9] The reduced perfusion and necrosis of the pancreas develop slowly over several days.[10] For this reason, necrosis cannot be accurately diagnosed in the initial stage of acute pancreatitis. In the first few days, decreased enhancement of the pancreas may simply reflect edema and, only when an area of decreased perfusion becomes well demarcated (usually after 72 hours) can it be diagnosed as necrosis. In the patient with peripancreatic necrosis alone, the pancreatic parenchyma enhances in a fashion similar to interstitial edematous pancreatitis, but morbidity and the need for intervention are much higher than in interstitial edematous pancreatitis.[11] Patients with parenchymal necrosis alone have a higher risk of organ failure and death than patients with peripancreatic necrosis alone.[12] Evolution of pancreatic necrosis is variable and may resolve over time, persist, become infected, remain solid, or liquefy. There is no direct correlation between extent of necrosis, symptoms, and risk of superinfection.[13]

Severity of Pancreatitis

According to the revised Atlanta classification, the severity of acute pancreatitis can be divided into mild, moderately severe, and severe (Table 1).[6] Classifying the degree of severity is important because of the difference in treatment of the various degrees of severity (eg, patients with suspected severe acute pancreatitis need aggressive treatment, whereas patients with mild acute pancreatitis do not). On CT, the various forms of acute pancreatitis are staged by the CT severity index (CTSI), which is an imaging grading system that combines grading of intrapancreatic and extrapancreatic inflammatory changes with extent of pancreatic necrosis (Table 2).[14,15] This grading system can help predict morbidity and mortality in patients with acute pancreatitis and guide treatment

planning. A recent retrospective study in 549 patients validated the revised Atlanta classification system for severity of acute pancreatitis and outcome.[16]

Table 1	
Grades of severity in acute pancreatitis	
Grade	**Definition**
Mild acute pancreatitis	No organ failure No local or systemic complications
Moderately severe acute pancreatitis	Transient organ failure for ≤48 h and/or local or systemic complications without persistent organ failure
Severe acute pancreatitis	Persistent organ failure for >48 h Single organ failure Multiple organ failure ± Local and/or systemic complications[a]

[a] Some patients with persistent organ failure may recover without local complications.[19]

Adapted from Banks PA, Bollen TL, Dervenis C, et al. Classification of acute pancreatitis—2012: revision of the Atlanta classification and definitions by international consensus. Gut 2013;62:108; with permission.

Table 2		
Computed tomographic severity index		
Characteristics	**Grade**	**Points**
Inflammation of the pancreas		
Normal pancreas	A	0
Pancreatic enlargement, focal or diffuse	B	1
Peripancreatic inflammation	C	2
Single peripancreatic fluid collection	D	3
Two or more peripancreatic fluid collections	E	4
Pancreatic parenchymal necrosis		
No necrosis	—	0
<30%	—	2
Between 30% and 50%	—	4
More than 50%	—	6

Points for pancreatic inflammation and necrosis are added for total CTSI score.

Adapted from Sakorafas GH, Tsiotos GG, Sarr MG. Extrapancreatic necrotizing pancreatitis with viable pancreas: a previously under-appreciated entity. J Am Coll Surg 1999;188:643–8; and Balthazar EJ. Acute pancreatitis: assessment of severity with clinical and CT evaluation. Radiology 2002;223:10.

Mild pancreatitis

Mild acute pancreatitis is present when no organ failure develops and systemic and local complications are absent. Patients with mild acute pancreatitis usually can be discharged in the first week and mortality is rare and associated with comorbidities.[17]

Moderately severe pancreatitis

Transient organ failure, local complications, and exacerbation of comorbid disease typify moderately severe acute pancreatitis. When transient organ failure transitions into persistent organ failure, the condition becomes severe acute pancreatitis. Local complications can consist of peripancreatic fluid collections that result in leukoytosis, fever, or abdominal pain over an extended period of time. Even inability to tolerate food orally can be caused by local complications. Systemic complications brought about by acute pancreatitis include increased symptoms from pre-existing disease (see later discussion under systemic complications). Moderately severe pancreatitis leads to increased morbidity and mortality compared with mild acute pancreatitis, but both are lower than seen in severe pancreatitis.[18] Moderately severe acute pancreatitis may resolve spontaneously or may require prolonged care.

Severe pancreatitis

Severe acute pancreatitis is characterized by persistent organ failure that may involve a single organ or multiple organs (see discussion of organ failure later). As mentioned earlier, SIRS brings about organ failure. SIRS carries an increased risk of persistent organ failure if it continues. Patients with persistent organ failure usually also develop local complications and have a high mortality if persistent organ failure develops early in the disease process.[19] Some patients with persistent organ failure may recover without local complications.[20] The mortality increases further with superinfection of necrosis.[21]

Complications

According to the revised Atlanta classification system, complications from acute pancreatitis can be divided into organ failure, systemic complications, and local complications.[6]

Organ failure

The respiratory, renal, and cardiovascular systems are used for determining organ failure. Organ failure is usually assessed based on the Marshall scoring system, which is a simplified and universally accepted system that can be used initially and repeated daily to gauge disease severity (Table 3).[6,22,23] Based on this system, a score of 2 or more for one of these 3 organ systems constitutes organ failure. Persistent multiorgan failure is defined as 2 or more organs failing over the same 3-day period.

Systemic complications

Besides persistent organ failure, other features that define severe acute pancreatitis include systemic complications, which are events that are triggered by acute pancreatitis and represent acute exacerbations of pre-existing comorbidities such as chronic lung disease and coronary artery disease.

Local complications

The term local complication was used in the original Atlanta classification and has been retained as useful to distinguish between acute edematous interstitial pancreatitis without complications and acute pancreatitis with local complications.[5] In the revised Atlanta classification, local complications consist of acute peripancreatic fluid collections (APFCs), pseudocysts, acute necrotic collections (ANCs), and walled-off necroses

Table 3
Marshall scoring system for acute pancreatitis

Organ System	Score				
	0	1	2	3	4
Respiratory (PaO$_2$/Fio$_2$)	>400	301–400	201–300	101–200	<101
Renal[a] (serum creatinine, mg/dL)	≤1.5	>1.5 to ≤1.9	>1.9 to ≤3.5	>3.5 to ≤5.0	>5.0
Cardiovascular (systolic blood pressure, mm Hg)	>90	<90 Fluid responsive	<90 Not fluid responsive	<90 pH < 7.3	<90 pH < 7.2

Organ failure is described as a score ≥2 for at least 1 of these 3 organ systems.
   Duration of organ failure is defined as transient (≤48 h) or persistent (>48 h) from the time of presentation.
   Persistent multiorgan failure is defined as 2 or more organs failing over the same 3-day period.
   [a] If pre-existing chronic renal failure is present, the score depends on further worsening of the baseline renal function.
Data from Refs.[6,22,23]

(WONs).[6] These various collections are defined by CT and are described in detail later under the heading "Imaging Findings." They may be sterile or infected. Other complications caused by necrotizing pancreatitis include pseudoaneurysm, splenic or portal vein thrombosis, obstruction or ileus of the gastrointestinal tract, contiguous inflammation of the colon, biliary stones, cholecystitis, pancreatic duct strictures, involvement of neighboring solid organs, ascites, and pleural effusions.[9] The description of local complications should include their locations and morphologic appearances, such as wall thickness, heterogeneity of the collection, and possible presence of extraluminal gas. Such local complications are suspected when there is a change in the clinical presentation, such as increased abdominal pain, fever, or increasing organ failure.

IMAGING TECHNIQUES
Computed Tomography

Imaging usually is not required in the initial phase of acute pancreatitis or in patients with acute pancreatitis who are rapidly improving clinically. However, imaging is recommended in the initial phase when the diagnosis is indeterminate clinically. Unless contraindicated related to renal function, contrast-enhanced CT (CECT) should be used in patients with SIRS, organ failure, or other clinical or biochemical predictors of severe acute pancreatitis and in patients who clinically are suspected to develop complications due to acute pancreatitis.[24] The best time for scanning these patients by CECT is after 72 hours from onset of symptoms. The patient should be re-examined with CECT when the clinical picture drastically changes for the worse, such as when fever suddenly develops, a drop in hematocrit is encountered, or sepsis ensues. A CECT also is useful for guidance of catheter placement to drain fluid collections and for determining the success of treatment in patients who have undergone percutaneous drainage or other interventions including surgical debridement. In addition, CECT is indicated to exclude a possible pancreatic neoplasm in patients who have a first episode of pancreatitis and are 40 years of age or older with no identifiable cause for pancreatitis.[25]

In assessing for acute pancreatitis, intravenous contrast is needed because the CT diagnosis of pancreatic necrosis relies on lack of enhancement in the necrotic area of the pancreas. Following initial scout images, the upper abdomen is scanned with a low-dose technique to look for stones, calcifications, and possible hemorrhage. At the University of California, San Francisco, a dual-phase pancreatic CECT is preferred for the initial study, which on follow-up studies can be reduced to a single-phase pancreas protocol at 70 to 80 seconds. Using a multidetector row CT, the dual-phase protocol is performed at 45 and 70 to 80 seconds extending from the diaphragm to the iliac crest at a slice thickness of 1.25 to 2.5 mm. Reformations in the coronal and sagittal planes also are performed. The coronal plane is particularly useful for assessing the extent of fluid collections in the abdomen. If the patient can tolerate it, neutral oral contrast (water or VoLumen; Bracco Diagnostics, Inc, Princeton, NJ, USA) is administered for improved visualization of the duodenal sweep and stomach. Dose reduction strategies should be used. In patients with renal insufficiency or contrast allergies, a nonenhanced CT or MR can be performed.[26–28] Subtraction color maps may be helpful for diagnosing pancreatic necrosis in the early stages of acute pancreatitis (within first 72 hours).[29]

Magnetic Resonance

MR generally is not the modality of choice for evaluating patients with acute pancreatitis but is useful in patients with impaired renal function or allergies to iodinated contrast, in young or pregnant patients, in patients with suspected choledocholithiasis not seen on CECT, and when assessment of the composition of a pancreatic fluid collection is needed to determine presence or absence of nonliquefied material (necrotic debris) or superinfection.[30–34] MR is more sensitive than CT for detecting hemorrhage and for demonstrating communication of a collection with the pancreatic duct. Although MR with diffusion-weighted sequences may be equivalent to iodinated contrast material–enhanced CT for the diagnosis of acute pancreatitis, it is superior to nonenhanced CT.[34]

For complete evaluation of the pancreatic duct and parenchyma, the following sequences are used at the University of California, San Francisco: in-phase and opposed-phase T1-weighted gradient echo in the axial plane, T2-weighted single-shot fast spin echo or turbo spin echo in the axial and coronal plane, T2-weighted fast recovery spin echo with fat suppression in the axial plane, and T1-weighted, 3-dimensional dynamic gradient echo before and after gadolinium with fat suppression in the axial plane. Diffusion-weighted MR imaging is added because it enables differentiation between different degrees of severity of acute pancreatitis and between sterile and infected collections associated with acute pancreatitis.[33,34] Heavily T2-weighted MRCP sequences may be added when needed as a slab or 3-dimensional technique in the coronal plane. Because MR protocols are persistently evolving, the details are not listed here. For more detailed information as a snapshot in time, please refer to the reviews by Barral and colleagues[34] and Tirkes and colleagues.[35]

IMAGING FINDINGS

Acute Interstitial Edematous Pancreatitis

On CECT, acute pancreatitis manifests itself as either focal or diffuse enlargement of the pancreas with homogeneous or slightly heterogeneous enhancement (Fig. 1). At times, very subtle inflammatory changes may be missed, especially when no previous CT studies are available. The peripancreatic fat may appear normal, particularly in mild cases, or demonstrate mild stranding (Fig. 2) or early peripancreatic fluid collections (described later under the heading "Pancreatic and peripancreatic collections") (Figs. 3 and 4). In the early stage of acute pancreatitis, pancreatic necrosis cannot be diagnosed with certainty. Decreased perfusion of the pancreatic parenchyma appears as diffuse or focal heterogeneity related to various degrees of edema that can be mistaken for pancreatic necrosis (Fig. 5). This finding is especially the case for areas of poor enhancement that are estimated to be less than 30% in the early phase.[14,15] A definitive diagnosis in these patients necessitates a follow-up study, because these findings should be considered indeterminate at this stage. Pancreatic necrosis cannot be diagnosed accurately before 72 hours from onset of acute pancreatitis and is best

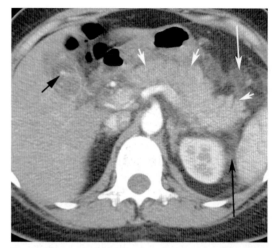

Fig. 2. Acute interstitial edematous pancreatitis, CTSI 2. A CT image in the axial plane of a 34-year-old woman with acute onset of epigastric pain for 48 hours depicts a pancreas that enhances heterogeneously (short white arrows) with peripancreatic stranding anterior to the pancreas (long white arrow) and in the left anterior pararenal space (long black arrow). CT also demonstrates gallstones (short black arrow).

assessed between 5 and 7 days after onset. Obtaining a CECT at the start of the late phase is recommended in patients with proven or suspected necrotizing pancreatitis to identify those patients who are increased risk for adverse outcomes.[36] Subtraction color maps have been shown to improve diagnostic results for pancreatic necrosis

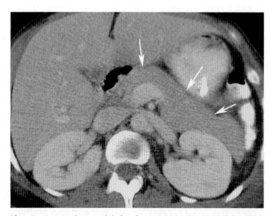

Fig. 1. Acute interstitial edematous pancreatitis, CTSI 1. This 45-year-old man suffered from acute onset of epigastric pain for 12 hours. Acute pancreatitis was diagnosed based on the clinical presentation and elevated lipase and amylase levels. CT shows a slightly enlarged pancreas (arrows) without peripancreatic stranding.

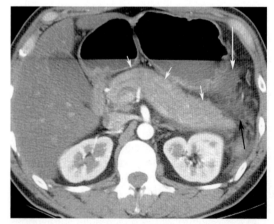

Fig. 3. Acute interstitial edematous pancreatitis with a single peripancreatic fluid collection, CTSI 3. A CT image in the axial plane of a 55-year-old woman demonstrates a swollen pancreas (short white arrows), which enhances heterogeneously. Peripancreatic stranding is evident (black arrow), and a single peripancreatic fluid collection (APFC) is identified next to the stomach (long white arrow).

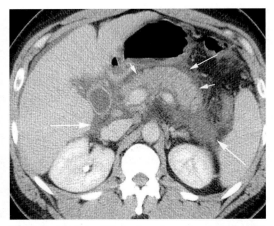

Fig. 4. Acute interstitial edematous pancreatitis with multiple fluid collections, CTSI 4. CT image in the axial plane of a 22-year-old man demonstrates an edematous pancreas (*short arrows*), and multiple fluid collections (APFCs) (*long white arrows*) are present anterior to the pancreas and in both anterior pararenal spaces.

within the first 72 hours,[29] but this has not found general use as yet.

With progression of acute pancreatitis, fluid collections develop around the pancreas, mostly in the lesser sac between the anterior pancreas and the posterior wall of the stomach and in the left pararenal space (see **Figs. 3** and **4**). These collections can persist, enlarge, and become encapsulated or resolve spontaneously. These collections

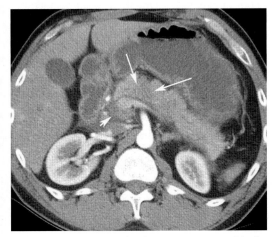

Fig. 5. Acute interstitial edematous pancreatitis for 24 hours. A CT image in the axial plane of a 22-year-old man shows a swollen and edematous pancreas with stranding and a small amount of APFC (*short arrow*). A focal area of decreased perfusion (*long arrows*) is identified in the body of the pancreas. This likely represents focal edema but could be confused with necrosis at this early stage. It should be considered indeterminate. A follow-up CT study after 7 days demonstrated absence of necrosis.

may be superinfected, or hemorrhagic, or they may produce mass symptoms.

Acute Necrotizing Pancreatitis

The presence of pancreatic necrosis, which CECT depicts as nonperfusion of the pancreatic parenchyma, constitutes necrotizing pancreatitis. It represents the most severe form of acute pancreatitis and occurs in 15% to 20% of patients with acute pancreatitis.[35] This necrotizing process distinguishes necrotizing pancreatitis from interstitial edematous pancreatitis. According to the revised Atlanta classification, 3 forms of acute necrotizing pancreatitis are discerned depending on location of the inflammatory process: involvement of the pancreatic parenchyma alone, the peripancreatic tissues alone, or both.[6] Peripancreatic necrosis generally appears as heterogeneous fluid except in the early stages when CECT may show a homogeneous collection (see later discussion). This characterization by location signifies a distinct change from the original Atlanta classification.[5]

Pancreatic parenchyma necrosis alone

Pancreatic parenchymal necrosis alone is the least common form of necrotizing pancreatitis (<5%).[36,37] Initially, CECT in patients with pancreatic necrosis shows a focally or diffusely enlarged pancreas with the necrosis seen as an area of mostly homogeneous nonenhancement, which over time changes into an area of more heterogeneous attenuation (**Fig. 6**). The changes seen on CECT are caused by the presence of nonviable tissue consisting predominantly of necrotic pancreatic parenchyma and some fat that slowly begins to liquefy. These areas of necrosis traditionally have been divided into 3 categories of involvement of the pancreas parenchyma: less than 30%, 30% to 50%, and greater than 50% (see **Table 2**).[14,15] A newer grading system, the modified CTSI, divided the necrosis into less than 30% and greater than 30% and added other manifestations (such as pleural effusion, ascites, vascular complications, or gastrointestinal complications) to it, but a later analysis did not demonstrate a clear benefit over the original Balthazar grading system.[15,38] Both CTSIs were found to diagnose clinically severe disease more accurately than clinical parameters and to correlate better with the risk of pancreatic infection and the need for intervention.[38]

Peripancreatic necrosis alone

Peripancreatic necrosis alone is the second most common form of necrotizing pancreatitis and may be seen in approximately 20% of patients.[36] It is important to recognize this type of necrosis because these patients have a better prognosis

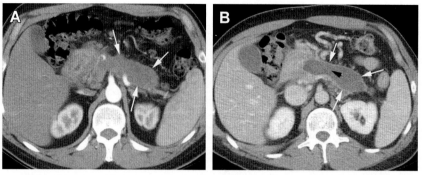

Fig. 6. Acute necrotizing pancreatitis: pancreas parenchyma alone. (*A*) CT image in the axial plane of a 38-year-old woman taken 7 days after onset shows an area of nonenhancement in the tail and body of the pancreas (*arrows*). The ANC is slightly heterogeneous. (*B*) Axial CT image of the same patient as **Fig. 6**A, 5 weeks later. The ANC has developed into a WON with an enhancing wall (*white arrows*) and septation (*black arrowhead*). It remains an area of heterogeneous attenuation.

than patients with pancreatic parenchymal necrosis.[39] Nonetheless, patients with peripancreatic necrosis alone have a higher morbidity than patients with interstitial edematous pancreatitis only.[17] Peripancreatic necrosis can be diagnosed on CECT when nonenhancing areas of heterogeneous attenuation (**Fig. 7**) are demonstrated in the lesser sac or retroperitoneum that include liquid and nonliquefied components. The presence or absence of necrotic material in peripancreatic collections can be difficult to determine by CECT, particularly in the early phase, and if clinical concern is strong enough, MR or ultrasound can be used to detect the nonliquefied necrotic components of the fluid collection. More recently it

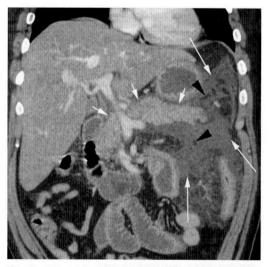

Fig. 7. Acute necrotizing pancreatitis: peripancreatic necrosis alone. A coronal CT image in a 24-year-old man shows an edematous but completely enhanced pancreas (*short white arrows*) with multiple ANCs (*long white arrows*) that are heterogeneous with islands of fat (*black arrowheads*) within the collections.

was found that a simple grading system based on the volume of extrapancreatic necrosis and using a threshold of 100 mL provided the best correlation with clinical outcome in patients with necrotizing pancreatitis (predicting organ failure and infection) and was superior to CTSI and measurements of the C-reactive protein level.[39]

Combination of pancreatic parenchymal with peripancreatic necrosis

The most common form of acute necrotizing pancreatitis involves necrosis of the pancreatic parenchyma and peripancreatic tissues. It can be seen in 75% to 80% of patients with acute necrotizing pancreatitis.[40] On CECT, a combination of the imaging findings described above for pancreatic parenchymal necrosis alone and peripancreatic necrosis alone (**Fig. 8**) can be seen.[9] Full-width necrosis of the pancreatic parenchyma may demonstrate a fistula with the main pancreatic duct and often is combined with a significant amount of peripancreatic necrosis.[41]

Pancreatic and Peripancreatic Collections

The revised Atlanta classification makes an important distinction between (i) fluid and (ii) collections with fluid and nonliquefied or only partially liquefied material (**Table 4**).[6] This distinction is largely new and based on morphologic characteristics depicted on CECT. The characteristics for the various fluid collections depend on the presence of interstitial edematous pancreatitis or necrotizing pancreatitis, location of the collection (peripancreatic or within the pancreas), presence or absence of a capsule, fluid content (fluid or fluid and nonliquefied necrotic material), presence or absence of superinfection, and history of prior intervention (necrosectomy). These fluid collections represent local complications in nonmild forms of acute

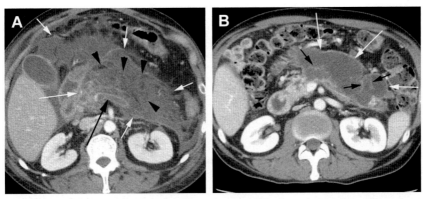

Fig. 8. Acute necrotizing pancreatitis: peripancreatic and parenchymal necrosis, 8 days after onset of symptoms. (*A*) An axial CT image in a 44-year-old woman with heavy EtOH abuse demonstrates necrosis of the pancreatic parenchyma with only the head of the pancreas partially enhancing (*long white arrow*) and extensive ANCs (*short white arrows*) containing areas of fat necrosis and heterogeneity (*black arrowheads*). Also note the splenic vein thrombosis (*long black arrow*). (*B*) Same patient as **Fig. 8**A 5 weeks later. The ANCs have matured into WONs involving the pancreas and peripancreatic areas with an enhancing capsule (*white arrows*) clearly demonstrated. Also, multiple loculations (*black arrows*) are seen.

Table 4
Computed tomographic criteria for local complications of acute pancreatitis based on the revised Atlanta classification

Fluid Collection	CT Features
Interstitial edematous pancreatitis	
APFC	Usually within the first 4 wk from onset **Homogeneous** collection with fluid attenuation Confined by normal peripancreatic fascial planes No fully definable wall surrounding the collection Adjacent to pancreas, no intrapancreatic extension
Pseudocyst (PC)	Usually after 4 wk from onset of symptoms **Homogeneous** collection (round or oval), fluid density Well-defined enhancing wall (complete encapsulation) Absence of nonliquefied material Adjacent to pancreas, no intrapancreatic extension
Necrotizing pancreatitis	
ANC	Usually within the first 4 wk from onset **Heterogeneous** collection with liquid and nonliquid components of various attenuation and varying degrees of loculations No fully definable wall surrounding the collection Located intrapancreatic and/or extrapancreatic
WON	Usually after 4 wk from onset of symptoms **Heterogeneous** collection with liquid and nonliquid components of various attenuations and varying degrees of loculations Well-defined enhancing wall (complete encapsulation) Located intrapancreatic and/or extrapancreatic[a]
Postnecrosectomy pseudocyst	Occurs after necrosectomy for necrotizing pancreatitis **Homogeneous** collection (round or oval), fluid density Well-defined enhancing wall (complete encapsulation) Absence of nonliquefied material Located intrapancreatic and/or extrapancreatic

Note: The term "pancreatic abscess" or "phlegmon" is no longer used.
[a] Often with irregular borders, extending to paracolonic gutters and increasing in size.
Data from Refs.[6,9,24,43]

pancreatitis and require supportive measures or interventional therapy. The original 1992 Atlanta classification distinguished 4 different types of local complications: APFC, pancreatic necrosis, pseudocyst, and pancreatic abscess.[5] The revised Atlanta classification distinguishes 5 types of pancreatic or peripancreatic collections (see Table 4). All of these collections can be sterile or infected. The term pancreatic abscess no longer is used because an abscess in the pancreas does not develop without pancreatic necrosis and the infected collection always consists of necrotic material and pus, which has different implications for drainage than a simple pus collection. Also the terms phlegmon and fluid collection are no longer used in describing findings in necrotizing pancreatitis because they are too ambiguous.

Acute peripancreatic fluid collection

In the acute phase of interstitial edematous pancreatitis, usually within the first 4 weeks and in the absence of necrosis, the acute collection is described as an APFC. It is a term new to the revised Atlanta classification. This fluid collection represents an exudate from the inflamed pancreas. It may be associated with rupture of a small peripheral pancreatic side branch duct. At times, there may be no connection to the pancreatic duct. These collections accumulate within the first few days and may resolve spontaneously within the first several weeks after onset of acute pancreatitis.[24] They contain only fluid without any necrotic components (please see Table 4 for additional morphologic features, see Figs. 3 and 4) and no intervention is needed (Table 5). APFCs should not be confused with ascites, which is located in the perihepatic and perisplenic areas (Fig. 9), in the paracolonic gutters, and in the pelvis.

Pseudocyst

In patients with interstitial edematous pancreatitis and APFC, over time, usually after 4 weeks, pancreatic pseudocysts may develop. This term pseudocyst remains unchanged from the original Atlanta classification. It denotes a fluid collection containing pancreatic juice with a high content of amylase and lipase and has a well-defined wall of granulation tissue (Fig. 10). For a detailed description, see Table 4. A pseudocyst does not contain any necrotic debris and appears as a homogeneous collection of high signal intensity on T2-weighted images (Fig. 11). Occasionally, a connection to the pancreatic duct can be visualized on CECT, particularly if a curviplanar reconstruction is obtained, but MR and endoscopic ultrasound are more accurate in performing this task. Ductal communication is not part of the revised Atlanta criteria for a pseudocyst, but it may be an important finding for deciding on the appropriate treatment (see Table 5). Pseudocysts are rare in acute pancreatitis in contrast to chronic pancreatitis. Infection of a pseudocyst is uncommon.

Table 5
Possible interventions in patients with acute pancreatitis and local complications

Type of Collection	Location	Infection	Drainage or Surgery
Interstitial edematous pancreatitis			
APFC	Adjacent to pancreas, extrapancreatic only	Extremely rare	None
Pseudocyst[a]	Adjacent or distant to pancreas	Rare	Rarely (only if symptomatic or infected)
Necrotizing pancreatitis			
Sterile ANC	Intrapancreatic and/or extrapancreatic	No	Based on clinical picture, percutaneous drainage at times, rarely endoscopic or surgical procedure
Infected ANC	Intrapacreatic and/or extrapancreatic	Yes	Percutaneous drainage, endoscopic procedure or surgery later if needed
Sterile WON	Intrapancreatic and/or extrapancreatic	No	Percutaneous drainage based on clinical picture, endoscopic procedure or surgery to follow if needed
Infected WON	Intrapancreatic and/or extrapancreatic	Yes	Percutaneous drainage, endoscopic procedure or surgery to follow if needed

Terminology based on references[6,9].
[a] Can be seen in disconnected duct syndrome and after necrosectomy.

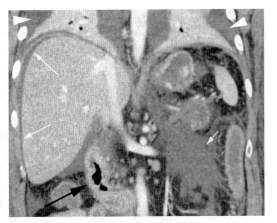

Fig. 9. Acute interstitial edematous pancreatitis with ascites and bilateral pleural effusions. The coronal CT image in this 53-year-old woman demonstrates an edematous duodenum (*black arrow*) and retroperitoneal APFC (*short white arrow*). Perihepatic ascites (*long white arrows*) and bilateral pleural effusions (*white arrowheads*) also are noted.

Acute necrotic collection

In the acute phase of necrotizing pancreatitis, usually within the first 4 weeks, the acute collection is described as ANC. All 3 types of necrotizing pancreatitis can be associated with ANC in the acute phase. The ANC represents a combination of parenchymal and fat necrosis mixed with exudates from the pancreas. The release of activated pancreatic enzymes into the peripancreatic and pancreatic areas leads to saponification of the fat and necrosis.

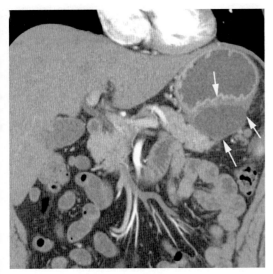

Fig. 10. Pancreatitis with pseudocyst. This coronal CT image demonstrates a well-defined fluid collection with an enhancing capsule (*arrows*) that represents a pseudocyst near the tail of the pancreas. The stomach is slightly elevated by the pseudocyst, and the gastric folds are mildly thickened (*downward arrow*).

Therefore, the collections contain necrotic material and pancreatic fluid to various degrees and within them septa are present that create loculations. Initially, the ANC may appear homogeneous but generally changes to heterogeneous due to the necrotizing process. Please see **Table 4** for the defining features (see **Figs. 6–8**; **Fig. 12**). The term ANC is new in the revised classification. CECT may miss the necrotic components and if a necrotizing process is clinically suspected, MR or ultrasound can be used to confirm the presence or absence of such necrotic material if considered relevant for treatment. Interventional treatment is based on the clinical picture (see **Table 5**). ANCs resolve spontaneously in 20% of patients, become superinfected in about 20%, and develop into sterile WONs (see later discussion) in approximately 60%.[42,43]

Walled-off necrosis

In the subacute phase of necrotizing pancreatitis, the ANC evolves over time into a WON. A thickened, nonepithelialized wall that surrounds the collection containing fluid and nonliquid material defines the interface between the viable fat and the necrosis. It represents the mature stage of an ANC and was known previously under the names necroma, organized pancreatic necrosis, and pseudocyst with necrosis. The term WON is new in the revised classification. It can involve the pancreas alone, the peripancreatic areas alone, or most commonly both, similar to ANC. Please see **Table 4** for a full description of the radiographic features (**Fig. 13**).

Because pseudocysts and WONs can have a similar appearance, they are often confused with each other. Unfortunately, the term pseudocyst often is given to any fluid-containing structure in or near the pancreas, including in some cases cystic pancreatic neoplasms, representing a major management problem. Pseudocysts occur only in patients with interstitial edematous pancreatitis (an exception is discussed later) and are always extrapancreatic. Pseudocysts are also more likely accompanied by a dilated pancreatic duct due to parenchymal compression, whereas with a WON, the pancreas fluid drains into the collection directly without ductal dilation. Pseudocysts do not need drainage unless they are symptomatic and, if needed, it can be a simple percutaneous drainage procedure or a cystogastrostomy placed endoscopically (**Fig. 14**). In WONs, necrotic material often needs to be removed percutaneously or endoscopically, which frequently is followed by surgical debridement (see **Table 5**).

Postnecrosectomy pseudocyst

Following necrosectomy for necrotizing pancreatitis, a pseudocyst can develop within the

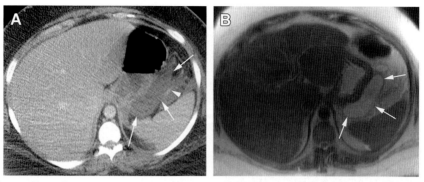

Fig. 11. Early pseudocyst formation in a patient with interstitial edematous pancreatitis. The 35-year-old woman with heavy EtOH abuse had transient organ failure and was not feeling well clinically. (*A*) The axial CT image demonstrates a fluid collection next to the stomach (*arrows*) that shows early partial rim enhancement indicative of early formation of a wall. The presence of nonliquefied material cannot be excluded. The arrowhead indicates the tip of the pancreatic tail. (*B*) Same patient as **Fig. 11A**. MR was obtained to assess if she had developed extrapancreatic necrosis. The axial T2-weighted single-shot fast spin echo MR image obtained a few days later depicts a homogeneous fluid collection of high signal intensity (*arrows*) with a thin early capsule but without evidence of nonliquefied material.

pancreas or in the peripancreatic tissue. It occurs in the so-called disconnected duct syndrome.[41] In these patients, necrosis develops in the body or neck of the pancreas while the tail remains viable. After removal of the necrotic debris via a necrosectomy, the viable pancreatic tail secretes pancreatic juice into the cavity created by the necrosectomy. Please see **Table 4** for complete description. A history of prior necrotizing pancreatitis with necrosectomy needs to be elicited for a correct diagnosis. This collection is called a post-necrosectomy pseudocyst[44] and represents a

long-term follow-up complication. A pseudocyst rarely develops after complete liquefaction of a WON or complete reabsorption of necrotic material.

Superinfection of fluid collections

All 5 types of pancreatic fluid collection can become superinfected, but overall infection of APFCs and pseudocysts is rare. Distinction between sterile and infected fluid collections is very

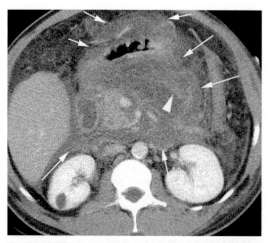

Fig. 12. ANC in necrotizing pancreatitis. The axial image in this 54-year-old woman shows a heterogeneous fluid collection (*long arrows*) without an enhancing capsule and high densities within (*white arrowhead*). The stomach wall is markedly thickened (*short white arrows*) from contiguous inflammation.

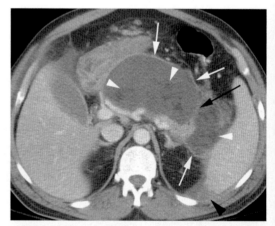

Fig. 13. WON in necrotizing pancreatitis. The axial CT image in this 27-year-old man demonstrates a large fluid collection with an enhancing capsule (*white arrows*) that involves the pancreatic parenchyma and extrapancreatic space. The collection contains areas of necrotic fat (*white arrowheads*) and septations (*black arrow*) and represents the combined form of necrosis after 6 weeks from onset of symptoms. Also, an extrapancreatic complication is seen in the form of a small splenic infarct (*black arrowhead*).

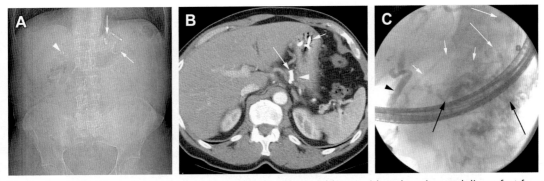

Fig. 14. Cystogastrostomy for a large pseudocyst. (*A*) This 40-year-old man with early satiety and discomfort from a large pseudocyst underwent an endoscopically placed cystogastrostomy. The scout view demonstrates the stent (*arrows*) with the superior coil in the stomach and the inferior coil in the pseudocyst. Surgical cholecystectomy clips (*arrowhead*) also are present. (*B*) Same patient as **Fig. 14A**. The axial CT image reveals the stent (*long arrow*) in the pseudocyst, which shows only a small residual fluid collection (*arrowhead*) following successful drainage. The portion of the stent located in the stomach (*short arrow*) also is seen. (*C*) Endoscopic retrograde cholangio-pancreatography (ERCP) in the same patient as **Fig. 14A**. The ERCP demonstrates filling of the pancreatic duct (*short white arrows*) without filling of a fluid collection, but communication with the stomach (*black arrows*) is readily identified demonstrating that the stent (*long white arrows*) is open. The common bile duct (*black arrowhead*) also is filled with contrast.

important because prognosis and management of these patients are very different[45] (see **Table 5**). Infection of pancreatic necrosis occurs in about 20% of patients and usually occurs between the second to fourth week from onset of symptoms of pancreatitis.[46] As previously mentioned, sterile fluid collections such as pseudocysts usually only need drainage when they become symptomatic. Patients with sterile necrosis usually do not require an intervention unless they have persistent pain, anorexia, or vomiting or are unable to resume oral feeding. In patients with suspected sterile pancreatic necrosis, CT is recommended in 7- to 10-day intervals to follow the evolution of these

fluid collections (increase in size, presence of air bubbles, or hemorrhage).[47,48] Superinfection of a pancreatic fluid collection can only be diagnosed on CT when air bubbles are present within the fluid collection (**Fig. 15**). Patients who clinically are suspected of having a superinfection but for whom CECT is negative without evidence of air bubbles within the collection (see differential diagnosis of air bubbles under Pitfalls in later discussion) may benefit from a fine-needle aspiration of the necrosis to rule out an infection (**Fig. 16**). Care must be taken to avoid contamination of the aspirate by passing through large or small bowel. Other possibly contaminating routes, such as

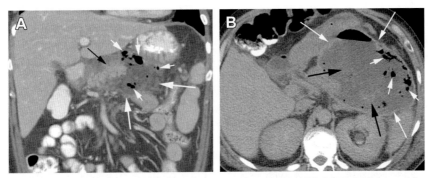

Fig. 15. Necrotizing pancreatitis with infected ANC (*A*) and infected WON (*B*). (*A*) This 20-year-old woman developed fever and sepsis and the CT demonstrates multiple air bubbles (*short white arrows*) in a fluid collection surrounding the edematous pancreas (*black arrow*), which represents the infected ANC. There is no evidence of a capsule but the collection is heterogeneous. (*B*) This 55-year-old man had been in the hospital for 6 weeks when his clinical picture deteriorated and a CT demonstrated multiple air bubbles (*short white arrows*) and an air-fluid level within an encapsulated fluid collection (*long white arrows*) that involved the pancreas and peripancreatic tissues. Also areas of increased attenuation (*black arrows*) are present within the WON.

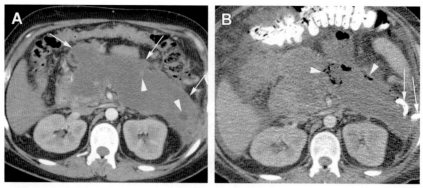

Fig. 16. Necrotizing pancreatitis with infected WON diagnosed with aspiration biopsy. (*A*) This 31-year-old man with a long history of EtOH abuse was diagnosed with necrotizing pancreatitis and became clinically much worse with fever and sepsis during the fifth week from onset. A CT showed a large WON with an enhancing rim (*arrows*) and heterogeneous fluid containing debris and necrotic fat (*arrowheads*) but no air. A CT-guided aspiration was performed that was gram-stain positive. (*B*) Same patient as **Fig. 16**A. Following placement of a percutaneous drainage tube (*long arrows*) by interventional radiology for infected WON, debris and air bubbles (*arrowheads*) are clearly identified. Several exchanges to larger-bore tubes were needed for complete drainage.

transgastric or transduodenal, also should be avoided.[49] A retroperitoneal route via the lateral flank is favored over an anterior approach through the peritoneum. Aspiration of fluid has a false negative rate of less than 10% for diagnosing infection.[45]

A recent study using PET/CT with fludeoxyglucose F 18 –labeled autologous leukocytes found increased tracer uptake in pancreatic fluid collections in 12 of 41 patients, among whom 10 had culture-proven infection with subsequent percutaneous drainage and 2 had unsuccessful aspirations.[50] In the same study, 29 patients with negative PET/CT scans had 25 proven negative cultures, and aspiration was unsuccessful in 4 cases. These results obtained with a noninvasive technique are promising but need to be confirmed in larger series.

Infection of pancreatic necrosis is associated with high morbidity and mortality (25%–70%).[43,51] Suspected superinfected fluid collection containing necrotic debris usually needs to be drained, but this is based on the clinical presentation (eg, presence or absence of clinical instability, such as organ failure, fever, sepsis, or hemorrhage) or the CT demonstration of air bubbles, increase in size, or hemorrhage within the collection. Many patients with infected necrosis can initially be treated with percutaneous catheter drainage as a temporizing measure, with endoscopic or surgical debridement at a later point (step-up approach).[43,51] Some patients may even undergo successful percutaneous drainage after surgical debridement. Several studies have shown that morbidity and mortality are increased with early surgical intervention in these patients.[47,51,52]

In some patients, percutaneous catheter drainage alone may be successful. One study suggested that the ultimate outcome may depend more on the presence of multisystem organ failure than on the presence of infection.[53]

DIFFERENTIAL DIAGNOSIS

Usually, the clinical picture combined with laboratory data is strong enough to suggest the correct diagnosis of acute pancreatitis. Clinically, the differential diagnosis of abdominal pain that could be confused with acute pancreatitis includes peptic ulcer disease, intestinal obstruction, abdominal aortic aneurysm, cholangitis or cholecystitis, choledocholithiasis, viral gastroenteritis, mesenteric ischemia, hepatitis, or myocardial infarction (**Box 1**). In all these cases, additional clinical history and the fact that the lipase and amylase are normal should prevent a

---

Box 1
Clinical differential diagnosis for acute pancreatitis

- Peptic ulcer disease
- Intestinal obstruction
- Abdominal aortic aneurysm
- Cholangitis and/or cholecystitis
- Viral gastroenteritis
- Mesenteric ischemia
- Hepatitis
- Myocardial infarction

misdiagnosis. In these cases, CECT should demonstrate a normal pancreas except in rare instances discussed under the section entitled Pitfalls. The amylase may be elevated in patients with acute abdominal pain and perforated viscus (**Fig. 17**) or mesenteric ischemia, but the amylase level will be less than that seen in acute pancreatitis. Mesenteric ischemia also shows elevation of lactic acid.

Occasionally, when a history of previous pancreatitis cannot be elicited, CT may misdiagnose a cystic neoplasm. In these cases, MR can help demonstrate necrotic debris with or without loculations to confirm that the cystic structure is related to previous acute pancreatitis (**Box 2, Fig. 18**).

PITFALLS

Mild acute pancreatitis can be missed on CECT if the patient is scanned on the first day of onset of symptoms because the findings of edema within the pancreas or stranding in the peripancreatic area are not yet evident. Also, necrosis may be missed or misdiagnosed when a patient suffering from acute pancreatitis is scanned with CECT in the first 72 hours because necrosis can be confused with diminished perfusion due to edema (see **Box 2, Fig. 5**).[15,54]

> ### Box 2
> **Imaging pitfalls for acute pancreatitis**
>
> *Early phase:*
> - FN for pancreatitis: if imaged within first 24 hours
> - FP: confusing pancreatic edema with necrosis
>
> *Late phase:*
> - FP for superinfection:
>   - Marsupialization
>   - Spontaneous fistula to gastrointestinal tract
>   - Previous intervention
> - Misdiagnosis of ANC as APFC in first 4 weeks
> - Misdiagnosis of WON as pseudocyst after ~4 weeks
> - Misdiagnosis of WON as cystic neoplasm
>
> *Mimickers:*
> - Perforated gastric or duodenal ulcer
> - Severe peptic ulcer disease
> - Mesenteric ischemia
> - Overhydration
> - Hypoalbuminemia
>
> *Abbreviations:* FN, false negative; FP, false positive.

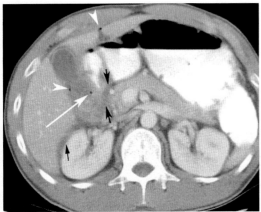

Fig. 17. Perforated duodenal ulcer mimicking acute pancreatitis. This 52-year-old woman came to the Emergency Room with acute onset of severe abdominal pain. The amylase was mildly elevated prompting the clinical diagnosis of acute pancreatitis. The axial CT image demonstrates fluid between the pancreatic head and the duodenum and stranding in the anterior pararenal space (*black arrows*), but the duodenal wall is thickened with free air next to it (*long white arrow*), in the gallbladder fossa, and in the falciform ligament areas (*white arrowheads*), indicative of a perforated duodenal ulcer. Surgery confirmed the perforated ulcer and absence of pancreatitis.

Resuscitation efforts with excessive rehydration can led to generalized edema, ascites, and edema in the pancreas that are associated with stranding and fluid in the retroperitoneum, which mimics acute pancreatitis. The severity of the pancreatic manifestations depends on the degree of hydration (**Fig. 19**). Similarly, hypoalbuminemia with ascites and generalized edema can mimic acute pancreatitis (**Fig. 20**).

Infection can be suggested on CECT if gas bubbles are present within the pancreatic collection due to the presence of gas-forming organisms (see **Figs. 15** and **16**).[55] Pitfalls for erroneously diagnosing a pseudocyst or necrosis as infected are caused by spontaneous drainage of the collection into the gastrointestinal tract. To avoid this diagnostic pitfall, the adjacent gastrointestinal walls need to be carefully analyzed. Marsupialization or other drainage procedures also can lead to the introduction of gas into a collection and erroneous interpretations (**Fig. 21**).

A perforated gastric or duodenal ulcer may be confused on CECT with pancreatitis because of stranding in the peripancreatic and duodenal

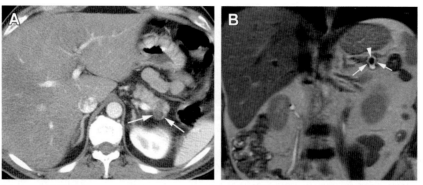

Fig. 18. Residual small WON after necrotizing pancreatitis confused with cystic neoplasm on CT. (*A*) This 77-year-old man presented with right lower quadrant pain, and a CT was performed to assess for acute appendicitis. CT confirmed acute appendicitis (not shown) but also noted a cystic mass (*arrows*) arising from the tail of the pancreas. The patient denied ever having had acute pancreatitis. A possible cystic neoplasm was diagnosed based on an oval-shaped structure of fluid density. For further more definitive evaluation, an MR was recommended. (*B*) Same patient as **Fig. 18**A. The MR imaging shows a well-encapsulated structure of high signal intensity (*arrows*) that contains an area of low signal intensity (*arrowhead*), which could represent hemosiderin or debris. A diagnosis of WON was made, and no intervention was recommended after the chart from a remote admission to an outside hospital confirmed previous necrotizing pancreatitis without intervention.

areas but usually detection of even small pockets of free intraperitoneal air prevents such an error (see **Fig. 17**). Clinically, elevated amylase in these patients adds to the diagnostic dilemma clinically, but the elevation is usually less marked than in acute pancreatitis.

Similarly, severe peptic ulcer disease caused by *Helicobacter pylori*, nonsteroidal anti-inflammatory drug use, or Zollinger-Ellison syndrome can produce enough stranding near the pancreatic bed that it could be confused with acute pancreatitis on CECT. Usually the gastric wall is thickened, the lipase and amylase are normal, and the epigastric pain does not generally radiate into the back, which should enable a correct diagnosis.

Mesenteric ischemia can produce an elevation of the amylase with a normal lipase. A history of atrial fibrillation or peripheral vascular disease in an elderly patient usually raises the index of suspicion for bowel ischemia, and CECT can be diagnostic without confusion with acute pancreatitis unless there is extensive mesenteric stranding in the upper abdomen.

REFERRING CLINICIAN: POINTS OF KNOWLEDGE

- The old Atlanta classification of acute pancreatitis from 1992 is no longer valid.
- Previous descriptions of pancreatic and peripancreatic fluid collection were confusing

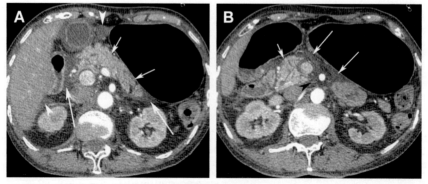

Fig. 19. Edematous pancreas after overhydration. (*A*) The pancreas is swollen and edematous (*short arrows*) with fluid and stranding in the peripancreatic area and between duodenum and head of pancreas (*long arrows*) mimicking acute pancreatitis. Ascites (*arrowheads*) is seen in Morrison pouch and surrounding the thick-walled gallbladder. (*B*) Same patient as **Fig. 19**A. Edema is shown in the head of pancreas (*short white arrow*) on this axial CT image with stranding and fluid in the lesser sac (*long white arrows*) and surrounding the superior mesenteric artery (*black arrowhead*), typically seen in excessive hydration.

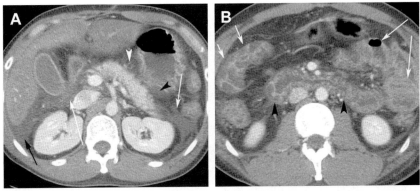

Fig. 20. Hypoalbuminemia in a 45-year-old woman with cirrhosis and diffuse edema. (*A*) The pancreas is mildly edematous with stranding and fluid in the peripancreatic space (*arrowheads*) and anterior pararenal spaces bilaterally (*long white arrows*). Ascites (*black arrow*) also is noted. (*B*) Same patient as **Fig. 20**A. Marked wall thickening is noted in the duodenum (*black arrowheads*), small bowel (*long white arrows*), and hepatic flexure (*short white arrows*) due to the low albumin.

and not used worldwide in a consistent manner.

- The revised Atlanta classification divides acute pancreatitis into interstitial edematous pancreatitis and necrotizing pancreatitis, outlines the clinical definition, defines early and late phases, assesses degrees of severity of pancreatitis, and depicts the definition of organ failure and its significance for outcome.
- Most importantly, the pancreatic fluid collections are now clearly defined based on CECT.
- Based on presence or absence of necrosis, 5 categories are described: APFC and ANC in

the first 4 weeks from onset; pseudocyst and WON after 4 weeks; and postnecrosectomy pseudocyst as a long-term complication after necrosectomy.

- The terms pancreatic abscess, phlegmon, or simply fluid collection are no longer used.
- In the first week after onset, only clinical parameters are relevant for treatment, whereas after the first week, morphologic criteria defined by CT are combined with clinical parameters to determine care.
- The revised Atlanta classification system provides a universally understandable and

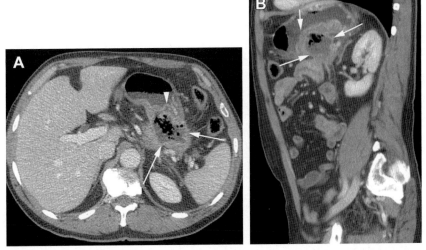

Fig. 21. Marsupialization of a pseudocyst. (*A*) The axial CT image demonstrates a fluid-filled structure with air bubbles and an enhancing rim (*white long arrows*) inseparable from the thickened gastric wall (*white arrowhead*). (*B*) Same patient as **Fig. 21**A. The sagittal CT image shows the same air-filled structure (*long white arrows*) with a communication to the lumen of the stomach (*short white arrow*) due to a marsupialization. This could be confused with infected pseudocyst or WON.

consistent categorization of acute pancreatitis and its complications that facilitates more objective communication between physicians and among institutions, which allows better treatment planning.

SUMMARY

Based on improved knowledge of the disease pathophysiology, superior diagnostic imaging, and expanded treatment options that include minimally invasive procedures, the revised Atlanta classification system provides a common language for clinicians, surgeons, and radiologists in diagnosing and staging acute pancreatitis. CT is declared the method of choice for imaging the pancreas with MR imaging or ultrasound used for clarification of the presence or absence of nonliquefied components within a fluid collection, for detection of gallstones not seen on CT, or when CT is contraindicated. The clinical presentation of acute pancreatitis is clearly defined and a precise description of pancreatic fluid collections is introduced. In the first week, only clinical parameters are used for treatment planning, whereas after the first week, morphologic criteria defined by CT combine with clinical parameters to determine care. Based on the presence or absence of necrosis, a new terminology based on CECT was introduced: ANC are distinguished from APFCs in the first 4 weeks after onset of acute pancreatitis, and WONs are distinguished from pseudocysts after the initial 4 weeks. The term postnecrosectomy pseudocyst in patients with disconnected pancreatic duct syndrome also was presented. These distinctions are important, because management of these patients is different based on the clinical and imaging findings.

REFERENCES

1. Bhatia M, Brady M, Shokuhi S, et al. Inflammatory mediators in acute pancreatitis. J Pathol 2000;190: 117–25.

2. Spanier BW, Dijkgraaf MG, Bruno MJ. Epidemiology, aetiology and outcome of acute and chronic pancreatitis: an update. Best Pract Res Clin Gastroenterol 2008;22:45–62.

3. Frossard J, Steer ML, Pastor CM. Acute pancreatitis. Lancet 2008;371:143–52.

4. Toouli J, Brooke-Smith M, Bassi C, et al. Guidelines for management of acute pancreatitis. J Gastroenterol Hepatol 2002;17:S15–39.

5. Bradley EL 3rd. A clinically based classification system for acute pancreatitis. Summary of the International Symposium on Acute Pancreatitis, Atlanta, GA, September 11 through 13, 1992. Arch Surg 1993;128:586–90.

6. Banks PA, Bollen TL, Dervenis C, et al. Classification of acute pancreatitis – 2012: revision of the Atlanta classification and definitions by international consensus. Gut 2013;62:102–11.

7. Yuan Y, Huang ZX, Li ZL, et al. Dual-source dual-energy computed tomography imaging of acute necrotizing pancreatitis–preliminary study. Sichuan Da Xue Xue Bao Yi Xue Ban 2011;42:691–4 [in Chinese].

8. Sing VK, Bollen TL, Wu BU, et al. An assessment of the severity of interstitial pancreatitis. Clin Gastroentrol Hepatol 2011;9:1098–103.

9. Thoeni RF. The revised Atlanta classification of acute pancreatitis: its importance for the radiologist and its effect on treatment. Radiology 2012;262:751–64.

10. Spanier BW, Nio Y, van der Hulst RW, et al. Practice and yield of early CT scan in acute pancreatitis: a Dutch observational multicenter study. Pancreatology 2010;10:222–8.

11. Sakorafas GH, Tsiotos GG, Sarr MG. Extrapancreatic necrotizing pancreatitis with viable pancreas: a previously under-appreciated entity. J Am Coll Surg 1999;188:643–8.

12. van Santvoort HC, Bakker OJ, Bollen TL, et al. A conservative and minimally invasive approach to necrotizing pancreatitis improves outcome. Gastroenterology 2011;141:1254–63.

13. Perez A, Whang EE, Brooks DC, et al. Is severity of necrotizing pancreatitis increased in extended necrosis and infected necrosis? Pancreas 2002;25: 229–33.

14. Balthazar EJ, Robinson DL, Megibow AJ, et al. Acute pancreatitis: value of CT in establishing prognosis. Radiology 1990;174:331–6.

15. Balthazar EJ. Acute pancreatitis: assessment of severity with clinical and CT evaluation. Radiology 2002;223:603–13.

16. Acevedo-Piedra NG, Moya-Hoyo N, Rey-Riveiro M, et al. Validation of the determinant-based classification and revision of the Atlanta classification systems for acute pancreatitis. Clin Gastroenterol Hepatol 2014;12:311–6.

17. Bruennler T, Hamer OW, Lang S, et al. Outcome in a large unselected series of patients with acute pancreatitis. Hepatogastroenterology 2009;56(91–92):871–6.

18. Vege SS, Gardner TB, Chari ST, et al. Low mortality and high morbidity in severe acute pancreatitis without organ failure: a case for revising the Atlanta classification to include "moderately severe acute pancreatitis". Am J Gastroenterol 2009; 104:710–5.

19. Johnson CD, Abu-Hilal M. Persistent organ failure during the first week as a marker of fatal outcome in acute pancreatitis. Gut 2004;53:1340–4.

20. de-Madaria E, Banks PA, Moya-Hoyo N, et al. Early factors associated with fluid sequestration and outcomes of patients with acute pancreatitis. Clin Gastroenterol Hepatol 2014;12:997–1002.

21. Petrov MS, Shanbhag S, Chakraborty M, et al. Organ failure and infection of pancreatic necrosis as determinants of mortality in patients with acute pancreatitis. Gastroenterology 2010;139:813–20.

22. Marshall JC, Cook DJ, Christou NV, et al. Multiple organ dysfunction core: a reliable descriptor of a complex clinical outcome. Crit Care Med 1995;23:1638–52.

23. Singh VK, Wu BU, Bollen TL, et al. A prospective evaluation of the bedside index for severity in acute pancreatitis score in assessing mortality and intermediate markers of severity in acute pancreatitis. Am J Gastroenterol 2009;104:966–71.

24. Lenhart DK, Balthazar EJ. MDCT of acute mild (nonnecrotizing) pancreatitis: abdominal complications and fate of fluid collections. AJR Am J Roentgenol 2008;190:643–9.

25. Mujica VR, Barkin JS, Go VL. Acute pancreatitis secondary to pancreatic carcinoma. Study Group Participants. Pancreas 2000;21:329–32.

26. Kim YK, Ko SW, Kim CS, et al. Effectiveness of MR imaging for diagnosing the mild forms of acute pancreatitis: comparison with MDCT. J Magn Reson Imaging 2006;24:1342–9.

27. De Waele JJ, Delrue L, Hoste EA, et al. Extrapancreatic inflammation on abdominal computed tomography as an early predictor of disease severity in acute pancreatitis: evaluation of a new scoring system. Pancreas 2007;34:185–90.

28. Spitzer AL, Thoeni RF, Barcia AM, et al. Early nonenhanced abdominal computed tomography can predict mortality in severe acute pancreatitis. J Gastrointest Surg 2005;9:928–33.

29. Tsuji Y, Takahashi N, Fletcher JG, et al. Subtraction color map of contrast-enhanced and unenhanced CT for the prediction of pancreatic necrosis in early stage of acute pancreatitis. AJR Am J Roentgenol 2014;202:W349–56.

30. Moon JH, Cho YD, Cha SW, et al. The detection of bile duct stones in suspected biliary pancreatitis: comparison of MRCP, ERCP, and intraductal US. Am J Gastroenterol 2005;100:1051–7.

31. Xiao B, Zhang XM, Tang W, et al. Magnetic resonance imaging for local complications of acute pancreatitis: a pictorial review. World J Gastroenterol 2010;16:2735–42.

32. Hirota M, Kimura Y, Ishiko T, et al. Visualization of the heterogeneous internal structure of so-called "pancreatic necrosis" by magnetic resonance imaging in acute necrotizing pancreatitis. Pancreas 2002;25:63–7.

33. Islim F, Salik AE, Bayramoglu S, et al. Non-invasive detection of infection in acute pancreatitis and acute necrotic collections with diffusion-weighted magnetic resonance imaging: preliminary findings. Abdom Imaging 2014;39:472–81.

34. Barral M, Taouli B, Guiu B, et al. Diffusion-weighted MR imaging of the pancreas: current status and recommendations. Radiology 2015;274:45–63.

35. Tirkes T, Menias CO, Sandrasegaran K. MR imaging for pancreas. Radiol Clin North Am 2012;50:379–93.

36. Brand M, Götz A, Zeman F, et al. Acute necrotizing pancreatitis: laboratory, clinical, and imaging findings as predictors of patient outcome. AJR Am J Roentgenol 2014;202:1215–31.

37. Isenmann R, Büchler M, Uhl W, et al. Pancreatic necrosis: an early finding in severe pancreatitis. Pancreas 1993;8:358–61.

38. Bollen TL, Singh VK, Maurer R, et al. Comparative evaluation of the modified CT severity index and CT severity index in assessing severity of acute pancreatitis. AJR Am J Roentgenol 2011;197:386–92.

39. Ashley SW, Perez A, Pierce EA, et al. Necrotizing pancreatitis: contemporary analysis of 99 consecutive cases. Ann Surg 2001;234:572–9.

40. Meyrignac O, Lagarde S, Bournet B, et al. Acute Pancreatitis: Extrapancreatic Necrosis Volume as Early Predictor of Severity. Radiology 2015;276:119–28.

41. Tann M, Maglinte D, Howard TJ, et al. Disconnected pancreatic duct syndrome: imaging findings and therapeutic implications in 26 surgically corrected patients. J Comput Assist Tomogr 2003;27:577–82.

42. Baron TH, Harewood GC, Morgan DE, et al. Outcome differences after endoscopic drainage of pancreatic necrosis, acute pancreatic pseudocysts and chronic pancreatic pseudocysts. Gastrointest Endosc 2002;56:7–17.

43. Shyu JY, Sainani NI, Sahni VA, et al. Necrotizing pancreatitis: diagnosis, imaging, and intervention. Radiographics 2014;34:1218–39.

44. Bollen TL. Imaging of acute pancreatitis; update of the revised Atlanta classification. Radiol Clin N AM 2012;50:429–45.

45. Büchler MW, Gloor B, Müller CA, et al. Acute necrotizing pancreatitis: treatment strategy according to the status of infection. Ann Surg 2000;232:619–26.

46. Triantopoulou C, Delis S, Dervenis C. Imaging evaluation of post-pancreatitis infection. Infect Disord Drug Targets 2010;10:15–20.

47. Segal D, Mortele KJ, Banks PA, et al. Acute necrotizing pancreatitis: role of CT-guided percutaneous catheter drainage. Abdom Imaging 2007;32:351–61.

48. Mortele KJ, Girshman J, Szejnfeld D, et al. CT-guided percutaneous catheter drainage of acute necrotizing pancreatitis: clinical experience and observations in patients with sterile and infected necrosis. AJR Am J Roentgenol 2009;192:110–6.

49. Linder JD, Geenen JE, Catalano MF. Cyst fluid analysis obtained by EUS-guided FNA in the evaluation of discrete cystic neoplasms of the pancreas: a prospective single-center experience. Gastrointest Endosc 2006;64:697–702.

50. Bhattacharya A, Kochhar R, Sharma S, et al. PET/CT with 18F-FDG-labeled autologous leukocytes for the diagnosis of infected fluid collections in acute pancreatitis. J Nucl Med 2014;55:1267–72.

51. van Santvoort HC, Besselink MG, Bakker OJ, et al. A step-up approach or open necrosectomy for necrotizing pancreatitis. Dutch Pancreatitis Study Group. N Engl J Med 2010;362:1491–502.

52. Schneider L, Büchler MW, Werner J. Acute pancreatitis with an emphasis on infection. Infect Dis Clin North Am 2010;24:921–41.

53. Guo Q, Li A, Xia Q, et al. The role of organ failure and infection in necrotizing pancreatitis: a prospective study. Ann Surg 2014;259:1201–7.

54. Bollen TL, van Santvoort HC, Besselink MG, et al. Update on acute pancreatitis: US, CT, and MRI features. Semin Ultrasound CT MR 2007;28:371–83.

55. Vege SS, Fletcher JG, Talukdar R, et al. Peripancreatic collections in acute pancreatitis: correlation between computerized tomography and operative findings. World J Gastroenterol 2010;16:4291–6.

The Acute Abdominal Aorta

Vincent M. Mellnick, MD*, Jay P. Heiken, MD

KEYWORDS

- Aorta • Aneurysm • Rupture • Penetrating atherosclerotic ulcer • Aortitis • Thrombosis
- Aortoenteric fistula

KEY POINTS

- Acute disorders of the abdominal aorta are potentially lethal conditions that require prompt evaluation and treatment and are primarily imaged with computed tomography (CT). MR imaging may be useful in select applications.
- Common subcategories of the acute abdominal aortic syndrome include unstable or ruptured aneurysm, dissection, penetrating atherosclerotic ulcer, and intramural hematoma, each of which has characteristic imaging features and distinct prognosis and management.
- Aortic inflammation and infection are less common acute aortic conditions with imaging features that often are better shown on portal venous rather than arterial phase CT or MR imaging.
- Acute traumatic injury of the abdominal aorta is rare, but should be evaluated with attention to direct and indirect imaging signs that help vascular surgeons grade injury severity and decide between observation and urgent repair.
- Aortic fistulas most commonly involve the duodenum after open aortic repair. Diagnosis of aortoenteric fistula is based primarily on observation of indirect, often subtle, imaging findings rather than active contrast extravasation.

INTRODUCTION

Acute disorders of the abdominal aorta are potentially lethal conditions that require prompt evaluation and treatment. Common subcategories of the acute abdominal aortic syndrome include unstable or ruptured aneurysm, dissection, penetrating atherosclerotic ulcer, and intramural hematoma (IMH). Inflammation, infection, traumatic injury, fistulization, and occlusion of the abdominal aorta are rare conditions that nevertheless warrant high clinical suspicion because of the potential catastrophic consequences of misdiagnosis. The clinical diagnosis of these diseases often is elusive because symptoms may be nonspecific, including abdominal pain, back pain, or hypotension. Consequently, imaging plays a vital role in guiding patient management.

The workhorse imaging method for evaluating acute conditions of the abdominal aorta is computed tomography (CT) because of its availability and rapid image acquisition capability, which enable inclusion of the entire abdomen and pelvis, thus allowing for possible alternative diagnoses. In addition, modern CT equipment and software provide for radiation dose reduction and high-quality multiplanar reconstruction. MR imaging is a helpful alternative imaging method for stable patients who have a contraindication to iodinated contrast. Although ultrasonography is useful in screening

Disclosures: None.
Mallinckrodt Institute of Radiology, Washington University School of Medicine, 510 South Kingshighway Boulevard, St Louis, MO 63110, USA
* Corresponding author. Mallinckrodt Institute of Radiology, Washington University School of Medicine, 510 South Kingshighway Boulevard, Box 8131, St Louis, MO 63110.
E-mail address: mellnickv@mir.wustl.edu

Radiol Clin N Am 53 (2015) 1209–1224
http://dx.doi.org/10.1016/j.rcl.2015.06.007

for and monitoring abdominal aortic aneurysms, it generally is not used in the setting of suspected acute aortic conditions. Therefore this article focuses on the CT and MR imaging features of acute conditions of the abdominal aorta and how these studies guide management.

NORMAL ANATOMY

The abdominal aorta extends from the diaphragmatic hiatus at T12 to the iliac bifurcation, following the curvature of the lumbar spine. It traditionally is divided into suprarenal, juxtarenal, and infrarenal segments based on the relationship with the renal arteries. The aortic wall consists of 3 layers: the endothelium or intima; the media, composed of smooth muscle; and the adventitia, the outermost connective tissue layer that provides structural support for the vessel. Normal abdominal aortic luminal diameter is approximately 2 cm, measured perpendicular to the long axis of the lumen.

IMAGING TECHNIQUE AND PROTOCOLS
Computed Tomography

CT, the most commonly used imaging method for evaluating the abdominal aorta, enables scanning of the entire abdomen and pelvis in 5 to 10 seconds with excellent z-axis resolution. When an acute aortic condition is suspected clinically, it is advisable to begin the CT examination with a noncontrast acquisition, which improves identification of critical findings, such as an IMH or high-attenuating crescent sign. Although abdominal aortic aneurysm rupture or impending rupture

may be diagnosed on the noncontrast images alone, postcontrast images usually are required in order to acquire preoperative aortic measurements for endoluminal stent graft repair. Oral contrast is contraindicated when evaluating the aorta, because it may obscure subtle findings, such as an aortoenteric fistula (AEF).[1]

The authors routinely acquire scans of the abdominal aorta in the arterial phase using a CT angiogram protocol, injecting 100 to 125 mL of iodinated contrast at a rate of 4 mL/s with bolus tracking over the descending thoracic aorta and a 15-second delay (Table 1). Images are obtained with 2-mm slice thickness and a reconstruction interval of 1 mm with a detector collimation varying from 0.6 to 1.2 mm depending on the scanner used. These settings typically allow for near-isotropic voxels and high-quality coronal and sagittal multiplanar reconstructions as well as three-dimensional (3D)–rendered maximum intensity projection (MIP) and shaded surface display images, all of which can aid in diagnosis and in depicting findings for surgeons. A delayed contrast phase may be acquired to evaluate for periaortic enhancement, to detect an endoleak after endoluminal stent graft repair, or for routine evaluation of the solid organs of the abdomen if another diagnosis is suspected.

Many modern scanners have software to aid in selecting an appropriate peak kilovoltage (kVp) for the clinical application and patient size. When possible, a lower kVp (100 or 80 kVp when possible) is advised for CT angiography to maximize the photoelectric effect of iodine and provide high-quality arterial opacification.[2] Dual-energy CT

Table 1
Imaging protocols: abdominal aorta

CT Angiography	MR Angiography
Noncontrast phase	ECG gated when possible
Arterial phase: 4 mL/s injection rate, bolus tracking off descending aorta + 15-s delay	Axial and coronal T2 FSE and SSFP images
No oral contrast	Contrast-enhanced axial FS 3D GRE with gadofosveset trisodium
Slice thickness, 2-mm; reconstruction interval, 1 mm	3D MRA to include abdominal aorta through femoral arteries
Sagittal and coronal MPRs, 3D postprocessing for endoluminal measurements	Noncontrast MRA: QISS or TOF imaging
Delayed images in select cases[a]	Delayed images in select cases[a,b]

Abbreviations: 3D, three dimensional; ECG, electrocardiogram; FS, fat-saturated; FSE, fast spin echo; GRE, gradient recalled echo; MPR, multiplanar reconstruction; QISS, quiescent-interval single-shot; SSFP, steady-state free precession; TOF, time of flight.
[a] If an endoleak, inflammatory aortic aneurysm, or aortitis is suspected.
[b] Aortic inflammation or infection should ideally be evaluated using a standard extracellular gadolinium-based contrast agent when imaged with MRI.

may be a useful adjunct in evaluating the abdomen because it permits the generation of virtual non-contrast images without the added time or radiation dose associated with conventional pre-contrast scanning.[3] When available, iterative reconstruction techniques also can be used to reduce the dose prospectively. However, radiation dose considerations should not compromise image quality because acute aortic conditions are potentially life-threatening and most commonly seen in older patients for whom radiation dose is not a primary consideration.

When endoluminal repair of an aortic aneurysm is being considered, it is important not only to report the maximum aortic diameter but also to provide measurements of the aorta at the proximal and distal attachment sites, the length and morphology of the aneurysm neck, and the diameter of the iliac and femoral arteries, all of which affect the approach and potential for endovascular repair.[4–6]

What the referring clinician needs to know: computed tomography for endovascular therapy planning

- Maximal aortic diameter
- Aortic diameter at proximal and distal attachment sites
- Aortic neck length and morphology
- Diameter and stenosis in the iliac and femoral arteries

MR Imaging

The use of MR for imaging the aorta continues to increase because of its excellent soft tissue contrast resolution, its improved imaging speed at higher magnetic field strengths, and lack of radiation exposure. Nevertheless, the applicability of MR imaging in the clinical setting of a suspected acute abdominal aortic condition remains limited. The length of scan time and the need for numerous breath holds, which require a substantial amount of patient cooperation, confine the role of MR angiography (MRA) to evaluating the acute aorta in stable patients in whom rupture has been excluded. With this limitation in mind, contrast-enhanced MRA is a reasonable consideration for patients with an increased serum creatinine level, but whose estimated glomerular filtration rate (eGFR) remains more than 30 mL/min/1.73 m^2.

In patients with eGFR less than 30 mL/min/1.73 m^2, intravenous gadolinium-based contrast agents are generally not advised because of concern for nephrogenic systemic fibrosis. However, noncontrast MRA techniques are available

that can accurately depict acute aortic conditions, most notably dissection, which otherwise would not be seen on noncontrast CT. The authors' non-contrast aorta MRA consists of electrocardiogram (ECG)-gated coronal and axial T2-weighted half-Fourier single-shot fast spin echo and balanced steady-state free precession (bSSFP) sequences, as well as axial volume-interpolated gradient recalled echo images (Table 1). In addition, depending on scanner availability, either ECG-gated quiescent-interval single-shot or time-of-flight MRA sequences are performed, the former having been shown to be a promising alternative to contrast-enhanced MRA.[7,8] ECG-gated cine bSSFP or similar sequences also may be used to show mobility of a dissection flap or adherent thrombus.[9]

When intravenous contrast is used for MRA, gadofosveset trisodium typically is used at our institution because of its albumin binding and prolonged circulation in the blood pool. After administration of contrast, axial volume-interpolated gradient recalled echo images are acquired. In addition, coronal 3D MRA is performed with high-resolution steady-state images of the abdominal aorta through the femoral arteries. Time-resolved MRA may be useful for assessing contrast flow through collaterals or within an endoleak. In the setting of suspected inflammatory aortic aneurysm or aortitis in which evaluation of the periaortic soft tissues also is of interest, gadofosveset trisodium is not the ideal contrast agent. Instead, use of a standard extracellular gadolinium-based contrast agent is advised (assuming GFR >30 mL/min/1.73 m^2) with acquisition of 5-minute delayed fat-saturated T1 images to evaluate for periaortic enhancement.

ACUTE AORTIC CONDITIONS
Abdominal Aortic Aneurysm

Aneurysms of the abdominal aorta (AAAs) most commonly involve the infrarenal segment and are typically true aneurysms that involve all 3 layers of the aortic wall. AAA is defined as having a diameter greater than 3 cm measured perpendicular to the long axis of the lumen.[10,11] Found in 2% to 4% of the population more than the age of 50 years, the prevalence of AAA increases with age and is most common in men.[12] Risk factors for developing AAA include positive family history, peripheral vascular disease, and smoking.

Rupture is the most lethal complication of an AAA, with morality rates ranging from 70% to 94%.[13–16] Risk of aneurysm rupture increases with AAA diameter, with less than a 0.5% annual risk of rupture for an aneurysm less than 4.0 cm in diameter, compared with a 30% to 50% risk of rupture within 1 year for an AAA greater than or equal to 8.0 cm.[17] In addition to size, other risk factors for AAA rupture include aneurysm expansion rate, smoking, and uncontrolled hypertension.[18] Hemorrhage from AAA rupture usually involves the retroperitoneum, with peritoneal involvement being much less common. Rupture into the inferior vena cava or gastrointestinal tract is rare. The classic clinical presentation consists of pain (abdominal, back, or flank), hypotension, and a pulsatile mass, but all of these signs and symptoms are not always present, necessitating a radiologic diagnosis.

Suspected AAA rupture is most commonly evaluated with CT. The primary imaging findings of AAA rupture often are obvious, and include a retroperitoneal hematoma extending directly from the aneurysm and active extravasation of contrast material (**Fig. 1**).[11] With impending or contained rupture, the findings may be much more subtle, including perianeurysmal soft tissue stranding (**Fig. 2**). Secondary CT findings associated with AAA rupture or impending rupture include the hyperattenuating crescent, draped aorta, and tangential calcium signs. In addition, rapidly increasing aneurysm diameter and focal discontinuity of intimal calcification within the wall of the aneurysm can be indications of impending rupture.

A hyperattenuating crescent refers to a crescentic area of high attenuation within the wall or mural thrombus of an aneurysm secondary to penetration of blood from the aneurysm lumen into the aortic wall or mural thrombus (see **Fig. 2**).[19] By definition, a hyperattenuating crescent has a higher CT attenuation than the luminal blood on unenhanced scans and a higher attenuation than skeletal muscle on postcontrast scans.[20] Although the reported prevalence of this finding in patients with AAA rupture ranges from 21% to 77%, the specificity has been reported to be as high as 93%.[20,21]

A draped aorta describes the appearance of an AAA wall that bulges posteriorly, either unilaterally or bilaterally, and has lost its fat plane with the adjacent psoas muscle and vertebra (**Fig. 3**). This finding is a sign of aortic wall insufficiency and impending rupture but also can be seen with a contained aortic leak.[22,23]

Focal discontinuity of intimal calcification within an AAA wall, particularly when shown to be a new finding compared with prior studies, has been shown to be a useful sign of acute or impending rupture.[20] The tangential calcium sign, defined as calcified atherosclerotic plaque adjacent to an area of focal calcium discontinuity that is divergent from the normal arc of the aorta, is another finding highly associated with AAA rupture (**Fig. 4**).[24]

Diagnostic signs of acute or impending rupture of aneurysms of the abdominal aorta

- Primary:
  - Retroperitoneal hematoma
  - Active contrast extravasation
  - Perianeurysmal stranding
- Secondary:
  - Hyperattenuating crescent sign
  - Draped aorta
  - Focal discontinuity of intimal calcification
  - Tangential calcium sign

PENETRATING ATHEROSCLEROTIC ULCER

A penetrating atherosclerotic ulcer (PAU) refers to an ulceration of atherosclerotic plaque that allows blood from the aortic lumen to contact the media of the aortic wall. Most common in older patients, PAU results from preexisting atherosclerotic disease and is most common in the middle and distal thirds of the thoracic aorta.[25,26] When PAU occurs

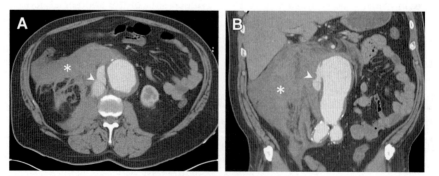

Fig. 1. Ruptured abdominal aortic aneurysm. Contrast-enhanced transaxial (*A*) and coronal (*B*) CT images show contained active extravasation (*arrowheads*). Note the large right-sided retroperitoneal hematoma (*asterisks*).

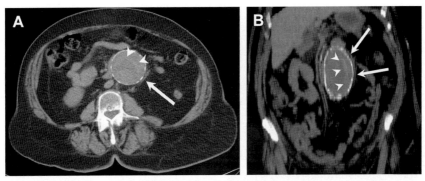

Fig. 2. Hyperattenuating crescent sign. Transaxial (*A*) and coronal (*B*) noncontrast CT images show an infrarenal aortic aneurysm with a crescent-shaped area of high attenuation in the mural thrombus (*arrowheads*), representing acute hematoma. There is also subtle stranding within the retroperitoneal fat (*arrows*). The patient expired from aneurysm rupture shortly after this scan was performed.

in the abdominal aorta, it may present clinically with pain, lower limb ischemia caused by embolism, or shock. Similar to AAA, the most lethal complication of PAU is rupture. The reported incidence of rupture from abdominal aortic PAU has ranged from 8% to 37%.[26,27] PAU also may resolve spontaneously, but can progress to an enlarging IMH, dissection, or subadventitial pseudoaneurysm.

On imaging studies, PAU presents as a focal outpouching of the aortic lumen with associated hematoma in the aortic media (**Fig. 5**). Although irregular atherosclerotic plaque without true penetrating ulceration may simulate a PAU and provide a potential pitfall, PAU may be differentiated from irregular plaque by the presence of a saccular outpouching deforming the outer contour of the aortic wall. Precontrast CT or T1-weighted MR imaging also may be useful to show IMH adjacent to the ulceration, which typically is shorter in length than with classic aortic dissection or a primary IMH.[26]

Penetrating Atherosclerotic Ulcer: Pearls, Pitfalls, and Variants

- Short-segment abnormality compared with dissection or IMH
- Deformity of outer aortic wall differentiates from ulcerated plaque
- Noncontrast images may show adjacent IMH
- May resolve spontaneously
- May progress to enlarging IMH, dissection, or pseudoaneurysm

ABDOMINAL AORTIC DISSECTION

Isolated acute dissection of the abdominal aorta is rare, accounting for less than 2% of all cases of aortic dissection.[28,29] Although the most commonly cited risk factor for aortic dissection is uncontrolled hypertension, other conditions, including Marfan syndrome, bicuspid aortopathy, vasculitis, cocaine use, and pregnancy, have

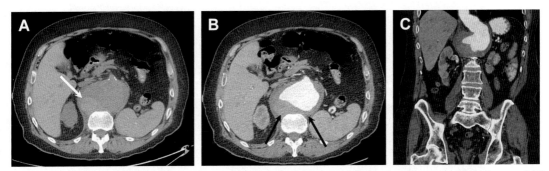

Fig. 3. Contained aortic rupture. Precontrast transaxial (*A*) and contrast-enhanced transaxial (*B*) and coronal (*C*) CT images show hyperattenuation within the aortic wall (*white arrow*), representing hematoma. Note the abnormal contour of the aortic lumen (*B, C*) and loss of the fat plane between the aorta and the vertebral body posteriorly (*black arrows*): the draped aorta sign.

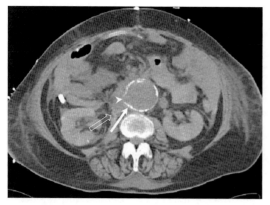

Fig. 4. Tangential calcium sign. Transaxial noncontrast CT shows an infrarenal aortic aneurysm with focal disruption of intimal calcification (*arrowhead*). The arc of the adjacent atherosclerotic calcification in the aortic wall (*solid arrow*) points at a tangent from the expected aortic circumference. Note the adjacent retroperitoneal stranding (*open arrow*).

been associated with aortic dissection.[14] Isolated abdominal aortic dissection most commonly originates in the infrarenal segment and in the setting of an accompanying AAA.[28] When dissection occurs more proximally in the abdominal aorta, it may involve the mesenteric and/or renal arteries, leading in some cases to end-organ ischemia and causing affected patients to present with abdominal and/or flank pain. Distal extension of the dissection flap also may occlude the iliac and/or femoral arteries, leading to lower extremity ischemia.

As with dissection in any segment of the aorta, abdominal aortic dissection appears on imaging studies as an intimal flap dividing the aorta into true and false lumens (**Fig. 6**). The true lumen typically is smaller than the false lumen, is surrounded by calcifications when present, and enhances

more rapidly than the false lumen. Identifying the dissection flap as well as the vessels supplied by each lumen on CT requires intravenous contrast. Although gadolinium-enhanced MR imaging similarly opacifies the aortic lumen, noncontrast MR imaging techniques also are capable of showing a dissection flap (**Fig. 7**). In particular, cine sequences can show pulsatile mobility of the flap throughout the cardiac cycle.

INTRAMURAL HEMATOMA

Aortic IMH often is described as an early-stage aortic dissection or dissection with a thrombosed false lumen. IMH is caused by spontaneous rupture of the vasa vasorum into the aortic media with resultant weakening of the aortic wall.[30,31] Although the clinical course, morbidity, and mortality of aortic IMH are similar to those of classic aortic dissection, the imaging features are distinct and the standard treatment less clear than that of classic dissection. IMH may resolve spontaneously, stabilize, or progress to classic dissection, focal aortic ulceration, or aortic aneurysm.[31,32] Factors that predict progression of an IMH to dissection or rupture include the presence of an aortic aneurysm or PAU, persistent symptoms after treatment, and progressive increase in aortic wall thickness and/or aneurysm diameter.[33,34] IMH most commonly occurs in the thoracic aorta, and rarely in the abdomen alone.

IMH is seen on CT and MR imaging as an eccentric, crescent-shaped collection of blood in the aortic wall. On CT, this feature is best seen as hyperattenuation (40–70 Hounsfield units) on precontrast images, particularly with the use of narrow window settings.[35] On MR imaging, precontrast T1-weighted or black blood images may be useful to show intramural blood products, which can be isointense or hyperintense to

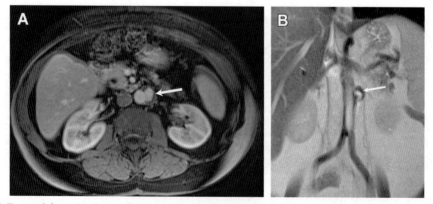

Fig. 5. PAU. Transaxial postcontrast volume-interpolated gradient recalled echo (*A*) and T2-weighted half-Fourier single-shot fast spin echo (*B*) MR images show a saccular outpouching from the infrarenal aorta (*arrows*).

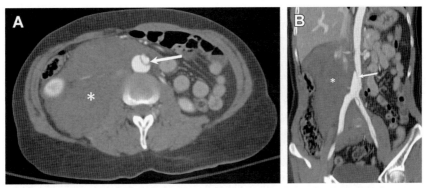

Fig. 6. Abdominal aortic dissection. Transaxial (*A*) and curved coronal (*B*) contrast-enhanced CT images show a dissection flap in the infrarenal aorta (*arrows*) extending into the iliac arteries. This isolated abdominal aortic dissection was complicated by aortic rupture, shown by a large retroperitoneal hematoma (*asterisks*).

skeletal muscle, depending on the age of the hematoma (**Fig. 8**).[36] Interpretation based on viewing postcontrast CT or MR images alone may be problematic because the IMH is less conspicuous adjacent to the brightly enhancing aortic lumen, thus potentially being confused for mural thrombus. Imaging features that support mural thrombus rather than an IMH include an irregular intraluminal surface (IMH typically is smoothly contoured); isolation to a dilated portion of the aorta (IMH is more common in normal-diameter aorta); and the presence of multiple, interrupted lesions.[31,36] Imaging features that help distinguish IMH from aortic dissection include lack of enhancement of IMH, whereas delayed images generally depict slow flow in the false lumen of a classic dissection.

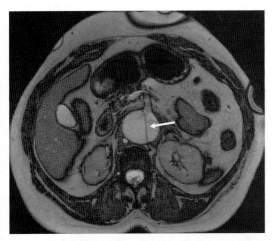

Fig. 7. Abdominal aortic dissection on noncontrast MRA. Transaxial balanced steady-state free precession MR image shows a dissection flap in the abdominal aorta (*arrow*). This sequence can be a useful noncontrast technique for showing a dissection flap, particularly on cine images.

Fixed, medial displacement of intimal atherosclerotic calcification rather than a spiraled appearance of displaced intimal calcium also favors an IMH rather than a classic aortic dissection.[37] An IMH also should not be confused for a hyperattenuating crescent sign in an unstable AAA.

Intramural Hematoma: Pearls, Pitfalls, and Variants

- Precontrast CT or MR imaging may more easily depict IMH, which may be confused for thrombus on postcontrast images alone.
- IMH: smoothly contoured, long segment, continuous. Mural thrombus: irregular contour, isolated to aneurysm, multiple interrupted lesions.
- Lack of contrast enhancement and fixed location of IMH differentiate it from enhancing, spiraling appearance of classic dissection false lumen.

ACUTE TRAUMATIC AORTIC INJURY

Most traumatic abdominal aortic injuries are caused by penetrating trauma, more commonly from gunshot wounds than from stab wounds.[38,39] Despite advances in medical care, mortality for these injuries remains very high, with estimates ranging from 52% to 72%.[40] Factors that predict survival include amount and distribution of hemorrhage: patients with free intraperitoneal bleeding show a higher mortality than those with bleeding confined to the retroperitoneum. In addition, an injury that is caused by a missile (as opposed to stabbing) and a low presenting blood pressure are negative prognostic indicators.[41]

Most blunt traumatic aortic injuries occur in the thorax, with injuries to the abdominal aorta comprising only 4% to 15% of cases.[42] Traumatic abdominal aortic injury most commonly involves

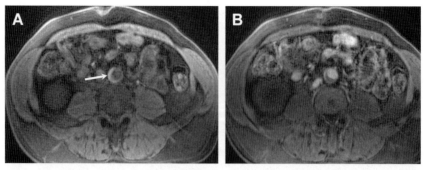

Fig. 8. IMH. Transaxial precontrast volume-interpolated gradient recalled echo MR image (*A*) shows a crescentic area of high signal intensity in the aortic wall (*arrow*). This area shows no enhancement or ulceration after intravenous gadolinium-based contrast administration (*B*).

the infrarenal portion and is postulated to be caused by a direct blow or anteroposterior crush injury rather than a deceleration injury, which is typical of traumatic thoracic aortic injury.[42,43] Blunt injury to the abdominal aorta is a life-threatening emergency, particularly when the aorta is transected with resultant hemorrhage into the retroperitoneum or peritoneum.

Patients who are hemodynamically stable typically are imaged with contrast-enhanced CT. Direct signs of abdominal aortic injury after blunt or penetrating trauma include an intraluminal flap, IMH, focal intimal injury, pseudoaneurysm, and active extravasation of contrast material. Indirect signs include retroperitoneal hematoma and periaortic retroperitoneal or mesenteric stranding (**Fig. 9**). In the setting of penetrating trauma, close attention to missile trajectory is critically important.

No universally accepted radiologic staging system for the classification of acute traumatic aortic injury (ATAI) exists. One system adopted by the Society of Vascular Surgery that is easily understood is based on the extent of injury to the

anatomic layers of the aortic wall: intimal tear (type I), IMH (type II), pseudoaneurysm (type III), and rupture (type IV).[44] Although precise classification of an ATAI into one of these types based on CT may be difficult, radiologists should be aware of this classification scheme because it can inform prognosis, guide treatment, and determine the need for follow-up imaging.[45]

What the Referring Clinician Needs to Know: Traumatic Aortic Injury Classification

- Type I: intimal tear
- Type II: IMH
- Type III: pseudoaneurysm
- Type IV: rupture

AORTIC OCCLUSION AND MOBILE THROMBUS

Acute aortic occlusion is a rare but catastrophic vascular condition that typically presents with lower extremity paralysis, cold extremities, and absent femoral pulses. The presence of lower

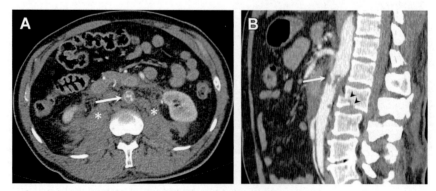

Fig. 9. Traumatic aortic transection. Transaxial (*A*) and sagittal (*B*) postcontrast CT images show intraluminal filling defects in the infrarenal aorta (*arrows*), representing an intraluminal flap and thrombus caused by traumatic aortic transection. Note the presence of retroperitoneal hematoma (*asterisks*) and an adjacent vertebral body fracture (*arrowheads*).

extremity paralysis may mislead emergency room physicians to suspect a neurologic diagnosis. Acute aortic occlusion may be caused by a large saddle embolus, such as from cardiac origin or thrombosis of a preexisting aortic abnormality. Without prompt treatment, the mortality of acute aortic occlusion is greater than 75%.[46]

Chronic aortoiliac occlusion (also known as Leriche syndrome) is more common than acute aortic occlusion, is typically seen in the elderly, and is caused by the deposition of atherosclerotic plaque, usually beginning at the aortic bifurcation. Clinically, this condition classically presents with claudication, absent or decreased femoral pulses, and impotence in men.[47] Readily diagnosed by contrast-enhanced CT or MR imaging, the chronicity of aortic occlusion may be assessed in part by the absence or presence of enlarged collateral vessels, which indicate a long-standing time course (**Fig. 10**).[48] Treatment of chronic Leriche syndrome usually is bypass of the occluded aortoiliac segments.

In addition to complete thrombosis, mobile nonocclusive thrombus also may be encountered in the abdominal aorta, although it is seen more commonly in the descending thoracic aorta.[49] Aortic thrombus typically arises from atherosclerotic plaque or within an aneurysm and may be a source of embolism to the lower extremities, migrating spontaneously or after an intra-arterial procedure. On occasion, an aortic thrombus may arise in an otherwise normal aorta in patients with hypercoagulability, smoking history, and/or endothelial injury.[50] Contrast-enhanced CT shows an eccentric, nodular filling defect in the aorta (**Fig. 11**). The mobility of an adherent thrombus may be shown with ultrasonography or cine MR imaging. Historically treatment has been anticoagulation, but endoluminal stent grafts have recently been used to cover the thrombus and prevent further embolism.[51]

AORTIC VASCULITIS

Inflammation of the aorta and its major branches is classified as large-vessel vasculitis and shows leukocyte infiltration into the vessel wall at pathology. Systemic symptoms and signs of aortic vasculitis include fever, malaise, arthralgias, myalgias, weight loss, and anemia. However, these clinical signs and symptoms are nonspecific, and diagnosis must be made in conjunction with imaging findings as well as inflammatory markers such as erythrocyte sedimentation rate (ESR) and C-reactive protein (CRP). The typical treatment of vasculitis is immunosuppression, commonly with corticosteroids. Specific disorders that may present with aortitis include Takayasu arteritis (TA) and giant cell (temporal) arteritis (GCA) (**Table 2**).

TA is most common in women in their second and third decades of life and has an increased incidence in Japan, southeast Asia, India, and Mexico.[52] Clinical presentations range from completely asymptomatic to severe neurologic impairment, but classically present with ocular disturbances and decreased pulses. Pertinent to the abdominal segment, involvement of the mesenteric or renal arteries may result in bowel ischemia or hypertension, respectively. The frequency of abdominal aortic involvement seems to decrease craniocaudally, with the suprarenal aorta involved in 72% of patients and the aorta below the inferior mesenteric artery involved in 35%.[53] Imaging findings of TA include periarterial fat stranding, wall thickening, stenosis, poststenotic dilatation, aneurysms, and arterial collaterals (**Fig. 12**).[54]

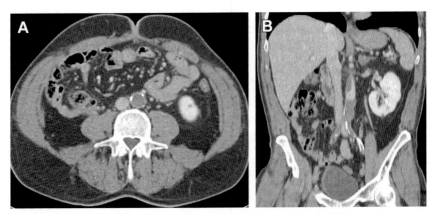

Fig. 10. Acute aortic occlusion. Sagittal (*A*) and coronal (*B*) contrast-enhanced CT images show complete thrombosis of the infrarenal aorta extending into the iliac arteries. Note the absence of collateral vessels, indicating acute timing of occlusion.

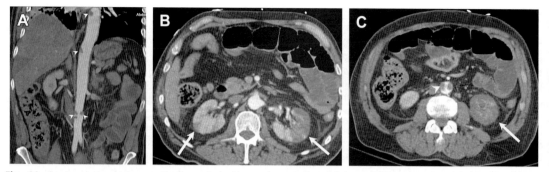

Fig. 11. Acute nonocclusive aortic thrombus. Coronal curved multiplanar (*A*) and transaxial (*B, C*) contrast-enhanced CT images show multiple nonocclusive thrombi in the lower thoracic and abdominal aorta (*arrowheads*). Areas of hypoattenuation in both kidneys (*arrows*) represent infarcts resulting from embolism.

In contrast with TA, GCA almost exclusively affects adults more than 50 years of age with the highest disease risk seen in patients aged 75 to 85 years. GCA is slightly more common in women and individuals of northern European descent.[52] It typically involves the extracranial branches of the carotid arteries (temporal arteritis), clinically manifesting with ophthalmoplegia, but can also involve the aorta, most commonly in the thorax, causing arm claudication.

In both TA and GCA, CT and MR imaging acquisition of delayed contrast-enhanced images can be helpful to show fibroinflammatory tissue around the aorta and to differentiate arteritis from IMH.[55]

In addition, inflammatory aortitis typically has uniform, circumferential involvement of the aortic wall with skip areas of vessel sparing compared with IMH, which more often is eccentric and involves a contiguous segment of the aorta.[31] Fluorodeoxyglucose (FDG)-PET can be useful to show the extent and activity of large-vessel vasculitis and to show response to steroid therapy.[56]

INFLAMMATORY ANEURYSM

Inflammatory AAA is a variant of abdominal aortic aneurysm in which there is inflammatory thickening of the aortic wall with perianeurysmal fibrosis, which may be adherent to the surrounding retroperitoneal structures. This subset accounts for 5% to 10% of all AAAs and is most commonly seen in the infrarenal abdominal aorta and in male patients.[57–59] Although the cause of inflammatory AAA is not known, histopathologic findings suggest that antigens, possibly lipids or products of lipid oxidation, are present in the arterial adventitia.[57,60–62] Some evidence also points to a possible autoimmune origin for this condition, with overlap in the imaging features of inflammatory AAA and retroperitoneal fibrosis. Several recent reports have shown the presence of immunoglobulin (Ig) G4–positive plasma cells in some inflammatory AAA.[63–66]

Clinically, most patients with inflammatory AAA have abdominal or back pain. When accompanied by more extensive retroperitoneal fibrosis, symptoms of ureteral, venous, or duodenal obstruction may be present. In addition, 20% to 50% of patients have constitutional symptoms of fever, malaise, and weight loss.[67] Markers of systemic inflammation such as ESR and CRP commonly are at increased levels. Rupture of an inflammatory AAA is uncommon, likely because of the extensive periaortic fibrosis. Treatment consists of corticosteroids for reducing inflammation and

Table 2	
Inflammatory aortitis: characteristic features	

TA	GCA
Young women	Older patients, slightly more common in women
Aortic involvement common, decreasing craniocaudally	Typically involves the extracranial branches of the carotid arteries, ophthalmoplegia
Periarterial inflammation, wall thickening, stenosis, poststenotic dilatation, aneurysms, and arterial collaterals	Abdominal aortic involvement rare
Uniform, circumferential involvement of the aortic wall with skip areas[a]	Uniform, circumferential involvement of the aortic wall with skip areas[a]

[a] Features seen in both.

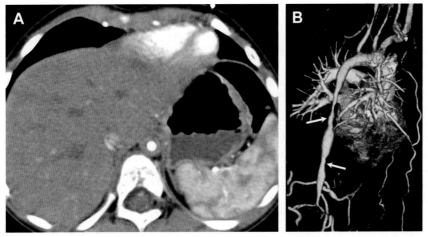

Fig. 12. TA. Transaxial contrast-enhanced (*A*) and 3D volume-rendered (*B*) contrast-enhanced CT images show marked luminal narrowing and wall thickening of the suprarenal abdominal aorta (*A*). Several segments of aortic narrowing can be seen (*B, arrows*).

consideration of surgical repair when size exceeds 5.5 cm.[57]

CT of an inflammatory AAA shows a thickened aortic wall with a surrounding mantle of soft tissue attenuation that shows delayed contrast enhancement (**Fig. 13**).[68] The fibrotic tissue surrounding the aorta typically has a smooth contour and spares the posterior aortic wall. The MR imaging appearance of the periaortic tissues varies depending on the degree of inflammation; increased T2 signal is seen with more acute inflammation, whereas more chronic fibrosis often is T2 hypointense compared with skeletal muscle.[69] MR imaging also may show diffusion restriction within the inflamed retroperitoneum, but this finding is nonspecific and should be correlated with ancillary imaging findings and followed closely to exclude an underlying malignancy.[70] Posterior aortic wall involvement, a lobular mass, and anterior displacement of the aorta from the adjacent

vertebrae are features that suggest a retroperitoneal mass rather than an inflammatory aneurysm.[14,71] In addition, PET-CT may show increased FDG uptake within the wall of an inflammatory AAA. Although this finding also is nonspecific, it may be useful to monitor treatment response.[72]

INFECTIOUS AORTITIS

Infectious aortitis can result from bacterial colonization of a preexisting aneurysm or formation of an infectious pseudoaneurysm (IPA). Traditionally these have been termed mycotic aneurysms, because of their funguslike shape. However, because this term is confusing (not many are caused by fungal organisms) and inaccurate (the wall abnormality often does not involve all 3 layers, as required for a true aneurysm), IPA or infectious aortitis is the preferred terminology. Most

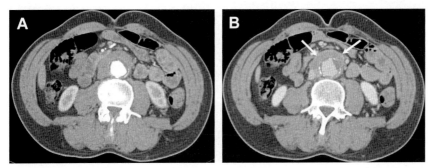

Fig. 13. Inflammatory aortic aneurysm. Transaxial arterial (*A*) and portal venous phase (*B*) CT images show an infrarenal aortic aneurysm with wall thickening and a rind of soft tissue anteriorly and laterally, sparing the posterior wall. Note that the rind of soft tissue shows enhancement on the delayed images (*arrows*). This patient had an increased serum IgG4 level.

commonly caused by bacteria, infection of the aorta can occur by direct inoculation, such as in the setting of trauma or lumbar discitis, or by hematogenous seeding, the latter mechanism being more common. Microorganisms with affinity for the arterial wall, namely *Staphylococcus* species as well as *Salmonella* and other gram-negative species, are the most common pathogens to cause an infectious pseudoaneurysm, although a diverse range of bacterial species has been identified in diseased aortic walls.[73–75] Predisposing factors for developing IPA include a compromised immune status as well as abnormal aortic endothelium, caused by either acute injury or atherosclerosis, including a preexisting AAA. Clinically, these patients present with a painful abdominal mass and evidence of infection such as fever, leukocytosis, and increased levels of inflammatory markers (eg, ESR, CRP). Blood cultures play a vital role in diagnosis and treatment, but may be negative in as many as 25% of patients because of early administration of antibiotics.[76]

On CT and MR imaging, IPA appears as a saccular, often bizarrely shaped, eccentric, arterially enhancing outpouching of the aortic lumen, often with no associated calcification or mural thrombus, helping differentiate it from a PAU (**Fig. 14**).[77–79] As with AAA, IPA most commonly occurs in the infrarenal segment of the abdominal aorta. Periaortic inflammation appears as stranding of the periaortic fat on CT or increased periaortic T2 signal on MR imaging and can be concentric or eccentric in distribution. In addition to surrounding inflammation, a well-defined inflammatory mass may be present, with variable enhancement that depends on the degree of necrosis.[79] Periaortic gas, in the absence of a recent procedure to explain it, is an uncommon feature of IPA.[79,80] A high index of suspicion should be

maintained for IPA because it has a much higher rate of expansion and rupture than classic atherosclerotic AAA. Standard care for IPA typically is a combination of antibiotic therapy, surgical excision, and bypass of the infected portion of the aorta. However, antibiotics followed by endovascular therapy may be options in select patients.[81] *Clostridium septicum* is a rare cause of aortitis but is of particular note because of its strong association with malignancy (most commonly colon cancer or hematologic malignancy).[82]

Pearls, Pitfalls, and Variants: Infectious Aortitis

- Infectious pseudoaneurysm is a more accurate term than mycotic aneurysm
- Most commonly occurs by hematogenous seeding but also can occur by direct inoculation
- Saccular, bizarrely shaped aortic outpouching
- More common in atherosclerotic, aneurysmal aorta or secondary to endothelial injury
- Blood cultures may be negative

AORTOENTERIC FISTULA

The transverse duodenum is the most common site for an AEF, owing to its proximity to the aorta in the retroperitoneum. AEF most frequently occurs in the setting of an abdominal aortic aneurysm, arising usually as a complication of surgical repair, and less commonly as a primary event.[83,84] Uncommonly, a fistula between the aorta and duodenum may result from vasculitis, radiation, or primary duodenal perforation, such as from malignancy, ulcer disease, or trauma.[84] Clinically, patients may present with abdominal pain; gastrointestinal bleeding; sepsis; and, in the setting of an aneurysm, a pulsatile mass. Affected

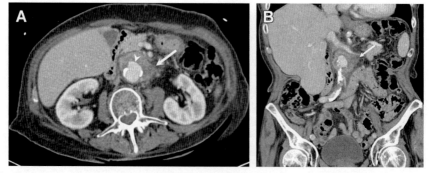

Fig. 14. Infectious aortic pseudoaneurysm. Transaxial (*A*) and coronal (*B*) contrast-enhanced CT images show a saccular, irregularly marginated outpouching of the infrarenal aorta. There is stranding of the periaortic fat (*arrows*) and thickening of the aneurysm wall, indicating inflammation. Note the lack of calcification in the expanded pseudoaneurysm wall (*arrowhead*).

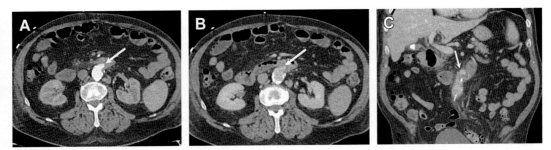

Fig. 15. AEF. Transaxial arterial (*A*), portal venous phase (*B*), and coronal portal venous phase (*C*) CT images show a focal outpouching of the aorta (*arrows*) that extends into the transverse duodenum, with loss of the intervening fat plane. The patient had a history of open aortic repair and presented with hematemesis. Note the absence of active contrast extravasation. An AEF was confirmed operatively.

patients may have a small-volume herald bleed preceding life-threatening, voluminous hemorrhage. Without operative intervention, the mortality approaches 100%. Therefore, a high index of suspicion is needed, particularly in patients who have undergone open AAA repair. Although diagnostic imaging options for AEF historically have included barium studies, aortography, and tagged red blood cell scintigraphy, these tests have substantial limitations compared with CT.[85] Upper gastrointestinal endoscopy also can play an important role in diagnosis.

CT findings of AEF include focal tethering of the duodenum to the aortic wall with duodenal wall thickening and loss of the intervening fat plane, and ectopic gas or fluid within the aortic wall or graft in a patient remote from the perioperative period (**Fig. 15**). Pseudoaneurysm formation and active contrast extravasation into the bowel lumen are seen much less commonly.[83,85] AEF and periaortic graft infection may be difficult to differentiate because of overlapping CT features. CT findings that correlate more strongly with AEF include ectopic gas, focal bowel wall thickening, breach of the aortic wall, and active contrast extravasation into the bowel lumen.[86,87] Although CT findings can be instrumental in enabling a diagnosis of AEF, a negative CT examination does not exclude an AEF.[86]

Aortoenteric Fistula: Clinical and Imaging Features

- Most common after open aortic aneurysm repair
- Focal tethering of duodenum to aortic wall
- Ectopic gas in aortic wall/graft
- Periaortic fluid
- Duodenal wall thickening
- Contrast extravasation into bowel lumen
- Negative CT examination does not exclude AEF

SUMMARY

Acute conditions of the abdominal aorta include a wide spectrum of diseases that may have serious consequences (most notably aortic rupture) if not diagnosed promptly. Imaging plays a critical role in diagnosis because clinical presentation is often nonspecific. Although CT is the imaging method of choice for acute abdominal aortic conditions because of its speed and accessibility, MR imaging plays an important role in stable patients, particularly those for whom iodinated contrast is contraindicated. Familiarity with these acute abdominal aortic conditions, their imaging features, and the appropriate CT and MR imaging protocols can lead to timely and accurate diagnoses, resulting in optimized patient care.

REFERENCES

1. Puvaneswary M, Cuganesan R. Detection of aortoenteric fistula with helical CT. Australas Radiol 2003;47(1):67–9.
2. Siegel MJ, Hildebolt C, Bradley D. Effects of automated kilovoltage selection technology on contrast-enhanced pediatric CT and CT angiography. Radiology 2013;268(2):538–47.
3. Sommer WH, Graser A, Becker CR, et al. Image quality of virtual noncontrast images derived from dual-energy CT angiography after endovascular aneurysm repair. J Vasc Interv Radiol 2010;21(3):315–21.
4. Arko FR, Filis KA, Seidel SA, et al. How many patients with infrarenal aneurysms are candidates for endovascular repair? The Northern California experience. J Endovasc Ther 2004;11(1):33–40.
5. Armerding MD, Rubin GD, Beaulieu CF, et al. Aortic aneurysmal disease: assessment of stent-graft treatment-CT versus conventional angiography. Radiology 2000;215(1):138–46.
6. Iezzi R, Cotroneo AR. Endovascular repair of abdominal aortic aneurysms: CTA evaluation of contraindications. Abdom Imaging 2006;31(6):722–31.

7. Edelman RR, Sheehan JJ, Dunkle E, et al. Quiescent-interval single-shot unenhanced magnetic resonance angiography of peripheral vascular disease: technical considerations and clinical feasibility. Magn Reson Med 2010;63(4):951–8.

8. Klasen J, Blondin D, Schmitt P, et al. Nonenhanced ECG-gated quiescent-interval single-shot MRA (QISS-MRA) of the lower extremities: comparison with contrast-enhanced MRA. Clin Radiol 2012; 67(5):441–6.

9. Minami H, Sugimoto T, Okada M. Evaluation of acute aortic dissection by cine-MRI. Kobe J Med Sci 1999; 45(1):1–11.

10. Scott RA, Ashton HA, Kay DN. Abdominal aortic aneurysm in 4237 screened patients: prevalence, development and management over 6 years. Br J Surg 1991;78(9):1122–5.

11. Rakita D, Newatia A, Hines JJ, et al. Spectrum of CT findings in rupture and impending rupture of abdominal aortic aneurysms. Radiographics 2007; 27(2):497–507.

12. Bengtsson H, Bergqvist D, Sternby NH. Increasing prevalence of abdominal aortic aneurysms. A necropsy study. Eur J Surg 1992;158(1):19–23.

13. Assar AN, Zarins CK. Ruptured abdominal aortic aneurysm: a surgical emergency with many clinical presentations. Postgrad Med J 2009;85(1003): 268–73.

14. Bhalla S, Menias CO, Heiken JP. CT of acute abdominal aortic disorders. Radiol Clin North Am 2003; 41(6):1153–69.

15. Johansen K, Kohler TR, Nicholls SC, et al. Ruptured abdominal aortic aneurysm: the Harborview experience. J Vasc Surg 1991;13(2):240–5 [discussion: 245–7].

16. Thomas PR, Stewart RD. Abdominal aortic aneurysm. Br J Surg 1988;75(8):733–6.

17. Brewster DC, Cronenwett JL, Hallett JW Jr, et al. Guidelines for the treatment of abdominal aortic aneurysms. Report of a subcommittee of the Joint Council of the American Association for Vascular Surgery and Society for Vascular Surgery. J Vasc Surg 2003;37(5):1106–17.

18. Aggarwal S, Qamar A, Sharma V, et al. Abdominal aortic aneurysm: a comprehensive review. Exp Clin Cardiol 2011;16(1):11–5.

19. Gonsalves CF. The hyperattenuating crescent sign. Radiology 1999;211(1):37–8.

20. Siegel CL, Cohan RH, Korobkin M, et al. Abdominal aortic aneurysm morphology: CT features in patients with ruptured and nonruptured aneurysms. AJR Am J Roentgenol 1994;163(5):1123–9.

21. Mehard WB, Heiken JP, Sicard GA. High-attenuating crescent in abdominal aortic aneurysm wall at CT: a sign of acute or impending rupture. Radiology 1994; 192(2):359–62.

22. Schwartz SA, Taljanovic MS, Smyth S, et al. CT findings of rupture, impending rupture, and contained rupture of abdominal aortic aneurysms. AJR Am J Roentgenol 2007;188(1):W57–62.

23. Halliday KE, al-Kutoubi A. Draped aorta: CT sign of contained leak of aortic aneurysms. Radiology 1996;199(1):41–3.

24. Wang L, Gratz B, Peterson C, et al. Abdominal aortic aneurysm rupture: diagnostic usefulness of secondary CT signs. Radiological Society of North America 2005 scientific assembly and annual meeting. Chicago, November 27-December 2, 2005.

25. Hayashi H, Matsuoka Y, Sakamoto I, et al. Penetrating atherosclerotic ulcer of the aorta: imaging features and disease concept. Radiographics 2000;20(4):995–1005.

26. Levy JR, Heiken JP, Gutierrez FR. Imaging of penetrating atherosclerotic ulcers of the aorta. AJR Am J Roentgenol 1999;173(1):151–4.

27. Batt M, Haudebourg P, Planchard PF, et al. Penetrating atherosclerotic ulcers of the infrarenal aorta: life-threatening lesions. Eur J Vasc Endovasc Surg 2005;29(1):35–42.

28. Borioni R, Garofalo M, De Paulis R, et al. Abdominal aortic dissections: anatomic and clinical features and therapeutic options. Tex Heart Inst J 2005; 32(1):70–3.

29. Roberts CS, Roberts WC. Aortic dissection with the entrance tear in abdominal aorta. Am Heart J 1991;121(6 Pt 1):1834–5.

30. Sawhney NS, DeMaria AN, Blanchard DG. Aortic intramural hematoma: an increasingly recognized and potentially fatal entity. Chest 2001;120(4):1340–6.

31. Chao CP, Walker TG, Kalva SP. Natural history and CT appearances of aortic intramural hematoma. Radiographics 2009;29(3):791–804.

32. Sueyoshi E, Matsuoka Y, Sakamoto I, et al. Fate of intramural hematoma of the aorta: CT evaluation. J Comput Assist Tomogr 1997;21(6):931–8.

33. Nienaber CA, Richartz BM, Rehders T, et al. Aortic intramural haematoma: natural history and predictive factors for complications. Heart 2004;90(4): 372–4.

34. von Kodolitsch Y, Csosz SK, Koschyk DH, et al. Intramural hematoma of the aorta: predictors of progression to dissection and rupture. Circulation 2003;107(8):1158–63.

35. Holden A. The value of narrow CT window settings in the recognition of subtle acute aortic intramural haematoma. Australas Radiol 2000;44(1):128–9.

36. Murray JG, Manisali M, Flamm SD, et al. Intramural hematoma of the thoracic aorta: MR image findings and their prognostic implications. Radiology 1997; 204(2):349–55.

37. Rubin GD. Helical CT angiography of the thoracic aorta. J Thorac Imaging 1997;12(2):128–49.

38. Asensio JA, Chahwan S, Hanpeter D, et al. Operative management and outcome of 302 abdominal vascular injuries. Am J Surg 2000;180(6): 528–34.

39. Deree J, Shenvi E, Fortlage D, et al. Patient factors and operating room resuscitation predict mortality in traumatic abdominal aortic injury: a 20-year analysis. J Vasc Surg 2007;45(3):493–7.

40. Lopez-Viego MA, Snyder WH III, Valentine RJ, et al. Penetrating abdominal aortic trauma: a report of 129 cases. J Vasc Surg 1992;16(3):332–6.

41. Bernstein MP, Mirvis SE. Penetrating trauma to the abdominal aorta: CT demonstration of active bleeding. Emerg Radiol 2001;8(1):43–7.

42. Mellnick VM, McDowell C, Lubner M, et al. CT features of blunt abdominal aortic injury. Emerg Radiol 2012;19(4):301–7.

43. Lassonde J, Laurendeau F, Page P. Ruptured abdominal aortic aneurysm. Can J Surg 1981; 24(4):420–2.

44. Lee WA, Matsumura JS, Mitchell RS, et al. Endovascular repair of traumatic thoracic aortic injury: clinical practice guidelines of the Society for Vascular Surgery. J Vasc Surg 2011;53:187–92.

45. Osgood MJ, Heck JM, Rellinger EJ, et al. Natural history of grade I-II blunt traumatic aortic injury. J Vasc Surg 2014;59(2):334–42.

46. Surowiec SM, Isiklar H, Sreeram S, et al. Acute occlusion of the abdominal aorta. Am J Surg 1998; 176(2):193–7.

47. Leriche R, Morel A. The syndrome of thrombotic obliteration of the aortic bifurcation. Ann Surg 1948;127(2):193–206.

48. Hardman RL, Lopera JE, Cardan RA, et al. Common and rare collateral pathways in aortoiliac occlusive disease: a pictorial essay. Am J Roentgenol 2011; 197(3):W519–24.

49. Spittell PC, Seward JB, Hallett JW Jr. Mobile thrombi in the abdominal aorta in cases of lower extremity embolic arterial occlusion: value of extended transthoracic echocardiography. Am Heart J 2000;139(2 Pt 1):241–4.

50. Habib H, Hsu J, Winchell PJ, et al. Mural thrombus in the normal-appearing descending thoracic aorta of a chronic smoker. Tex Heart Inst J 2013;40(5): 619–22.

51. Lohrmann GM, Peters F. Thoracic endovascular aortic repair in a patient with mobile aortic thrombosis. Case Rep Vasc Med 2014;2014:4.

52. Weyand CM, Goronzy JJ. Medium- and large-vessel vasculitis. N Engl J Med 2003;349(2):160–9.

53. Chung JW, Kim H-C, Choi YH, et al. Patterns of aortic involvement in Takayasu arteritis and its clinical implications: evaluation with spiral computed tomography angiography. J Vasc Surg 2007;45(5): 906–14.

54. Matsunaga N, Hayashi K, Sakamoto I, et al. Takayasu arteritis: protean radiologic manifestations and diagnosis. Radiographics 1997;17(3):579–94.

55. Nastri MV, Baptista LPS, Baroni RH, et al. Gadolinium-enhanced three-dimensional MR angiography of Takayasu arteritis. Radiographics 2004;24(3): 773–86.

56. Papathanasiou ND, Du Y, Menezes LJ, et al. (18) F-Fludeoxyglucose PET/CT in the evaluation of large-vessel vasculitis: diagnostic performance and correlation with clinical and laboratory parameters. Br J Radiol 2012;85(1014):e188–94.

57. Hellmann DB, Grand DJ, Freischlag JA. Inflammatory abdominal aortic aneurysm. JAMA 2007; 297(4):395–400.

58. Pennell RC, Hollier LH, Lie JT, et al. Inflammatory abdominal aortic aneurysms: a thirty-year review. J Vasc Surg 1985;2(6):859–69.

59. Hill J, Charlesworth D. Inflammatory abdominal aortic aneurysms: a report of thirty-seven cases. Ann Vasc Surg 1988;2(4):352–7.

60. Tang T, Boyle JR, Dixon AK, et al. Inflammatory abdominal aortic aneurysms. Eur J Vasc Endovasc Surg 2005;29(4):353–62.

61. Parums DV. The spectrum of chronic periaortitis. Histopathology 1990;16(5):423–31.

62. Parums DV, Chadwick DR, Mitchinson MJ. The localisation of immunoglobulin in chronic periaortitis. Atherosclerosis 1986;61(2):117–23.

63. Kasashima S, Zen Y. IgG4-related inflammatory abdominal aortic aneurysm. Curr Opin Rheumatol 2011;23(1):18–23.

64. Kasashima S, Zen Y, Kawashima A, et al. A new clinicopathological entity of IgG4-related inflammatory abdominal aortic aneurysm. J Vasc Surg 2009; 49(5):1264–71 [discussion: 1271].

65. Kasashima S, Zen Y, Kawashima A, et al. Inflammatory abdominal aortic aneurysm: close relationship to IgG4-related periaortitis. Am J Surg Pathol 2008; 32(2):197–204.

66. Sakata N, Tashiro T, Uesugi N, et al. IgG4-positive plasma cells in inflammatory abdominal aortic aneurysm: the possibility of an aortic manifestation of IgG4-related sclerosing disease. Am J Surg Pathol 2008;32(4):553–9.

67. Walker DI, Bloor K, Williams G, et al. Inflammatory aneurysms of the abdominal aorta. Br J Surg 1972; 59(8):609–14.

68. Iino M, Kuribayashi S, Imakita S, et al. Sensitivity and specificity of CT in the diagnosis of inflammatory abdominal aortic aneurysms. J Comput Assist Tomogr 2002;26(6):1006–12.

69. Cronin CG, Lohan DG, Blake MA, et al. Retroperitoneal fibrosis: a review of clinical features and imaging findings. Am J Roentgenol 2008;191(2): 423–31.

70. Orta Kilickesmez K, Kilickesmez O. Clear depiction of inflammatory abdominal aortic aneurysm with diffusion-weighted magnetic resonance imaging. Cardiovasc Intervent Radiol 2010;33(2):379–82.

71. Degesys GE, Dunnick NR, Silverman PM, et al. Retroperitoneal fibrosis: use of CT in distinguishing among possible causes. AJR Am J Roentgenol 1986;146(1):57–60.

72. Blockmans D, Van Moer E, Dehem J, et al. Positron emission tomography can reveal abdominal periaortitis. Clin Nucl Med 2002;27(3):211–2.

73. Brown SL, Busuttil RW, Baker JD, et al. Bacteriologic and surgical determinants of survival in patients with mycotic aneurysms. J Vasc Surg 1984;1(4):541–7.

74. Johnson JR, Ledgerwood AM, Lucas CE. Mycotic aneurysm. New concepts in therapy. Arch Surg 1983;118(5):577–82.

75. Marques da Silva R, Caugant DA, Eribe ER, et al. Bacterial diversity in aortic aneurysms determined by 16S ribosomal RNA gene analysis. J Vasc Surg 2006;44(5):1055–60.

76. Jaffer U, Gibbs R. Mycotic thoracoabdominal aneurysms. Ann Cardiothorac Surg 2012;1(3):417–25.

77. Gonda RL Jr, Gutierrez OH, Azodo MV. Mycotic aneurysms of the aorta: radiologic features. Radiology 1988;168(2):343–6.

78. Gomes MN, Choyke PL. Infected aortic aneurysms: CT diagnosis. J Cardiovasc Surg 1992;33(6):684–9.

79. Macedo TA, Stanson AW, Oderich GS, et al. Infected aortic aneurysms: imaging findings. Radiology 2004;231(1):250–7.

80. Vogelzang RL, Sohaey R. Infected aortic aneurysms: CT appearance. J Comput Assist Tomogr 1988;12(1):109–12.

81. Kan C-D, Lee H-L, Yang Y-J. Outcome after endovascular stent graft treatment for mycotic aortic aneurysm: a systematic review. J Vasc Surg 2007; 46(5):906–12.

82. Rucker CM, Menias CO, Bhalla S, et al. *Clostridium septicum* infrarenal aortitis secondary to occult cecal adenocarcinoma. AJR Am J Roentgenol 2004;183(5):1316–8.

83. Vu QD, Menias CO, Bhalla S, et al. Aortoenteric fistulas: CT features and potential mimics. Radiographics 2009;29(1):197–209.

84. Peck JJ, Eidemiller LR. Aortoenteric fistulas. Arch Surg 1992;127(10):1191–3 [discussion: 1193–4].

85. Pickhardt PJ, Bhalla S, Balfe DM. Acquired gastrointestinal fistulas: classification, etiologies, and imaging evaluation. Radiology 2002;224(1):9–23.

86. Hughes FM, Kavanagh D, Barry M, et al. Aortoenteric fistula: a diagnostic dilemma. Abdom Imaging 2007;32(3):398–402.

87. Low RN, Wall SD, Jeffrey RB Jr, et al. Aortoenteric fistula and perigraft infection: evaluation with CT. Radiology 1990;175(1):157–62.

Bowel Obstruction

Richard M. Gore, MD*, Robert I. Silvers, MD, Kiran H. Thakrar, MD,
Daniel R. Wenzke, MD, Uday K. Mehta, MD, Geraldine M. Newmark, MD,
Jonathan W. Berlin, MD

KEYWORDS

- Small bowel obstruction • Large bowel obstruction • Bowel ischemia • Bowel strangulation
- Closed loop obstruction • Volvulus • Intussusception

KEY POINTS

- Mechanical bowel obstruction is responsible for 15% of hospital admissions for the acute abdomen in the United States.
- Clinical features and plain abdominal radiographic findings are insufficiently accurate for the diagnosis of intestinal obstruction and its complications, such as ischemia and strangulation.
- Multidetector computed tomography has emerged as the best single imaging examination for the diagnosis of mechanical bowel obstruction and its complications and can help triage patients to either conservative or operative management.

INTRODUCTION

Mechanical bowel obstruction comprises 15% of all emergency admissions for abdominal pain and constitutes more than 300,000 admissions annually in the United States.[1] It is an important cause of morbidity and mortality, responsible for nearly 30,000 deaths and direct costs of more than $3 billion in medical care annually.[2] The clinical diagnosis of bowel obstruction can be challenging because results of physical examination, clinical presentation, and laboratory values are often nonspecific and nondiagnostic.

Small bowel obstruction (SBO) and large bowel obstruction (LBO) account for approximately 20% of cases of acute abdominal surgical conditions.[1,2] There are a number causes and degrees of bowel obstruction (Box 1, Fig. 1, Table 1) and the role of the radiologist is to answer several key questions: Is obstruction present? What is the level of the obstruction? What is the cause of the obstruction? What is the severity of the obstruction? Is the obstruction simple or closed loop? Is strangulation, ischemia, or perforation present?[3] In this presentation, the radiologic approach to and imaging findings of patients with known or suspected bowel obstruction are presented.

PATHOPHYSIOLOGY

Bowel obstruction causes distention of the gut through the accumulation of both gas and fluid. The gas that accumulates proximal to the obstruction is primarily swallowed air, reflected by its high nitrogen content (70%–80%) and the contribution of bacterial gas is thought to be small. The fluid and gas cause increased intraluminal pressure and distention of the bowel that also affect the motility of the intestine: initially causing increased peristalsis and then leading to decreased peristalsis and relaxation.

This decrease in motility and stasis caused by the obstruction itself promote bacterial overgrowth, markedly increasing the normally low levels of both gram-negative enteric and anaerobic organisms found in the small intestine. Obstruction leads to increased translocation of bacteria and endotoxins to both mesenteric lymph nodes and

Department of Radiology, Evanston Hospital, North Shore University Health System, 2650 Ridge Avenue, Evanston, IL 60201, USA
* Corresponding author.
E-mail address: rgore@uchicago.edu

Radiol Clin N Am 53 (2015) 1225–1240
http://dx.doi.org/10.1016/j.rcl.2015.06.008
0033-8389/15/$ – see front matter © 2015 Elsevier Inc. All rights reserved.

Box 1
Causes of intestinal obstruction

Extrinsic bowel lesions
Adhesions
Hernias
Volvulus
Carcinomatosis
Abscess
Endometriosis

Intrinsic bowel lesions
Inflammatory
   Diverticulitis
   Appendicitis
   Inflammatory bowel disease
Intussusception
Ischemic
Radiation injury
Chemical
Postanastomotic
Obturation
   Polypoid neoplasms
   Gallstones
   Foreign bodies
   Bezoars

Table 1
Classification of mechanical bowel obstruction

Classification	Division
Etiology	Intraluminal Intramural Extrinsic
Location	Small bowel (proximal or distal) Colon
Speed of onset	Acute Subacute Chronic
Degree	Partial Complete
Progression	Open vs closed loop Simple vs strangulated

obstruction in which both the afferent and efferent limbs of an obstructed segment of bowel are occluded. The intraluminal pressure rises rapidly, impairing first the venous drainage and then the arterial supply to the bowel wall. Ischemia and gangrene of the bowel permit the escape of enteric organisms and their toxins into the portal and systemic circulation, adding to the clinical picture of sepsis.[1–4]

The cecum has the largest diameter of the gastrointestinal (GI) tract, and therefore its wall develops the highest tension according to the Laplace law (wall tension = intraluminal pressure × radius). The increased pressure may cause separation of the muscle fibers, leading to cecal "diastatic" perforation. Dissection of air into the wall results in pneumatosis, which may precede frank perforation. The risk of perforation increases when the cecum reaches a diameter of 9 cm. The duration and rapidity of onset of the distention are also important. The intraluminal pressure needed to produce perforation is between 20 and 55 mm Hg. Ischemia and bacterial overgrowth also play a role in GI tract perforation

possibly the systemic circulation, which may be responsible for some of the systemic septic consequences of bowel obstruction.[1–4]

With continued bowel obstruction, if the intraluminal pressure continues to rise, perfusion of the bowel wall may be impaired, which promotes the development of ischemia, necrosis, and perforation. This most commonly occurs in closed loop

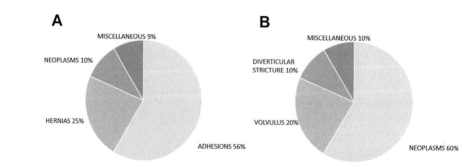

Fig. 1. Causes of bowel obstruction. (*A*) Leading causes of SBO. (*B*) Leading causes of LBO.

and the systemic effects seen with strangulating obstruction.[4]

Simple obstruction implies that the lumen is partially or completely occluded, but that blood flow is preserved. *Strangulation* or *strangulated obstruction* means that blood flow is compromised, leading to bowel wall edema, intestinal ischemia, and, if left untreated, necrosis and perforation. A simple obstruction can be *complete* (ie, no fluid or gas passes beyond the site of obstruction) or *incomplete* (ie, some fluid and gas does pass beyond the site of obstruction). In *open loop obstruction*, intestinal flow is blocked distally, but the proximal loops are *open* and can be decompressed by vomiting or nasogastric intubation. In *closed loop obstruction*, both flow into and flow out of the closed loop are blocked, resulting in progressive accumulation of fluid and gas within the isolated loop, placing it at risk for ischemia, volvulus, and perforation.[3,4]

CLINICAL FEATURES

The cardinal symptoms of bowel obstruction are pain, nausea and vomiting, abdominal distension, and decreased stool and flatus. The pain is classically colicky in nature, reflecting increased peristaltic activity as the bowel distends in response to the obstruction. The initial increase in motility is later replaced by reduced activity as the bowel relaxes and dilates, so the colicky pain may be replaced by a more constant pain. If the obstruction is more proximal, the pain may be relieved by vomiting.[5,6]

The pain of simple obstruction often increases slowly and may remain constant in severity. In closed loop obstruction, the pain may continue to increase until the bowel perforates. There then may be a brief paradoxic decrease in the pain as the distention is relieved, until the signs of peritonitis develop. Pain out of proportion to physical examination suggests strangulation.[5-7]

Nausea and vomiting are common symptoms, with vomiting being more likely and profuse the more proximal the obstruction. Abdominal distension is more pronounced the more distal the obstruction. LBO typically produces significant distention, whereas SBO may produce less distention due to decompressive vomiting.[5,6]

The final symptom of bowel obstruction is decreased passage of flatus and stool. The lack of liquid or solid stool is less specific because the bowel distal to the obstruction may continue to produce mucous and other secretions and the colon may contain an appreciable amount of fecal material that may continue to pass for some time.[5,6]

RADIOLOGIC EVALUATION OF BOWEL OBSTRUCTION
Plain Abdominal Radiographs

The plain radiograph of the abdomen has traditionally been used as the first radiologic study in the workup of acute abdominal pain and suspected bowel obstruction (**Box 2**). These radiographs may confirm the diagnosis, locate the site of obstruction, and, in some cases, identify the nature of the obstructing lesion. The bowel is usually dilated proximal to the obstruction; however, depending on the competency of the ileocecal valve, proximal LBO can mimic SBO (**Fig. 2**).[8]

Air-fluid levels may traverse the entire lumen of the obstructed bowel loops or be trapped as bubbles between folds at the top of a fluid-filled bowel loop, resulting in a "string of pearls" sign (**Fig. 3**). Fluid-filled loops may not be seen on supine radiographs but may be recognized on erect or cross-table lateral decubitus radiographs.[8] Plain abdominal radiographs have only a moderate sensitivity of between 40% and 80% for the diagnosis of SBO.[8-10]

A gasless abdomen can be seen in the setting of bowel obstruction and ischemia in which the gut is completely filled with fluid (**Fig. 4**). Fluid-filled loops may not be visible, leading to a false-

---

Box 2
Plain radiographic and computed tomography (CT) findings in bowel obstruction

Small bowel obstruction

1. Dilated gas or fluid-filled small bowel: greater than 3 cm (KUB), greater than 2.5 cm CT

2. Air-fluid levels greater than 2.5 cm

3. Air-fluid levels at disparate levels within the same loop

4. String of pearls sign

5. Gastric distension

6. Small bowel dilated out of proportion to colon

7. Paucity of colorectal gas

8. Gasless abdomen

Large bowel obstruction

1. Colonic distension

2. Colon collapsed beyond obstruction

3. Small bowel dilation depending on the duration of the obstruction and the competency of the ileocecal valve

Abbreviation: KUB, Plain abdominal radiograph.

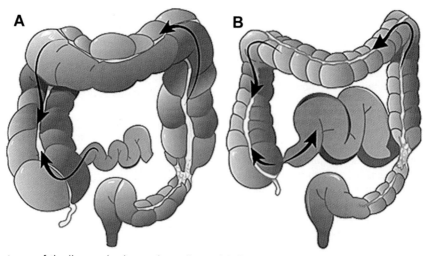

Fig. 2. Importance of the ileocecal valve to the radiographic findings of LBO. (*A*) If the ileocecal valve is competent, pronounced right side colonic distention can occur. (*B*) An incompetent ileocecal valve allows retrograde decompression of gas and fluid into the small bowel that can simulate an SBO.

negative diagnosis or erroneous interpretation of the level of obstruction.[11] Plain abdominal radiographs are poor at suggesting the diagnosis of closed loop, ischemic, or strangulating obstruction.

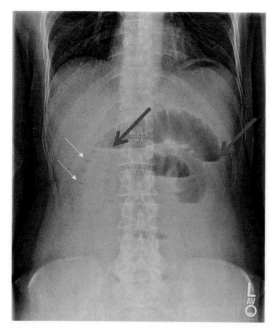

Fig. 3. High-grade distal SBO due to adhesive disease. Upright plain abdominal radiograph shows air-fluid levels at different levels within the same loop (*red arrows*). Portions of the predominantly fluid-filled obstructed small bowel may show only small gas bubbles, producing the so called "string of pearls" appearance (*yellow arrows*).

Plain abdominal radiographs are helpful in the diagnosis of cecal and sigmoid volvulus (**Fig. 5**).

Intraluminal Contrast Material

Positive oral contrast material is not essential in the diagnosis of obstruction on computed tomography (CT) because the intraluminal fluid and gas already present within the obstructed bowel serve as excellent contrast agents. If positive oral contrast material has been given in patients with SBO, a delayed abdominal radiograph can assess if the contrast material has progressed to the colon, indicating partial obstruction.

Computed Tomography

By virtue of its ability to provide a global perspective of the gut, vasculature, mesenteries, omenta, peritoneum, retroperitoneum, and subperitoneum, multidetector CT (MDCT) has become the imaging modality of choice in patients with known or suspected obstruction. CT is most valuable when there are systemic signs suggesting infection, bowel infarction, or an associated palpable mass. CT identifies bowel obstruction as distended bowel loops (>2.5–3 cm) seen proximal to collapsed loops and can reveal the cause of obstruction, such as tumor, volvulus, appendicitis (**Fig. 6**A), or diverticulitis (see **Fig. 6**B). The transition zone should be carefully evaluated for masses.[12–21]

CT can accurately predict the etiology of obstruction in 70% to 95% of patients and can often suggest superimposed ischemia and intestinal perforation.[22,23] The CT finding of pneumatosis

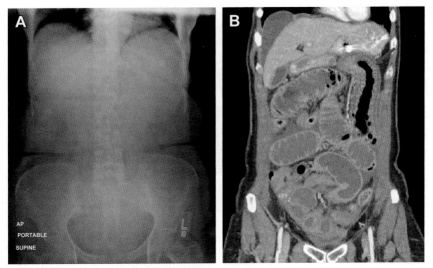

Fig. 4. Gasless abdomen in the setting of high-grade SBO and bowel ischemia. (*A*) Plain abdominal radiograph shows a gasless abdomen. (*B*) Coronal reformatted CT images obtained several hours later demonstrates distended and fluid-filled bowel. Note the mesenteric fluid and ascites. The mural thickening with submucosal edema of one jejunal loop (*arrow*) is suspicious for ischemia.

(**Fig. 7**) indicates breakdown in the mucosal integrity of the bowel wall and is strongly suggestive of ischemia; however, the CT finding of pneumatosis does not always predict irreversible ischemia at surgery. The CT findings of free intraperitoneal gas or portomesenteric gas have a much greater likelihood of irreversible transmural necrosis than pneumatosis alone.[22,23]

Ultrasonography and MR imaging

Although CT is the best overall examination for evaluating patients with suspected bowel obstruction, it uses ionizing radiation. Accordingly, in children (**Fig. 8**) and pregnant women, ultrasonography and MR imaging should be considered as an alternative examination for evaluating these patients.[24]

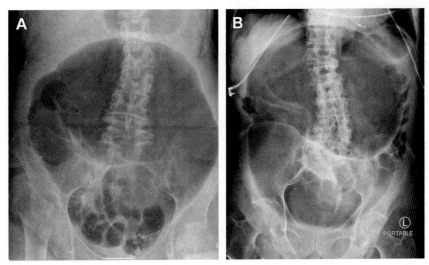

Fig. 5. Colonic volvulus: plain abdominal radiographic features. (*A*) Cecal volvulus. The dilated cecum, which extends to the left of the midline, produces a coffee-beanlike appearance with its hilum directed toward the right lower quadrant. (*B*) Sigmoid volvulus. There is massive distension of the sigmoid colon that extends superiorly to the diaphragm, the so called "northern exposure sign."

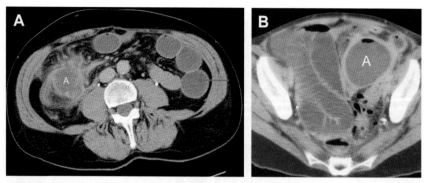

Fig. 6. Infectious-inflammatory causes of bowel obstruction: CT features. (*A*) Appendicitis with abscess (*A*) formation causing SBO (*arrow*). (*B*) Diverticulitis of the sigmoid colon with abscess (*A*) formation and associated SBO.

SMALL BOWEL OBSTRUCTION
Adhesions

Adhesions are the most common cause of SBO, accounting for approximately two-thirds of cases. The incidence of SBO from adhesions has increased during the past 30 years because of the increasing number of laparotomies. Although adhesions form in more than 90% of patients who have undergone laparotomy, only approximately 5% of abdominopelvic surgeries are complicated by SBO. They develop in 0.05% of

patients with cesarean delivery, in 1% of patients after appendectomy, and up to 10% of patients who have had colorectal surgery. Ten percent to 15% of adhesions are attributed to previous or concurrent inflammation. A small fraction of adhesions are thought to be congenital in origin.[1,5]

Approximately 1% of patients will develop an SBO in the immediate postoperative period. Approximately 90% of these early postoperative obstructions are caused by adhesions, 7% by hernias, and the remainder are related to abscess formation, intussusception, or technical factors.[1,5]

The most important radiographic finding in the diagnosis of SBO is the abrupt transition from dilated to nondilated small intestine at the site of obstruction. Adhesions are not usually seen on CT. The small bowel feces sign (**Fig. 9**) is often seen proximal to the point of obstruction.[25,26]

The CT diagnosis of adhesions is a diagnosis of exclusion: there is an abrupt transition from dilated to collapsed small intestine without apparent

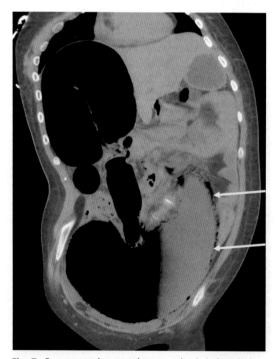

Fig. 7. Pneumatosis secondary to colonic ischemia in a patient with sigmoid volvulus. Coronal reformatted CT scan shows a markedly distended sigmoid colon with pneumatosis (*arrows*).

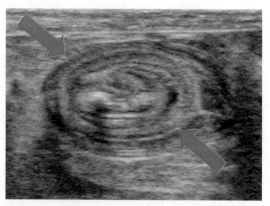

Fig. 8. Intussusception: sonographic findings in an infant. Transverse sonogram reveals a mass (*arrows*) with a swirled appearance of multiple alternating hyperechoic and hypoechoic small bowel loops producing the loop within a loop or target appearance.

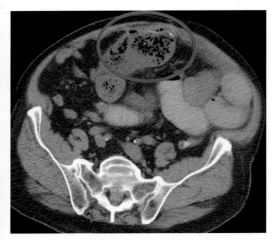

Fig. 9. Adhesive disease causing SBO. Axial CT image shows SBO with the small bowel feces sign (*circle*) due to adhesive disease at the anastomosis in this patient with previous small bowel resection.

cause. The transition zone may appear rounded or beaklike. Other abnormalities can cause a transition zone without apparent cause on CT, including small primary tumors, such as carcinoid tumor; small intraperitoneal metastases; and short inflammatory, ischemic, or drug-related strictures. The CT diagnosis of adhesion is supported by a history of previous laparotomy in the absence of a history of a tumor with a predilection for peritoneal spread (eg, ovarian carcinoma) or a known history of inflammatory bowel disease. The CT diagnosis of adhesions is accurate in 70% to 95% of patients.[27,28]

In one study of adhesion-related SBO, an anterior parietal adhesion, the presence of a small bowel feces sign, and the lack of a beak sign were associated with successful nonsurgical treatment, whereas 2 beak signs or more, a whirl sign, a C-shaped or U-shaped appearance of the bowel loop, and a high degree of obstruction were associated with nonsurgical treatment failure.[27]

In another study, when intraperitoneal fluid, high-grade or complete obstruction, mesenteric fatty stranding, and an absent small bowel feces sign were present, MDCT had a high sensitivity of 98.4% and specificity of 90.9% for the predicting the need for surgery.[28]

Closed Loop Obstruction and Strangulation

The most common causes of closed loop obstruction are single adhesive bands, internal or external hernias, or rents in the mesentery. The trapped loop or loops become progressively dilated and fluid-filled. The vessels feeding the trapped intestine may be compressed by the band or hernia

orifice or occluded by twisting of the mesentery; either process resulting in strangulation. Both dilatation and the risk of strangulation of the trapped-loops depend on the stage and degree of compression or twisting.[29]

The radiographic findings (**Boxes 3** and **4**) of strangulation vary depending on the level of trapping and twisting. Initially, the closed loop may not be dilated. In the usual patient, however, the closed loop is dilated and fluid-filled, with little or no intraluminal gas. If the closed loop(s) are parallel to the plane of reconstruction on CT, they appear in a C-shaped or U-shaped configuration. If the loops are imaged perpendicular to the plane of reconstruction, they appear in a radial configuration, with the trapped mesentery pointing toward the band or hernia opening (**Fig. 10**). The loops that enter and exit the closed loop lay side by side and are narrowed or tapered at the level of the band or mesenteric rent. The entry or exit site may have a beaklike appearance when imaged in cross-section. Small intestine proximal to the closed loop may be dilated and fluid-filled, whereas the small intestine distal to the closed loop is collapsed. The mesenteric vessels radiate to the point of obstruction.[28–32]

With a strangulated obstruction, there is a continuum from bowel wall edema, to mild to moderate ischemia, to transmural infarction, and finally, to perforation. CT has a sensitivity of approximately 80% to 90% in the diagnosis of strangulation in patients with closed loop obstruction. CT may reveal circumferential bowel wall thickening of low, normal, or high attenuation. Following intravenous contrast material administration, the obstructed segment of bowel may be normal or have increased thickness and may show normal enhancement, delayed enhancement, diminished enhancement, or no enhancement. On unenhanced CT scans, high-attenuation bowel wall

---

Box 3
CT findings of closed-loop obstruction ischemia

1. C-shaped, U-shaped, or coffee bean configuration of the bowel loop with converging toward the site of torsion

2. Beak or whirl sign at the site of obstruction

3. Radial configuration of bowel loops when vertically oriented

4. Convergence of mesenteric vessels to a single point

5. Close proximity of afferent and efferent limbs, often at the site of mesenteric convergence

Box 4
CT findings of bowel ischemia

1. Circumferential mural thickening >3 mm
2. Target or halo sign (submucosal edema)
3. Focal loss of mural enhancement (impaired arterial flow)
4. Persistent mural enhancement (impaired venous outflow)
5. Mural hemorrhage or haziness on NCCT
6. Pneumatosis
7. Perforation

Abbreviation: NCCT, Non contrast CT scan.

thickening implies hemorrhage with ischemia. Diminished or lack of contrast enhancement (**Fig. 11**) is very suspicious for vascular compromise.[22,29–32]

A mural stratification pattern (see **Fig. 4**B) with low attenuation of the submucosa, reflecting submucosal edema, may indicate a spectrum of pathology ranging from bowel wall edema to full-thickness infarction. Pneumatosis (see **Fig. 7**) in the wall of the closed loop indicates a rent in the mucosa and strangulation. Sloughed mucosa or debris in lumen may have the appearance of feces. If the closed loop is twisted, its mesentery also will appear twisted or whirled. Fluid in the leaves of the small bowel mesentery (see **Figs. 10**B and **11**B) is suggestive but not specific for ischemia, because intraperitoneal fluid can occur in simple SBOs. However, strangulation is implied by haziness of the mesenteric fat (**Fig. 12**) and large mesenteric vessels, findings reflecting mesenteric edema and venous engorgement, respectively, related to compression or twisting of mesenteric vessels.[22,29–32]

Volvulus is implied by twisting of the folds at the point of obstruction. Smooth, thick valvulae conniventes in a partially closed loop imply edema with possible ischemia.[33]

Hernias

Hernias occur at predictable sites of weakness in the abdominal wall where there is only fascia and peritoneum between the viscera and skin. A wide variety of internal hernias occur at sites of mesenteric and omental weakness, normal openings of the peritoneal surface, or under adhesive or congenital bands. Before the era of laparotomy, hernias were the most common cause of SBO.[34]

Inguinal hernias (**Fig. 13**) comprise approximately 80% of anterior abdominal wall hernias; femoral hernias comprise only approximately 5%. Inguinal hernias are more common in men than women (7:1), whereas femoral hernias are more common in women than men (1.8:1). Most patients with an inguinal hernia have a patent processus vaginalis as the cause of the inguinal hernia. These hernias usually result from elevated abdominal pressure related to pregnancy, coughing, constipation, obesity, prostatism, or physical exertion. Inguinal hernias may be caused by weakening of muscular aponeurosis and fascia due to age, cigarette smoking, or collagen deficiency.[3,34]

Weakness in the linea alba at the umbilicus leads to *umbilical/paraumbilical hernia*. Most pediatric umbilical hernias close spontaneously, but persistent umbilical hernias may require surgery.

Epigastric hernias also occur in defects in the linea alba. These hernias are more frequent in men. Multiple hernias are seen in 20% of patients. Epigastric hernias usually contain incarcerated preperitoneal fat and do not contain a peritoneal sac. Gastric herniation is uncommon.[3,34]

Complications in *parastomal hernias* are uncommon. However, peritoneal herniation develops in more than 50% of patients who have had a colostomy for at least 5 years.[3,34]

Spigelian hernias occur below the line of Spigel (semilunar line) because the junction of the rectus abdominis and lateral flank muscles is weak owing to the lateral abdominal wall muscle aponeurosis passing only anterior to the rectus. A Spigelian hernia is usually small (1–2 cm) and intraparietal,

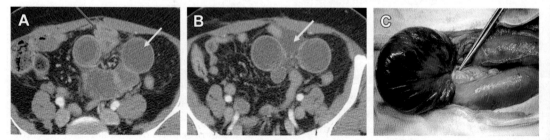

Fig. 10. Closed loop obstruction. (*A*) Axial CT shows distended small bowel loops with mural thickening (*yellow arrow*) converging to the exit and entry site (*red arrow*). (*B*) There is fluid (*arrow*) in the adjacent mesentery very suspicious for ischemia. (*C*) By the time of surgery, this bowel had become necrotic.

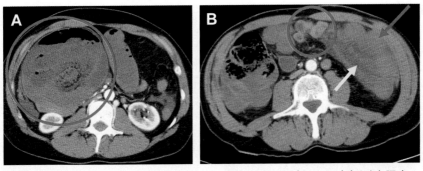

Fig. 11. Closed loop obstruction with ischemia due to internal hernias: CT features. (*A*) Axial CT shows a cluster of poorly enhancing (*circle*) jejunal loops in a right paraduodenal internal hernia. Note the twisted, edematous mesentery. (*B*) CT shows clustering of small bowel loops (*circle*) entering and exiting a transomental hernia. Note the thickened, poorly enhancing jejunal loops in the hernia sac (*red arrow*) and the hemorrhage in the small bowel mesentery (*yellow arrow*).

rarely penetrating the fascia of the external oblique muscle. Spigelian hernias contain omentum, small bowel, or colon. Incarceration and strangulation are common complications.[3,34]

CT and barium studies may reveal smooth, tapered compression of the bowel loops entering and exiting the hernia, with the degree of narrowing determined by the width of the luminal opening. Dilatation of the small bowel proximal to the hernia indicates obstruction at the entry site due to compression or twisting. Dilatation of loops with the hernia itself suggests obstruction at the outflow loop.[3,4,34]

Internal hernias

Internal hernias are becoming increasingly common and are well-described complications of gastric bypass surgery and liver transplantation. Roux-en-Y laparoscopic gastric bypass surgery predisposes to 3 major types of internal hernias: transmesocolic (through the defect in the transverse mesocolon made when performing a retrocolic anastomosis), retroanastomotic (**Fig. 14**) (behind the jejunal-jejunal anastomosis), and Petersen defect (behind the Roux loop).[30]

In transmesocolic internal hernias, CT shows multiple clumped jejunal loops superior to the transverse mesocolon between the stomach and

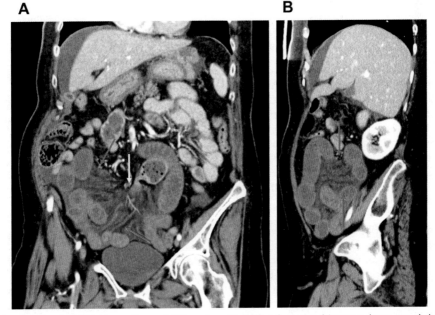

Fig. 12. Ischemic bowel: CT features. Coronal (*A*) and sagittal (*B*) reformatted images show mural thickening of obstructed bowel with mesenteric edema (*arrows*).

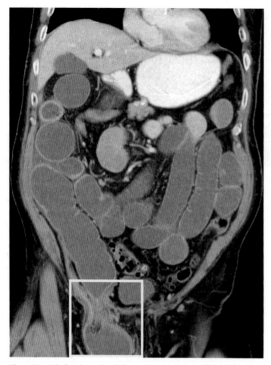

Fig. 13. Right inguinal hernia causing SBO. Coronal reformatted image shows an indirect inguinal hernia (*square*) causing distal ileal obstruction.

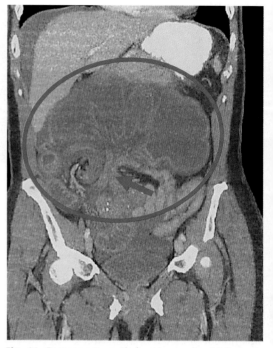

Fig. 14. Retroanastomotic hernia causing high-grade proximal SBO in a patient who had undergone a prior Roux-en-Y gastric bypass procedure. Coronal reformatted CT image demonstrates distended jejunum with a mushroom shape (*circle*). The stem (*arrow*) of the mushroom shows the mesenteric defect that allows the hernia to develop.

spleen, a high position of the distal jejunal anastomosis, an ascending course of tightly clustered vessels in the jejunal mesentery, and a dilated efferent jejunal loop. On CT, Petersen defect hernias show mesenteric swirling associated with a mushroom shape of the mesentery.[30]

Extrinsic Tumors of the Mesentery and Omentum

A variety of neoplastic, inflammatory, or vascular extraluminal masses may cause SBO. These masses compress the bowel lumen and distort the lumen by a desmoplastic reaction involving the mesentery and peritoneal surfaces of the bowel. Spread of inflammation from appendicitis (see **Fig. 6**A) or diverticulitis (see **Fig. 6**B) can secondarily affect the small bowel. The inflammatory process may cause an adynamic ileus or SBO.[3]

Carcinomatosis involving the small bowel mesentery is most frequently caused by ovarian carcinoma (**Fig. 15**) in women and by carcinomas arising from organs adjacent to the peritoneum (including stomach, pancreas, colon, and liver) in men and women. Carcinomatosis is frequently multifocal, occurring at dependent sites in the peritoneal cavity in which ascitic fluid accumulates,

including the mesenteric border of the distal ileum, medial base of the cecum, sigmoid mesentery, pararectal fossae, and rectovesical or rectouterine space. CT may demonstrate ascites or peritoneal implants on the surface of the liver, peritoneum, omentum, or mesentery. CT may also reveal the underlying malignant tumor responsible for the ascites.[3]

Carcinoid tumors, mycobacterial infection, and desmoid tumors may mimic intraperitoneal metastases. Metastases or lymphoma in retroperitoneal lymph nodes may secondarily infiltrate the small bowel mesentery, causing SBO. Retroperitoneal nodal invasion also may resemble intraperitoneal metastases, with mass effect and desmoplastic tethering of the adjacent bowel.[3]

Primary Small Bowel Tumors

Adenocarcinoma of the small intestine has a predilection for the second to fourth portions of the duodenum and the proximal jejunum. When patients with small bowel adenocarcinoma present with clinical signs of obstruction, these tumors are almost always at an advanced stage.

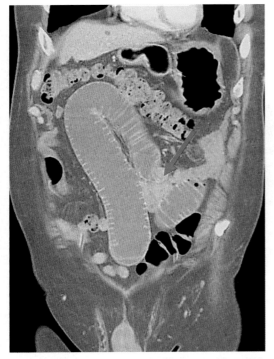

Fig. 15. Recurrent ovarian carcinoma causing SBO. Coronal reformatted CT scan shows a solid serosal tumor implant (*arrow*) causing the bowel obstruction.

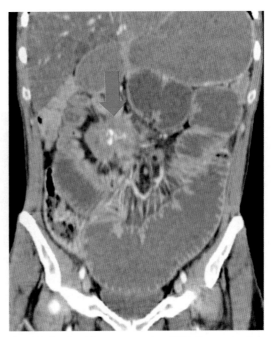

Fig. 16. Carcinoid tumor causing SBO. Coronal reformatted CT scan demonstrates a partially calcified, speculated mesenteric mass (*arrow*) that is causing ileal obstruction.

Small carcinoid tumors typically appear as smooth-surfaced submucosal masses 1 to 2 cm in diameter. Once carcinoid tumors infiltrate the deep layers of the small bowel wall or the adjacent mesentery, however, they may be indistinguishable from intraperitoneal metastases. CT (**Fig. 16**) demonstration of a large central mesenteric nodal metastasis (with calcification in 50%) is virtually diagnostic of carcinoid tumor.[3]

Crohn Disease

Fibrostenotic Crohn disease (**Fig. 17**) may cause recurrent episodes of partial SBO. Although high-grade obstructions are uncommon, SBO is the most frequent indication for surgery in patients with Crohn disease. Severe luminal narrowing has been termed "the string sign." Obstruction is diagnosed on barium studies or CT by delayed passage of contrast medium through the diseased segment with proximal small bowel dilatation.[35,36]

Intraluminal Causes

Gallstones, bezoars, foreign bodies, meconium, and tangles of Ascaris worms may obturate the small bowel and less commonly the colonic lumen, causing obstruction. Gallstone-induced SBO (**Fig. 18**), also known as gallstone ileus,

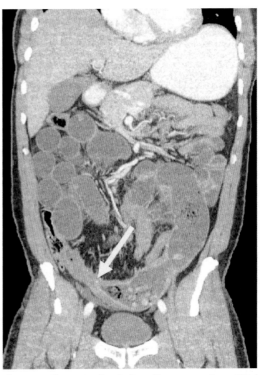

Fig. 17. Fibrostenotic Crohn disease causing distal SBO. Coronal reformatted CT image shows mural thickening and lumen narrowing of the distal ileum (*arrow*).

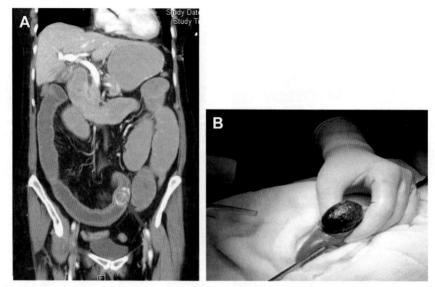

Fig. 18. Gallstone ileus. (*A*) There is a lamellated, calcified obstructing gallstone (*arrow*) identified on this coronal reformatted CT image. (*B*) The stone was surgically removed through a small bowel enterotomy.

usually occurs in elderly patients, especially women. A gallstone can erode through the wall of the gallbladder or bile duct into the small bowel or colon. Most fistulas extend from the gallbladder fossa to the duodenum. Passage of gallstones through the gastrointestinal tracts may result in large gallstones becoming trapped in the narrowest segments of bowel: the terminal ileum and sigmoid colon. The classic Rigler triad of a calcified gallstone, gas in a shrunken gallbladder or biliary tract, and SBO is seen in only a minority of patients on plain radiographs, but is better depicted on CT.[37]

Intussusception

Various extrinsic, intrinsic, and intraluminal processes result in small bowel intussusception. A loop of small intestine with part of its mesentery invaginates into the lumen of the bowel segment distal to it. The inner, advancing segment is termed the *intussusceptum* and the outer receiving segment the *intussuscipiens*. Most intussusceptions are nonobstructive, transient intussusceptions without a lead-point that are detected on abdominal CT performed for other reasons. Nonobstructive, transient intussusceptions also are seen in small bowel disorders associated with dysmotility, such as scleroderma or celiac disease.[38]

Benign or malignant polypoid tumors are the most common causes of small bowel intussusception in adults presenting with SBO. In postoperative patients, intussusceptions may be related to suture lines, adhesions, or intestinal tubes.[3,39]

If the intussusception is of the ileocolic or colocolic variety, the pathognomonic "crescent" sign may be seen. This sign is produced when the intussuscipiens invaginates into the intussusceptum and stretches the outer wall. Intraluminal gas trapped between the 2 intestinal surfaces can appear as a semilunar lucency lacking haustral septa or valvulae conniventes. This lucent crescent is wider than normal bowel in diameter and often superimposed on a round soft tissue density representing the mass created by the intussusception. A more central and less distinct lucency may be seen, representing gas trapped in the lumen of the intussuscipiens.[3]

On CT, intussusceptions appear as 3 different patterns, which reflect their severity and duration: (1) the "target" sign (**Fig. 19**), (2) a sausage-shaped mass with alternating layers of low and high attenuation, and (3) a reniform mass.[3,39]

Small bowel intussusception may be manifested on CT by a pair of concentric rings of soft tissue with an eccentrically located area of fat attenuation inside the outer ring. The outer ring of soft tissue represents the intussuscipiens, whereas the inner ring of soft tissue represents the wall of the intussusceptum. The eccentrically located fat represents the mesentery of the intussusceptum. Vessels in the invaginating mesentery may be visible as punctate dots or thin, undulating strands of soft tissue or intravenous contrast attenuation. If the wall of the intussuscipiens is thickened, the possibility of bowel wall edema and ischemia should be considered. Obstruction is implied by dilatation of small bowel proximal to the

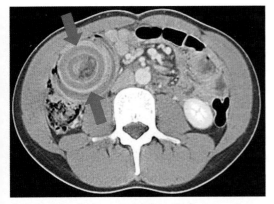

Fig. 19. Ileocolic intussusception: CT features. A mass with concentric rings of bowel (*arrows*) produces a target appearance on this CT image. The outer ring represents the intussuscipiens and the inner ring represents the wall of the intussusceptum. Mesenteric fat is at the center of the target. These loops show mural thickening with submucosal edema suspicious for ischemia that was confirmed at surgery.

intussusception associated with collapsed small bowel distally.[38,39]

Ultrasound shows a targetlike lesion (see **Fig. 8**) in which the hypoechoic halo is produced by the mesentery and the edematous wall of the intussuscipiens, and the hyperechoic center is produced by multiple interfaces of compressed mucosal, submucosal, and serosal surfaces of the intussusceptum. Multiple concentric rings, best seen on transverse scans, are also characteristic. The corresponding appearance on longitudinal scans is that of multiple, thin, parallel, hypoechoic, and echogenic stripes.[38,39]

LARGE BOWEL OBSTRUCTION

Mechanical LBO is 4 to 5 times less common than SBO and differs significantly in terms of etiology, pathophysiology, therapy, and prognosis. Colon obstruction is most often the result of a neoplasm, whereas most SBOs are due to adhesions (see **Fig. 1, Table 1**).[6]

Carcinoma of the Colon

LBO is caused by intrinsic colon carcinoma (**Fig. 20**) in approximately 55% of cases. Nearly 20% of colon cancers are complicated by some degree of obstruction; 5% to 10% are complicated by complete obstruction that requires emergent surgical intervention. The mortality rate is high (10%–30%) in patients requiring emergency surgery, regardless of the site of tumor. The location of obstruction in one series was as follows: cecum, 11%; right colon, 5%; hepatic flexure, 3%;

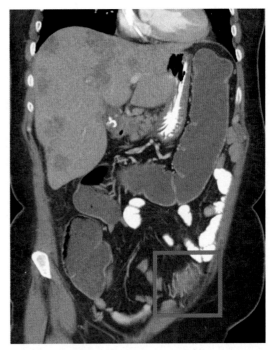

Fig. 20. Carcinoma of the junction of the sigmoid and descending colon causing LBO. There is a distal colonic mass (*square*) causing obstruction identified on this coronal reformatted CT image. The ileocecal valve is competent so no small bowel dilation is present. Note the multiple hepatic metastases.

transverse colon, 11%; splenic flexure, 12%; descending colon, 10%; sigmoid colon, 35%; and rectum, 13%. Obstructing colon cancers typically manifest as a soft tissue mass, often large, at the site of obstruction.[6]

Diverticulitis

Colon obstruction is the result of diverticular disease in approximately 12% of cases. Diverticulitis can cause both SBO and LBO. Partial colonic obstruction can complicate acute diverticulitis as a consequence of edema and pericolic inflammation or abscess formation. High-grade obstruction is uncommon; it is far more frequently caused by carcinoma of the colon. More commonly, obstruction follows recurrent attacks of diverticulitis with marked fibrosis of the colon wall leading to narrowing and eventually stricture formation. The site of obstruction is usually in the sigmoid colon, near the site of inflammation. Obstruction of the transverse or right colon due to diverticulitis is rare.[6]

Volvulus

Colonic volvulus accounts for approximately 10% of LBOs and can affect the sigmoid colon, cecum, transverse colon, and, rarely, the splenic flexure. Symptoms are caused by narrowing and obstruction of the gut, strangulation of the blood vessels, or both.[33]

The major predisposing factors necessary for colonic volvulus are a segment of redundant mobile colon on a mesentery or mesocolon and a fixed point around which rotation can occur. The sigmoid colon (see **Fig. 5**A) is therefore the most frequent site of colonic volvulus, especially in patients older than 60 years. Cecal (see **Fig. 5**B) or ascending colon volvulus occurs in patients with a congenital defect in attachment of the right colon or postpartum ligamentous laxity and a mobile cecum. Anything that causes colon distention, including pseudo-obstruction, distal tumor, endoscopy, enemas, or postoperative ileus, may precipitate cecal volvulus in susceptible individuals.[6,33]

On CT, a "whirl" sign (**Fig. 21**) has been described in volvulus. The whirl is constituted by the afferent and efferent limbs leading into the volvulus. Tightly twisted mesentery and bowel compose the central portion of the whirl. The distended and redundant sigmoid colon may overlie the liver and extend superior to transverse colon, producing the so-called "northern exposure" sign.[6,33,40]

Adult Intussusception

Intussusception accounts for only 1% to 3% of mechanical intestinal obstruction in adults and a demonstrable cause is found in 80% of adult cases. Colonic intussusception is usually due to a primary colon cancer, whereas small bowel intussusception is generally related to a benign tumor and less often to a malignancy, most commonly a metastatic lesion.[39]

Benign lesions that can serve as lead points in colonic intussusception include adenomatous polyps, lipomas, gastrointestinal stromal tumors, appendiceal stump granulomas, and villous adenomas of the appendix. The normal appendix may transiently intussuscept, although clinically significant appendiceal intussusception usually occurs in the setting of appendiceal inflammation, infestation, neoplasm, or endometriosis deposition. The colonic CT features of intussusception are similar to those observed in the small bowel (see earlier in this article).

Adhesions

Adhesional LBO is unusual because the colon is characteristically fixed and of large caliber and has thick walls. The small bowel, in contrast, has an inherently small caliber and a high degree of mobility and is therefore very prone to obstruction by adhesions.

Folding of the cecum on itself, the "cecal bascule," often occurs at the site of an adhesive band. The ascending colon can be obstructed by congenital bands or adhesions caused by inflammatory changes after colonoscopy and polypectomy. Inflammation of the appendices epiploicae can rarely cause obstruction in the rectosigmoid, and ischemia and inflammation of the greater omentum can rarely cause obstruction in the transverse colon.[4,8]

Hernias

Hernias cause LBO less often than SBO because of the relatively fixed nature of the colon and its larger caliber. Inguinal, femoral, umbilical, spigelian, incisional, lumbar, and diaphragmatic hernias can all contain colon and cause LBO. Internal hernias, such as through the foramen of Winslow, can contain colon and cause obstruction as well.[41]

Obturation Obstruction

The terminal ileum is the narrowest portion of the gut and, as a result, is the most common site of

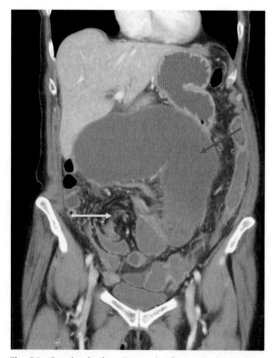

Fig. 21. Cecal volvulus. Coronal reformatted CT image shows a markedly distended, fluid-filled cecum (*red arrow*) that extends to the left of the midline. Note the whirled (*yellow arrow*) appearance of the adjacent ileocolic mesentery.

obturation obstruction. The sigmoid colon, measuring 2.5 cm in diameter, only slightly larger than the distal ileum, is the narrowest portion of the colon, followed by the hepatic and splenic flexures. These are the most likely points of colonic impaction of an intraluminal object. Three percent to 5% of patients with gallstone ileus have colonic obstruction.

Elderly, inactive, debilitated, and mentally challenged patients; drug addicts in methadone maintenance programs; transplantation and hemodialysis patients; and individuals with adult Hirschsprung disease are at risk for developing fecal impaction. The most common sites are the rectum (70%) and sigmoid colon (20%). Obstruction, volvulus, stercoral ulceration, perforation, rectal prolapse, and rectal fissure are potential complications of fecalomas.[4]

SUMMARY

The diagnosis and management of patients with bowel obstruction has been revolutionized over the past 2 decades by cross-sectional imaging. Although ultrasound, MR, plain abdominal radiographs and contrast enemas, and small bowel examinations can be useful in certain circumstances, MDCT has evolved as the premier imaging test for patients with known or suspected bowel obstruction. CT findings can be very helpful in determining which patients may benefit from a trial of conservative therapy and those patients who need prompt surgical intervention.

REFERENCES

1. Taylor MR, Lalani N. Adult small bowel obstruction. Acad Emerg Med 2013;20:528–44.
2. Cappell MS, Batke M. Mechanical obstruction of the small bowel and colon. Med Clin North Am 2008; 92(3):575–97.
3. Rubesin SE, Gore RM. Small bowel obstruction. In: Gore RM, Levine MS, editors. Textbook of gastrointestinal radiology. 4th edition. Philadelphia: Elsevier-Saunders; 2015. p. 806–26.
4. Gore RM, Szucs RA, Wolf EL, et al. Miscellaneous abnormalities of the colon. In: Gore RM, Levine MS, editors. Textbook of gastrointestinal radiology. 4th edition. Philadelphia: Elsevier-Saunders; 2015. p. 1102–33.
5. Tavakkoli A, Ashley SW, Xinner MJ. Small intestine. In: Brunicardi F, editor. Schwartz's principles of surgery. 10th edition. New York: McGraw Hill; 2014. p. 987–1066.
6. Bullard Dunn KM, Rothenberger DA. Colon, rectum, anus. In: Brunicardi F, editor. Schwartz's principles of surgery. 10th edition. New York: McGraw Hill; 2014. p. 1067–158.
7. Umphrey H, Cannon CL, Lockhart ME. Differential diagnosis of Crohn's disease. Surg Clin North Am 2013;93(1):167–85.
8. Messner JM, Levine MS. Gas and soft tissue abnormalities. In: Gore RM, Levine MS, editors. Textbook of gastrointestinal radiology. 4th edition. Philadelphia: Elsevier-Saunders; 2015. p. 178–96.
9. Gore RM, Thakrar KH, Wenzke DR, et al. The acute abdomen. In: Gore RM, Levine MS, editors. Textbook of gastrointestinal radiology. 4th edition. Philadelphia: Elsevier-Saunders; 2015. p. 2255–70.
10. Maglinte DD, Kelvin FM, Rowe MG, et al. Reliability and role of film radiography and CT in the diagnosis of small bowel obstruction. AJR Am J Roentgenol 1996;167(6):1451–5.
11. Thompson WM. Gasless abdomen in the adult: what does it mean? AJR Am J Roentgenol 2008;191(4): 1093–9.
12. Santillan CS. Computed tomography of small bowel obstruction. Radiol Clin North Am 2013;51:17–27.
13. Masselli G, Gualdi G. CT and MR enterography in evaluating small bowel diseases: when to use which modality? Abdom Imaging 2013;38(2):249–59.
14. Manchanda SD, Prasad A, Sachdev N, et al. Multi detector computed tomography (MDCT) evaluation of small bowel obstruction: pictorial review. Trop Gastroenterol 2010;31(4):249–59.
15. Silva AC, Pimenta M, Guimarães LS. Small bowel obstruction: what to look for. Radiographics 2009; 29(2):423–39.
16. Katz DS, Yam B, Hines JJ, et al. Uncommon and unusual gastrointestinal causes of the acute abdomen: computed tomographic diagnosis. Semin Ultrasound CT MR 2008;29:386–98.
17. Desser TS, Gross M. Multidetector row computed tomography of small bowel obstruction. Semin Ultrasound CT MR 2008;29:308–21.
18. Ros PR, Huprich JE. ACR Appropriateness Criteria on suspected small-bowel obstruction. J Am Coll Radiol 2006;3:838–41.
19. Filippone A, Cianci R, Storto ML. Bowel obstruction: comparison between multidetector-row CT axial and coronal planes. Abdom Imaging 2007;32:310–6.
20. Mak SY, Roach SC, Sukumar SA. Small bowel obstruction: computed tomography features and pitfalls. Curr Probl Diagn Radiol 2006;35:65–74.
21. Nicoloaou S, Kai B, Ho S, et al. Image of acute small bowel obstruction. AJR Am J Roentgenol 2005; 184(4):1036–44.
22. Hayakawa K, Tanikake M, Yoshida S, et al. CT findings of small bowel strangulation: the importance of contrast enhancement. Emerg Radiol 2013;20:3–9.
23. Brown CV. Small bowel and colon perforation. Surg Clin North Am 2014;94(2):471–5.

24. Beddy P, Keogan MT, Sala E, et al. Magnetic resonance imaging for the evaluation of abdominal pain in pregnancy. Semin Ultrasound CT MR 2010; 31(5):433–41.

25. Belabrousse E, Baulard R, Sarlieve P, et al. Value of small bowel feces sign in CT of adhesive small bowel obstruction. J Radiol 2005;86(4):393–8.

26. Lazarus DE, Slywotsky C, Bennett GL, et al. Frequency and relevance of the small bowel feces sign on CT in patients with small bowel obstruction. AJR Am J Roentgenol 2004;183(5):1361–6.

27. Millet I, Ruyer A, Alili C, et al. Adhesive small bowel obstruction: value of CT in identifying findings associated with the effectiveness of nonsurgical management. Radiology 2014;273(2):425–32.

28. Chang WC, Koh H, Lin CS, et al. Features on MDCT that predict surgery in patients with adhesive-related small bowel obstruction. PLoS One 2014;9(2):e89604.

29. Paulson EK, Thompson WM. Review of small bowel obstruction: the diagnosis and when to worry. Radiology 2015;275(2):332–42.

30. Lockhart ME, Tessler RN, Cannon CL, et al. Internal hernias after gastric bypass. AJR Am J Roentgenol 2007;188(3):745–50.

31. Geffroy Y, Boulay-Coletta I, Julies MC, et al. Increased unenhanced bowel-wall attenuation at multidetector CT is highly specific of ischemia complicating SBO. Radiology 2014;270(1):159–67.

32. Hongo N, Mori H, Matsumoto S, et al. Internal hernias after abdominal surgeries: MDCT features. Abdom Imaging 2011;36:349–62.

33. Lepage-Saucier M, Tang A, Billiard JS, et al. Small and large bowel volvulus: clues to early recognition and complications. Eur J Radiol 2010;74:60–6.

34. Gore RM, Ghahremani GG, Donaldson CE, et al. Hernias and abdominal wall pathology. In: Gore RM, Levine MS, editors. Textbook of gastrointestinal radiology. 4th edition. Philadelphia: Elsevier-Saunders; 2015. p. 2053–76.

35. Luk C, Hunt SR. Surgical management of Crohn's disease. Surg Clin North Am 2013;93(1):167–85.

36. Baker ME, Gore RM. Crohn's disease of the small bowel. In: Gore RM, Levine MS, editors. Textbook of gastrointestinal radiology. 4th edition. Philadelphia: Elsevier-Saunders; 2015. p. 725–55.

37. Luu MB, Deziel DJ. Unusual complications of gallstones. Surg Clin North Am 2014;94(2):377–94.

38. Feinstein KA, Fernbach SK. Diseases of the pediatric colon. In: Gore RM, Levine MS, editors. Textbook of gastrointestinal radiology. 4th edition. Philadelphia: Elsevier-Saunders; 2015. p. 2164–79.

39. Amr MA, Polites SF, Alzahari M, et al. Intussusception in adults and the role of evolving CT technology. Am J Surg 2015;209(3):580–3.

40. Javors BR, Baker SR, Miller JA. The northern exposure sign: a newly described finding in sigmoid volvulus. AJR Am J Roentgenol 1999;173(3):571–4.

41. Murphy KP, O'Connor OJ, Maher MM. Adult abdominal hernias. AJR Am J Roentgenol 2014;202(6):W506–11.

Radiological Evaluation of Bowel Ischemia

Harpreet S. Dhatt, MD, Spencer C. Behr, MD, Aaron Miracle, MD, Zhen Jane Wang, MD, Benjamin M. Yeh, MD*

KEYWORDS

- Computed tomography • Bowel ischemia • Intestinal ischemia • Oral contrast • Bowel infarction
- Mesenteric ischemia • Pneumatosis intestinalis • Mesenteric artery occlusion

KEY POINTS

- Choice of computed tomography (CT) technique affects the visibility of CT findings. Positive oral contrast may improve the detection of fluid collections, hematomas, and bowel leakage. Neutral oral contrast improves visualization of bowel wall hypoenhancement or hyperenhancement.
- Findings of bowel ischemia include mural hypoenhancement associated with adjacent mesenteric edema, pneumatosis, and free fluid.
- Hyperemia (shock bowel) may be seen adjacent to segments of acute pale ischemia.
- Evaluation of the arteries and veins leading to and from diseased bowel can reveal the cause of bowel ischemia as embolic, dissection, thrombosis, inflammation, or malignant.

PATHOPHYSIOLOGY AND PRESENTATION

Intestinal ischemia has diverse causes and presentations.[1,2] Mesenteric ischemia is classified into 2 forms, acute and chronic, which are differentiated on the timing of symptom onset and extent of decreased blood flow. Mesenteric ischemia is further subdivided by cause: arterial, venous, and nonocclusive. In a general sense, intestinal ischemia frequently presents with nonspecific clinical symptoms. The classic triad of abdominal pain, hematochezia, and fever is seen in only 1 out of 3 patients.[3] More commonly, nonspecific symptoms are seen and include diarrhea, vomiting, and bloating.

ACUTE MESENTERIC ISCHEMIA

Acute mesenteric ischemia (AMI) occurs from arterial embolic or thrombotic obstruction, mesenteric venous thrombosis, or a nonocclusive cause.[4] The mean age of patients with acute mesenteric arterial occlusive ischemia (embolic and thrombosis)

is 70 years. However, patients younger than 50 years may also form occlusive emboli in the setting of atrial fibrillation.[5] Arterial emboli from a cardiac[6] or septic source are the most common causes of AMI and compose 40% to 50% of the cases. Patients often present with abrupt onset of abdominal pain, diarrhea, and vomiting.[7]

Thrombotic arterial ischemia may be acute or chronic and occurs in patients with a preexisting atherosclerotic lesion in a mesenteric artery with superimposed thrombosis formation. The major risk factors in these patients include atherosclerotic disease, aortic dissection and aneurysm, arteritis, and dehydration. These patients undergo gradual progression of arterial occlusion. Therefore, many present with abdominal angina, a syndrome of postprandial pain lasting up to 3 hours. This syndrome results in food fear, early satiety, and weight loss. In the acute setting, however, the clinical symptoms are similar to those found in patients with the arterial embolic disease.[5]

Chronic arterial bowel ischemia presents with subacute and even less specific symptoms.

Department of Radiology and Biomedical Imaging, University of California San Francisco, 505 Parnassus Avenue, San Francisco, CA 94143-0628, USA
* Corresponding author.
E-mail address: Ben.Yeh@ucsf.edu

Radiol Clin N Am 53 (2015) 1241–1254
http://dx.doi.org/10.1016/j.rcl.2015.06.009
0033-8389/15/$ – see front matter © 2015 Elsevier Inc. All rights reserved.

Although chronic bowel ischemia may present with abdominal pain, it may also present with weight loss or food fear.[3] Although chronic mesenteric ischemia remains rare, occurring in 1 out of 1000 hospital admissions, it has a high mortality, with death rates ranging from 30% to 90%.[7] Chronic bowel ischemia generally presents in patients older than 60 years and is 3 times more common in women.[8]

This syndrome occurs in the setting of long-standing mesenteric arterial atherosclerotic disease resulting in constant decreased blood flow, especially in the postprandial state. Patients may present with significant weight loss secondary to postprandial pain lasting up to 90 minutes. These patients often report prior such episodes of intestinal angina clueing the clinician to the diagnosis. However, 15% to 20% of these patients demonstrate no symptoms. Over time, as the vascular obstructive process progresses, chronic, dull abdominal pain ensues.[9]

In contrast, mesenteric venous ischemic, although a less common cause of AMI, has a more variable patient population presentation and occurs in younger patients, often less than 50 years old.[3] It can commonly occur because of segmental bowel strangulation or thrombosis. Pertinent medical history is also critical for diagnosis as other risk factors for venous thrombosis include hypercoagulable predispositions, such as pregnancy, protein C and S or antithrombin deficiencies, polycythemia vera, malignancy, infection, portal hypertension, or venous trauma.[10] Patients may present with acute or subacute abdominal pain. They may have symptoms of AMI over a prolonged period with gradual progression.[11]

Nonocclusive mesenteric ischemia (NOMI), occurring in 10% to 20% of AMI cases, is most common in elderly patients with severe systemic illnesses that reduce cardiac output. It most commonly occurs in the postoperative intensive care unit setting. The clinical diagnosis can be challenging because of the diminished mental state of these patients. These patients may have nonspecific symptoms that can range from abdominal pain and nausea to ileus. Other predisposing factors include trauma, cocaine use, ergot ingestion, digoxin, alpha-adrenergic medications, cardiac failure, myocardial infarction, abdominal surgery, and aortic insufficiency.[12–14]

Ischemic bowel may result as a complication of other underlying intra-abdominal comorbidities. For example, the identification of bowel obstruction on computed tomography (CT) should always prompt the search for the complication of bowel ischemia because rapid triage to surgery may be necessary to prevent an abdominal catastrophe from bowel perforation.[15] Other underlying processes, such as embolic disease or vascular dissection, are important to identify so that long-term treatment can be directed toward future prevention of complications.[16] **Tables 1** and **2** summarize the major CT findings and reformations useful for diagnosis of bowel ischemia.

LABORATORY TESTS AND ADDITIONAL CONSIDERATIONS

In patients with abdominal pain, physicians are faced with a broad differential diagnosis that includes pancreatitis, cholelithiasis, diverticulitis, and appendicitis. Physical examination findings and laboratory values can be suggestive of a bowel cause but are generally nonspecific.[15] Elevated lactic acid levels, leukocytosis, and the presence of an anion gap may or may not be present. Elevated serum lactate levels indicate anaerobic metabolism in the setting of ischemic bowel but are also associated with other pathologic conditions.

Given the frequent ambiguous clinical presentation of intestinal ischemia, only one-third of patients are diagnosed accurately preoperatively.[17] CT imaging has been shown to outperform all other laboratory and physical examination findings for the detection of bowel ischemia.[15] Catheter-angiography, providing both diagnosis and treatment, has improved mortality over the last 40 years but is an invasive test.[7]

Multidetector CT (MDCT) provides reliable imaging of bowel in the acute setting. Particular benefits of MDCT over magnetic resonance and ultrasound include the rapid speed of image acquisition, which minimizes bowel motion artifact, large field of view

Table 1 CT findings or reformations that may be highlighted or be obscured by the use of positive bowel contrast agent	
Possibly highlighted	**Possibly obscured**
Intra-abdominal abscess*	Bowel wall nonenhancement*
Enteric fistula or leak*	Bowel wall hyperenhancement*
Extraluminal tumor	CT angiogram reformation
Hematomas	Active gastrointestinal bleed

The presence of these frequently coexisting conditions (* often occur together) is usually not known until after the CT scan is done. The choice to administer positive bowel contrast is based on clinical best guess and institution-based expertise.

Table 2
Major clinical and CT findings of bowel ischemia

Features	Arterial Ischemia	Venous Ischemia	Nonocclusive Ischemia
Incidence	60%–70%	5%–10%	20%–30%
Acuity	Acute or chronic	Acute or chronic	Acute or chronic
Clinical risk factors	Cardiovascular disease: atrial fibrillation, post-myocardial infarction, aortic injury, atherosclerosis, septic emboli, systemic vasculitis	Bowel strangulation, hypercoagulable state, portal hypertension, venous trauma, infection	Hypotension, heart failure, recent surgery or trauma, medications, including recreational
Vasculature	Arterial filling defect, severe arterial narrowing, dissection, aneurysm	Venous filling defect, often with enlarged venous diameter	Nonspecific
Bowel wall Thickness	May be thin acutely but may be thickened and involved with hematoma, edema, or inflammation	Thickened and edematous	Generally thickened
Bowel wall Enhancement	Variable; diminished or nonenhancement in regions of pale ischemia; hyperenhancement in areas of reperfusion	Diminished enhancement of mucosa and serosa, target appearance	Diminished enhancement
Mesentery/fat	Mesenteric fat stranding with free fluid associated with the territory of ischemia	Mesenteric fat stranding with free fluid associated with the territory of ischemia	Mesenteric fat stranding with free fluid associated with the territory of ischemia

and territory of coverage, ability to image through gas and many metals with minimal artifact, and excellent patient tolerance. Potential risks of CT are low but include risks associated with the ionizing radiation dose and nephrotoxicity or reactions to iodinated intravenous contrast material. Conventional angiography is a second-line imaging modality that can be extended to relieve areas of obstruction in the mesenteric arteries.

COMPUTED TOMOGRAPHY ORAL CONTRAST: POSITIVE OR NEUTRAL?

Generally, approximately 800 to 1200 mL of oral fluid is given to distend the bowel before CT scanning. A fundamental decision for CT scanning in patients with suspicion of bowel ischemia is whether or not to administer positive versus neutral oral contrast material. Unfortunately, each choice provides certain benefits and drawbacks. In the emergency setting, urgency may prevent oral contrast administration and CT may be obtained with intravenous contrast material alone. In these cases, the bowel may be poorly distended at imaging and may be more difficult to evaluate.

Contrast agents that provide CT numbers greater than 50 Hounsfield units (HU) are considered to be *positive* agents, and those with CT numbers near water (−20 to +20 HU) are generally considered to be *neutral* agents. All positive oral contrast agents use tri-iodinated compounds or barium sulfate to block X rays and effectively mark the lumen of bowel. Positive oral contrast agents improve the ability of CT to distinguish abscess, hematoma, and nonbowel masses from opacified segments of bowel and help confirm the presence of a bowel leak or fistula. In the setting of bowel obstruction, diminishing oral contrast intensity is generally seen in close proximity to the bowel transition point than in more upstream segments of bowel. Positive oral contrast material may also be valuable to detect bowel wall thickening when intravenous contrast material cannot be given.

A limitation with the use of positive oral contrast is that bright intraluminal contrast material may interfere with the evaluation of hypoenhancement or hyperenhancement of the bowel wall, which may be seen with various forms of bowel ischemia. Also, positive oral contrast may interfere with

3-dimensional reformations of the vasculature by maximum-intensity projection and volume-rendered reformations.

Neutral oral contrast material, such as water or sorbitol solutions with 0.1% barium sulfate, are non-Food and Drug Administration approved agents that can distend the bowel with fluid that has CT numbers between −20 and +20 HU. Neutral oral contrast agents, used in conjunction with intravenous contrast agents, allow visualization of bowel wall hypoenhancement or hyperenhancement and may allow visualization of intraluminal active extravasation of intravenous contrast material.

Three-dimensional reformations of the vasculature are generally possible when neutral contrast agents are used. The major drawback of neutral oral contrast is its resemblance to other bodily fluids: abscesses, free fluid, and, to a lesser extent, hematomas and tumors. Fistula and leakage of enteric contents may be less vivid or more difficult to identify with neutral than with positive oral contrast agents. Negative oral contrast agents, such as gases and oils, are rarely used for the evaluation of mesenteric ischemia.

COMPUTED TOMOGRAPHY SCAN PARAMETERS

The CT scan acquisition techniques should be tailored to the clinical need. A noncontrast phase is not essential but helps to assess for intramural hemorrhage and serves as a baseline for subsequent intravenous contrast-enhanced images. In the authors' institution, a 150-mL bolus of 350 mg iodine per milliliter of intravenous contrast material is injected at 3 mL/s via a power injector. If an arterial phase is deemed necessary, the injection rate is increased to 5 mL/s and a bolus threshold trigger is used. A region of interest is drawn over the proximal aorta, and scanning of the abdomen and pelvis is obtained once a 150-HU threshold is reached. For all scans, a portal venous phase is acquired at 80-seconds delay and reformatted into 2.5-mm axial, 2.5-mm sagittal, and 3.0-mm coronal images. When available, dual-energy CT imaging is used with the 80-seconds delay to assist with the detection of bowel enhancement abnormalities.[18]

ANATOMY

To accurately diagnose mesenteric ischemic disease, interpreting physicians must be acquainted with both mesenteric arterial and venous anatomy of the bowel. There are 3 major arteries that supply the small and large bowel (**Figs. 1** and **2**). The celiac trunk generally supplies the distal esophagus to the second portion of the duodenum. The superior mesenteric artery (SMA), located at the level of first lumbar vertebral body, supplies the third and fourth portions of the duodenum via the superior and inferior pancreaticoduodenal arteries, and supplies the jejunum, ileum, and the colon to level

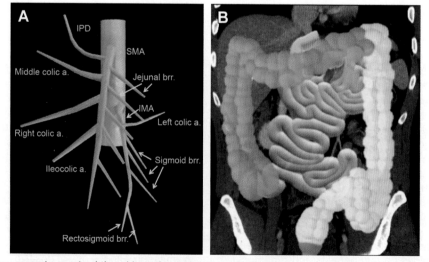

Fig. 1. The mesenteric arteries (*A*) and bowel segments supplied by mesenteric arteries (*B*). a, artery; brr, branch artery; IMA, inferior mesenteric artery; IPD, inferior pancreaticoduodenal artery; SMA, superior mesenteric artery. The duodenum, jejunum, ileum, and colon proximal to the splenic flexure is supplied by the superior mesenteric artery (*bowel with orange color*), and the descending and sigmoid colon and upper rectum are supplied by the inferior mesenteric artery (*bowel in yellow color*). The distal most rectum is supplied by the middle and inferior rectal arteries from the internal iliac artery (*bowel in purple color*).

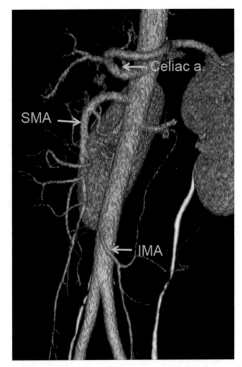

Fig. 2. Volume-rendered oblique sagittal reformation of normal CT angiogram shows the major mesenteric arteries. a, artery; IMA, inferior mesenteric artery; SMA, superior mesenteric artery.

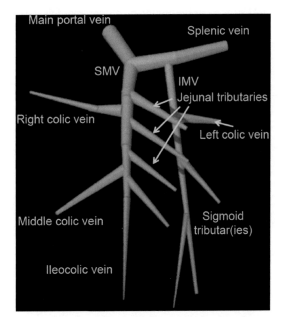

Fig. 3. Normal major mesenteric veins. IMV, inferior mesenteric vein; SMV, superior mesenteric vein.

of the splenic flexure. The inferior mesenteric artery (IMA), located at the level of the third lumbar vertebral body, supplies the distal colon from the level of the distal transverse portion to the upper rectum. Branches of the internal iliac arteries and the middle and inferior rectal arteries supply the distal rectum.

There are numerous important mesenteric collateral pathways that provide a rich vascular safety net for mesenteric blood supply. The gastroduodenal artery is the first branch of the common hepatic artery and provides a collateral pathway between the celiac artery and the SMA. The marginal artery of Drummond and the arcade of Riolan connect the SMA and IMA. Four arcades of anastomosis are formed between the IMA and lumbar arteries arising from the aorta, sacral, and internal iliac arteries. In addition, the peripheral small mesenteric vessels are anatomically arranged in a parallel series configuration that supplies the mucosa, submucosa, and muscularis propria of bowel.[19]

The superior and inferior mesenteric veins run parallel to the arteries and drain the respective part of the bowel (Fig. 3). The inferior mesenteric vein joins the superior mesenteric vein (SMV) after emptying into the splenic vein to form the main portal vein.

Numerous collateral venous pathways exist or can form between the mesenteric and systemic veins, including gastric and esophageal, renal, lumbar, and pelvic veins. They tend to be more robust than those seen with the mesenteric arteries.

STAGES OF ISCHEMIA

Although understanding the anatomy allows localization of the disease process, familiarity with disease states helps the radiologist provide a better evaluation of abnormal gut. Acute bowel ischemia is characterized by 3 stages, specifically based on the extent of bowel wall involvement. Stage I (reversible disease) is pathologically characterized by necrosis, erosions, ulcerations, edema, and hemorrhage localized to the mucosa.[20,21] Stage II represents necrosis extending into the submucosal and muscularis propria layers. Finally, the high-mortality stage III disease involves all 3 layers (transmural necrosis).[22–24] In addition, superinfection of postmucosal breakdown in the colon may facilitate further necrosis and perforation.

ARTERIAL ISCHEMIA: BLOOD VESSEL EVALUATION

The most common cause of acute ischemic colitis and associated necrosis is arterial embolic disease, which composes 60% to 70% of cases.[11,23,25] The primary systemic risk factors include atrial fibrillation,[6,16] post–myocardial infarction cardiac wall motion abnormalities, emboli from aortic injury or atherosclerosis, and rarely cholesterol and postaortic surgery embolism. Emboli preferentially affect SMA because of its small takeoff angle compared with those of the celiac and IMA. Although thrombi and large emboli may occlude the proximal SMA and ostia of major mesenteric vessels resulting in extensive small bowel and colon ischemia, smaller emboli may lodge in the distal portions of the vessel and cause smaller regions of segmental ischemia.[11,23,25]

Acute arterial thrombi and emboli may appear as obvious low-attenuation filling defects in the SMA, its branches, or other major mesenteric arteries[26] (**Figs. 4** and **5**). The presence of emboli involving other visceral organs may help the radiologist suggest this diagnosis.

Systemic vasculitides causing vascular occlusions uncommonly affect mesenteric vasculature and ultimately the bowel. However, when involved, polyarteritis nodosa is most commonly (50%–70%) the underlying cause. Polyarteritis nodosa may cause small arterial aneurysms as well as occlusions. Systemic lupus erythematous (SLE), Henoch-Schönlein purpura, Wegener granulomatosis, Churg-Strauss disease, Buerger disease, and hemolytic uremic syndrome may also occlude small mesenteric arteries and intramural

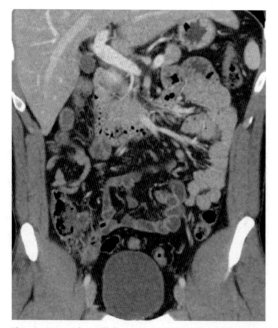

Fig. 4. Normal small bowel on CT: Coronal image of normal small bowel. Notice the relative increased enhancement of the jejunum in the left upper quadrant compared with the ileum in the right lower quadrant. The apparent jejunal hyperenhancement is caused by the higher-fold density of the valvulae conniventes in collapsed jejunum than ileum.

mesenteric veins. Takayasu arteritis and giant cell arteritis primarily affect the large vessels.

Although the clinical symptoms may overlap with other forms of bowel ischemia, arteritis tends to affect younger patients. An appropriately elicited medical history may focus the clinician to the correct diagnosis.[27] Additionally, the associated ischemia and extensive wall thickening may involve unusual sites, such as the stomach, duodenum, occasionally jejunum, ileum, and rectum.[27] The associated gastrointestinal complications can be devastating, ranging from regional gangrene to hemorrhage and perforation.[28]

Aortic dissection with extension into or occlusion of the mesenteric arteries may result in bowel ischemia and hemorrhage.[11] Isolated dissection of the superior mesentery artery is an exceedingly rare occurrence resulting in acute ischemia and may be associated with underlying fibrous dysplasia of the mesenteric artery.

Another rare cause of mesenteric ischemia is a mesenteric aneurysm, which may rupture and cause pain and hemorrhage. Most splanchnic true and pseudoaneurysms are found in asymptomatic patients on cross-section imaging or autopsy (0.01%–0.25%), with SMA involved 6% of the times.[11]

The development of intestinal ischemia from an arterially obstructing lesion also depends on the location of the obstruction, patients' collateral vasculature, and the acuity and degree of the obstruction. The presence of 2 collateral arcades, the first connecting the celiac artery and the SMA via the pancreaticoduodenal and gastroduodenal arteries and the second connecting SMA to IMA via the arch of Riolan and marginal artery of Drummond, allow bidirectional flow that can bypass obstructing lesions. In the presence of obstructions involving all 3 major arteries (celiac, SMA, and IMA), the phrenic, lumbar, and pelvic collateral arteries may dilate to provide accessory visceral blood flow. However, if the lesion is distal to the point of collateral flow, the collateral supply is ineffective and ischemia is more likely to ensue.[29] Additionally, if there is rapid development of obstruction from an embolus or vasculitis, patients may not be able to develop sufficient collaterals in time to provide perfusion. Patients with diabetes or severe diffuse atherosclerotic disease may have limited ability to develop collaterals, which places diabetic patients at high risk for bowel ischemia from even mild lesions.[29]

ARTERIAL ISCHEMIA: BOWEL WALL EVALUATION

Abnormal intestinal mural enhancement is critical to assess when there is a suspicion of bowel

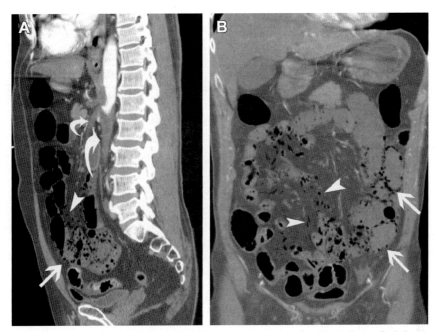

Fig. 5. Arterial ischemia from SMA thrombosis. Elderly man presented with 3 days of abdominal pain and anorexia. Sagittal (*A*) and coronal (*B*) CT images show pneumatosis intestinalis (*white arrows*) and mesenteric venous gas (*white arrowheads*) associated with extensive clot in the aorta (*large curved white arrow*) extending into the celiac trunk and SMA (*small curved white arrow*).

ischemia. The intensity of bowel wall enhancement varies depending on the cause of the ischemia. Normal small and large bowel show homogenous mural enhancement, particularly in the venous phase of enhancement. During the early phase of arterial occlusion, a key finding is substantially diminished bowel mural enhancement (**Fig. 6**)[15,30,31] and has been termed *pale ischemia*. Alternatively, in the postreperfusion period after arterial injury, hyperenhancement of the bowel is

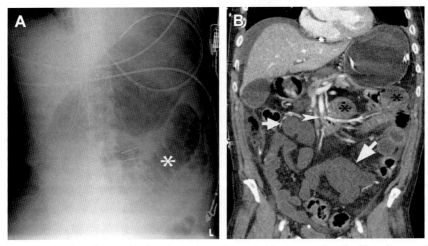

Fig. 6. Plain radiograph of small bowel ischemia. Plain radiograph (*A*) shows a focally dilated paper-thin segment of small bowel (*white asterisk*) that had persisted over several consecutive examinations. Subsequent coronal re-formatted CT image (*B*) of the same patient shows the corresponding dilated segment (*black asterisk*) as well as other fluid-filled segments of small bowel with absent mural enhancement (*white arrows*) and clot in the SMA (*white arrowhead*). At laparotomy, 220 cm of dead bowel was found.

present (**Fig. 7**),[30] much like shock bowel. Commonly, shock bowel may be seen immediately adjacent to pale ischemia because of the development of collateral pathways in acute bowel ischemia.

Pneumatosis intestinalis, which is the presence of locules of air within or a contiguous line of gas dissecting between bowel layers, is commonly described as a finding of transmural bowel ischemia (**Fig. 8**). When pneumatosis intestinalis is present along with portomesenteric gas, the specificity approaches approximately 100% for ischemic bowel. However, it is critical to note that, in the absence of clinical signs or symptoms of ischemia, the finding of isolated pneumatosis intestinalis should not trigger a definite diagnosis of intestinal ischemia.[32–34] Pneumatosis intestinalis is not a specific finding of intestinal ischemia and may occur in a wide range of nonemergent benign scenarios (**Fig. 9**). When found, however, bowel ischemia must be excluded first and foremost.

In exclusively arterial occlusive mesenteric ischemia, the presence of segmental mesenteric fat stranding and free fluid interleaved between the mesenteric folds associated with the poorly enhancing bowel is highly suggestive of transmural infarction.[35–38] Although the severity of bowel ischemia is variable, perforation and peritonitis are high-mortality complications of infarction.

Assessing the mural thickness of the gut for findings of intestinal ischemia may be problematic

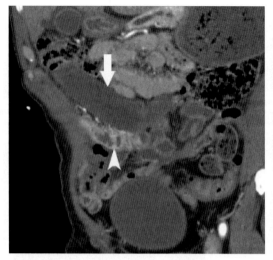

Fig. 8. Coronal contrast-enhanced CT shows pale arterial ischemia with absent mural enhancement in a segment of small bowel (*white arrow*). An adjacent segment of small bowel shows mural hyperenhancement (*white arrowhead*), indicating bowel reperfusion injury.

because bowel wall thickness depends on the cause, site, extent, duration, and superimposed complications of intestinal disease. Furthermore, there is significant variation in thickness of large bowel depending up on distention. Typically, gas or fluid-filled normal small bowel wall thickness measures 1 to 2 mm, whereas the wall of partially collapsed bowel may measure 2 to 3 mm in the ileum and colon. Normal partially collapsed jejunum may have an even greater apparent thickness than 3 mm.[27,39,40]

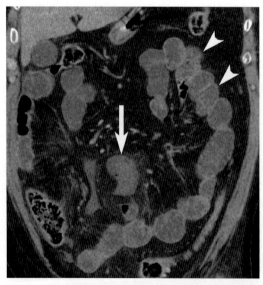

Fig. 7. A 54 year old with SMA thrombus causing arterial bowel ischemia. Thin hypoenhancing bowel wall (*white arrow*) and associated subtle mesenteric fat stranding is seen on coronal contrast-enhanced CT image. Mural enhancement of nonischemic jejunum (*white arrowheads*) is seen in the left upper abdomen.

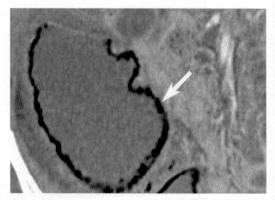

Fig. 9. Coronal CT showing pneumatosis intestinalis. Gas within the bowel wall (*white arrow*) can be suggestive of bowel ischemia and infarction in the appropriate clinical setting. In the absence of other concerning CT findings, clinical signs, or symptoms of bowel ischemia, a benign cause pneumatosis should be considered.

In the setting of primary arterial occlusion resulting in ischemia or transmural infarction, small bowel may become dilated with a classic paper-thin wall appearance (see **Fig. 5**B). This appearance occurs as a result of loss of bowel wall tissue, vasculature, and muscular tone. However, in cases of reversible ischemia, mild bowel thickening may be noted.[27,40] When acute arterial occlusion results in intramural hemorrhage, edema, and/or superimposed infection, abnormal bowel wall thickening up to 15 mm of the small and large intestines is commonly demonstrated (**Fig. 10**).[35]

VENOUS ISCHEMIA: MESENTERIC VEIN EVALUATION

Mesenteric venous occlusion composes up to 10% of bowel ischemia cases and is usually associated with mechanical obstruction but can be caused by venous thrombosis.[38] The latter may occur in patients with hypercoagulable syndromes, such as sickle cell disease, antiphospholipid antibody syndrome, polycythemia vera, and protein C/S deficiency, or in hypercoagulable states, such as pregnancy and with the use of oral contraceptives. Underlying inflammatory diseases, such a vasculitis (eg, SLE), also result in occlusion of small intramural mesenteric veins. Infectious causes, albeit rare, such as enterocolic lymphocytic phlebitis, have also been known to occlude small intramural colonic veins leading to ischemia.[2,11,23]

Venous circulation can also be compromised in association with bowel strangulation, typically observed in volvulus, intussusception, and closed-loop obstructions. Bowel ischemia occurs in 10% of small bowel obstructions; initially the low-pressure venous outflow is compressed with subsequent loss of arterial inflow. The strangulated segments of bowel are usually fluid filled, distended, and edematous with ascites[28,41] (**Figs. 11** and **12**). The enhancement is usually variable depending on the duration of obstruction. Early

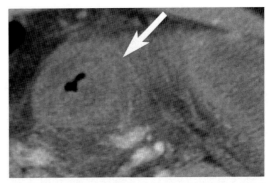

Fig. 11. Abnormally thickened bowel (*white arrow*) with mesenteric fat stranding and slightly decreased mural enhancement is nonspecific; causes include bowel ischemia, edema, intramural hemorrhage, and/or superimposed infection.

obstruction, with only venous compromise, may demonstrate hyperenhancement. Subacute findings with compromise of arterial supply demonstrate diminished or absent mural enhancement (see **Fig. 11**). CT has high sensitivity and specificity for diagnosis of strangulation, 83% to 100% and 61% to 93%, respectively. Among all the findings, decreased mural enhancement, segmental mesenteric fat stranding, and adjacent ascites interleaved between folds of the mesentery are the most specific for bowel ischemia.[42–45]

Thrombosis within the mesenteric veins may appear as a low-attenuation filling defect on contrast-enhanced CT and can be visualized in approximately 90% of cases of venous bowel ischemia (**Fig. 13**).[46,47] In addition, because of venous outflow obstruction, engorged mesenteric veins are typically observed. The venous obstruction elevates hydrostatic pressure in the bowel wall because high-pressure arterial inflow may continue despite venous occlusion. The vascular engorgement and edema of the bowel wall in turn lead to leakage of extravascular fluid into the

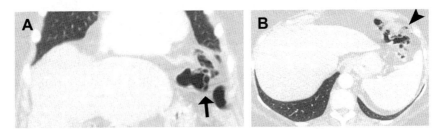

Fig. 10. Benign pneumatosis. CT images in lung window of a patient who presented with abdominal pain after trauma. Coronal image (*A*) shows pneumatosis cystoids coli (*black arrow*), whereas the axial image (*B*) shows small volume of pneumoperitoneum (*black arrowhead*). Patient was admitted for observation and discharged without any intervention as his pain resolved spontaneously.

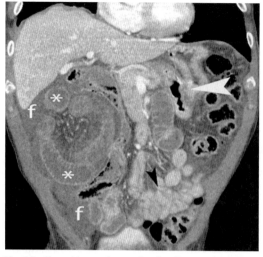

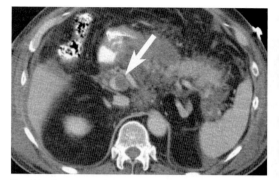

Fig. 14. Contrast-enhanced CT shows low-attenuation clot within SMV (*white arrow*) in a patient with pancreatitis.

Fig. 12. Closed loop obstruction leading to mesenteric ischemia. CT scan of a patient who presented with sudden abdomen pain and nausea. A focally dilated segment of ischemic small bowel (*white asterisk*) with collapsed proximal (*white arrowhead*) and distal (*black arrowhead*) small bowel is seen. The dilated ischemic bowel shows less enhancement than the collapsed segments of normal small bowel. The presence of adjacent free fluid (f) and mesenteric edema is also concerning for early ischemia.

bowel wall and mesentery (**Fig. 14**). The resultant edematous bowel may have a halo or target appearance caused by mild mucosal enhancement, submucosal and muscularis propria nonenhancement, and mild serosal/subserosal enhancement. This finding is easily identified on CT, and the wall may measure up to 1.5 cm in

thickness (**Fig. 15**).[28,38] The impaired venous drainage ultimately results in loss of arterial supply resulting in ischemia and infarction with CT findings as described earlier. In these cases, bowel enhancement is significantly diminished or absent (**Figs. 16 and 17**). The presence of mesenteric edema and fluid may be more prominent in venous ischemia than in arterial ischemia.

NONOCCLUSIVE MESENTERIC ISCHEMIA

NOMI is usually multifactorial in cause. Depending on the definition, NOMI may compose up to 20% to 30% of all acute mesenteric ischemic syndromes and may be associated with high mortality, ranging from 30% to 93%.[48] There has been an overall decrease in incidence of this syndrome with improved management of hemodynamic

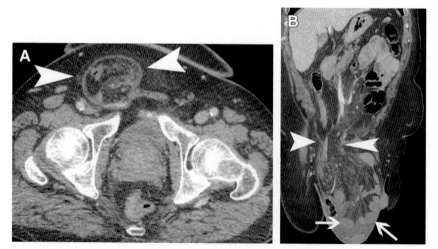

Fig. 13. Strangulated small bowel. Axial (*A*) and coronal (*B*) CT images of incarcerated small bowel (*white arrows*) in a large right inguinal hernia (*white arrowheads*). CT findings include hypoenhancement of the small bowel wall (*white arrows*) with adjacent fluid and fat stranding of the associated mesentery in the hernia sac.

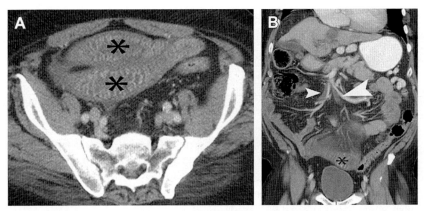

Fig. 15. Venous bowel ischemia from SMV thrombosis. Axial (*A*) and coronal reformatted (*B*) CT images of a patient with history of cirrhosis presenting with abdominal pain. Axial CT image shows marked bowel wall thickening with hyperenhancement and mesenteric edema (*asterisks*). Coronal image shows thrombosis of the SMV (*arrowheads*). Venous ischemia presents with marked bowel thickening and may show some bowel wall enhancement, unlike arterial ischemia, which often shows normal to thinned wall thickness and absent mural enhancement.

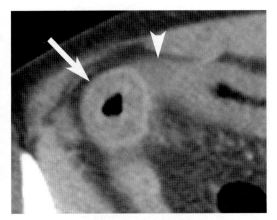

Fig. 16. Target-appearance of bowel. Venous occlusion resulting in bowel edema with hyperenhancement (*white arrow*) of serosal/subserosal layers, mesenteric stranding, and small adjacent free fluid (*white arrowhead*).

instability. In the setting of septic, hemorrhagic, or cardiogenic shock, a profound decrease of systemic blood pressure results in reflexive mesenteric arterial vasoconstriction with diversion of blood flow to the brain and heart. Other causes of reduced mesenteric blood flow include blunt abdominal trauma, overdose of digitalis, and the use of amphetamines, cocaine, ergotamine, or other agents resulting in vasoconstriction.[28,48,49] Classic CT findings of shock bowel include diffuse small bowel wall thickening and mural hyperenhancement with relative sparing of the colon and mesenteric ascites (**Figs. 18** and **19**). However, one must also be familiar the normal differences in small bowel enhancement, such as jejunal hyperenhancement compared with ileum, because of the higher density of valvulae conniventes (**Fig. 18**). The ischemic injuries range from localized superficial mucosa damage to the watershed

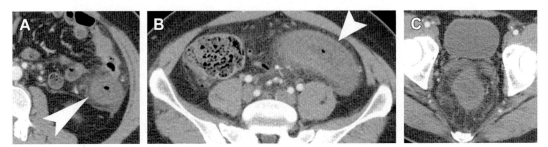

Fig. 17. Venoocclusive disease. Three axial CT images (*A–C*) show marked bowel wall thickening with poor enhancement of the colon (*white arrowhead*) continuously from the descending colon to the rectum. Associated mesenteric fat stranding is seen.

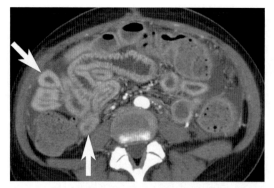

Fig. 18. Shock bowel. Mucosal hyperenhancement of thick walled small bowel (*white arrows*) and ascites suggests recent hypotension.

regions (splenic flexure, rectosigmoid region) with sparing of the right colon (**Fig. 20**). In severe cases, the entire bowel may be affected.[48–50] The diagnosis of NOMI may be challenging because CT findings overlap with other forms of bowel disease, such as infectious and inflammatory enteritis and colitis. The pattern of bowel enhancement is quite variable and may include absent, decreased, or hyperenhancement.[38,51,52] In addition, hypoperfusion may lead to extravascular leakage of fluid resulting in bowel edema, mesenteric stranding, and ascites (see **Fig. 11**).

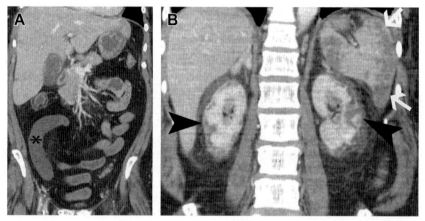

Fig. 19. (*A, B*): Shock bowel from hypotension. Coronal CT images of an elderly man with sepsis and hypotension. The first image (*A*) shows nonenhancement of a small bowel segment (*black asterisk*) compatible with small bowel ischemia. Additional image (*B*) shows evidence of global hypotension and shock with renal cortical necrosis (*black arrowheads*) and splenic infarcts (*white arrows*).

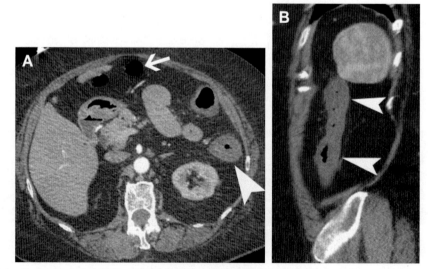

Fig. 20. Watershed colonic ischemia. Axial (*A*) and sagittal (*B*) CT images of a patient with hypotension show segmental bowel wall thickening and poor mural enhancement of the descending colon (*white arrowheads*) with sparing of the transverse colon (*white arrow*).

SUMMARY

Radiologists play a critical role in diagnosis and appropriate triage of patients with mesenteric ischemia. MDCT is an invaluable imaging test for patients with suspected mesenteric ischemia and outperforms all other medical tests. Because mesenteric ischemia may present with many different radiological appearances, an understanding of intestinal vascular and mesenteric anatomy as well as the pathophysiology of mesenteric ischemic disease helps improve the diagnosis of this challenging disease. The variable and overlapping appearance of various forms of mesenteric ischemia can be confusing; however, recognition of these findings is important for accurate diagnosis (**Table 2**).

REFERENCES

1. Cartwright SL, Knudson MP. Evaluation of acute abdominal pain in adults. Am Fam Physician 2008; 77(7):971–8.

2. Ruotolo RA, Evans SR. Mesenteric ischemia in the elderly. Clin Geriatr Med 1999;15(3):527–57.

3. Kumar S, Sarr MG, Kamath PS. Mesenteric venous thrombosis. N Engl J Med 2001;345(23):1683–8.

4. Stamatakos M, Stefanaki C, Mastrokalos D, et al. Mesenteric ischemia: still a deadly puzzle for the medical community. Tohoku J Exp Med 2008; 216(3):197–204.

5. Huang HH, Chang YC, Yen DH, et al. Clinical factors and outcomes in patients with acute mesenteric ischemia in the emergency department. J Chin Med Assoc 2005;68(7):299–306.

6. Barajas RF Jr, Yeh BM, Webb EM, et al. Spectrum of CT findings in patients with atrial fibrillation and non-traumatic acute abdomen. AJR Am J Roentgenol 2009;193(2):485–92.

7. Schoots IG, Levi MM, Reekers JA, et al. Thrombolytic therapy for acute superior mesenteric artery occlusion. J Vasc Interv Radiol 2005;16(3):317–29.

8. Kougias P, Lau D, El Sayed HF, et al. Determinants of mortality and treatment outcome following surgical interventions for acute mesenteric ischemia. J Vasc Surg 2007;46(3):467–74.

9. Hohenwalter EJ. Chronic mesenteric ischemia: diagnosis and treatment. Semin Intervent Radiol 2009; 26(4):345–51.

10. Agaoglu N, Turkyilmaz S, Ovali E, et al. Prevalence of prothrombotic abnormalities in patients with acute mesenteric ischemia. World J Surg 2005;29(9): 1135–8.

11. Levine JS, Jacobson ED. Intestinal ischemic disorders. Dig Dis 1995;13(1):3–24.

12. Mitsuyoshi A, Obama K, Shinkura N, et al. Survival in nonocclusive mesenteric ischemia: early diagnosis by multidetector row computed tomography and early treatment with continuous intravenous high-dose prostaglandin E(1). Ann Surg 2007;246(2): 229–35.

13. Angel W, Angel J, Shankar S. Ischemic bowel: uncommon imaging findings in a case of cocaine enteropathy. J Radiol Case Rep 2013;7(2):38–43.

14. Barrett T, Upponi S, Benaglia T, et al. Multidetector CT findings in patients with mesenteric ischaemia following cardiopulmonary bypass surgery. Br J Radiol 2013;86(1030):20130277.

15. Jancelewicz T, Vu LT, Shawo AE, et al. Predicting strangulated small bowel obstruction: an old problem revisited. J Gastrointest Surg 2009;13(1):93–9.

16. Hunt SJ, Coakley FV, Webb EM, et al. Computed tomography of the acute abdomen in patients with atrial fibrillation. J Comput Assist Tomogr 2009; 33(2):280–5.

17. Mamode N, Pickford I, Leiberman P. Failure to improve outcome in acute mesenteric ischaemia: seven-year review. Eur J Surg 1999;165(3):203–8.

18. Potretzke TA, Brace CL, Lubner MG, et al. Early small-bowel ischemia: dual-energy CT improves conspicuity compared with conventional CT in a swine model. Radiology 2015;275:119–26.

19. Rosenblum JD, Boyle CM, Schwartz LB. The mesenteric circulation. Anatomy and physiology. Surg Clin North Am 1997;77(2):289–306.

20. Haglund U, Bergqvist D. Intestinal ischemia – the basics. Langenbecks Arch Surg 1999;384(3): 233–8.

21. Longo WE, Ballantyne GH, Gusberg RJ. Ischemic colitis: patterns and prognosis. Dis Colon Rectum 1992;35(8):726–30.

22. Ball WS Jr, Seigel RS, Goldthorn JF, et al. Colonic strictures in infants following intestinal ischemia. Treatment by balloon catheter dilatation. Radiology 1983;149(2):469–71.

23. Brandt L, Boley S, Goldberg L, et al. Colitis in the elderly. A reappraisal. Am J Gastroenterol 1981; 76(3):239–45.

24. Whitehead R. The pathology of ischemia of the intestines. Pathol Annu 1976;11:1–52.

25. Inderbitzi R, Wagner HE, Seiler C, et al. Acute mesenteric ischaemia. Eur J Surg 1992;158(2): 123–6.

26. Kirkpatrick ID, Kroeker MA, Greenberg HM. Biphasic CT with mesenteric CT angiography in the evaluation of acute mesenteric ischemia: initial experience. Radiology 2003;229(1):91–8.

27. Wiesner W, Khurana B, Ji H, et al. CT of acute bowel ischemia. Radiology 2003;226(3):635–50.

28. Rha SE, Ha HK, Lee SH, et al. CT and MR imaging findings of bowel ischemia from various primary causes. Radiographics 2000;20(1):29–42.

29. Cognet F, Ben Salem D, Dranssart M, et al. Chronic mesenteric ischemia: imaging and percutaneous

treatment. Radiographics 2002;22(4):863–79 [discussion: 879–80].

30. Klein HM, Lensing R, Klosterhalfen B, et al. Diagnostic imaging of mesenteric infarction. Radiology 1995;197(1):79–82.

31. Taourel PG, Deneuville M, Pradel JA, et al. Acute mesenteric ischemia: diagnosis with contrast-enhanced CT. Radiology 1996;199(3):632–6.

32. Antonopoulos P, Siaperas P, Troumboukis N, et al. A case of pneumoperitoneum and retropneumoperitoneum without bowel perforation due to extensive intestinal necrosis as a complication to chemotherapy: CT evaluation. Acta Radiol Short Rep 2013;2(7). 2047981613498723.

33. Lee HS, Cho YW, Kim KJ, et al. A simple score for predicting mortality in patients with pneumatosis intestinalis. Eur J Radiol 2014;83(4):639–45.

34. Milone M, Di Minno MN, Musella M, et al. Computed tomography findings of pneumatosis and portomesenteric venous gas in acute bowel ischemia. World J Gastroenterol 2013;19(39):6579–84.

35. Horton KM, Fishman EK. Multidetector CT angiography in the diagnosis of mesenteric ischemia. Radiol Clin North Am 2007;45(2):275–88.

36. Ho LM, Paulson EK, Thompson WM. Pneumatosis intestinalis in the adult: benign to life-threatening causes. AJR Am J Roentgenol 2007;188(6):1604–13.

37. Kernagis LY, Levine MS, Jacobs JE. Pneumatosis intestinalis in patients with ischemia: correlation of CT findings with viability of the bowel. AJR Am J Roentgenol 2003;180(3):733–6.

38. Wiesner W, Mortele KJ, Glickman JN, et al. Pneumatosis intestinalis and portomesenteric venous gas in intestinal ischemia: correlation of CT findings with severity of ischemia and clinical outcome. AJR Am J Roentgenol 2001;177(6):1319–23.

39. Macari M, Balthazar EJ. CT of bowel wall thickening: significance and pitfalls of interpretation. AJR Am J Roentgenol 2001;176(5):1105–16.

40. Macari M, Megibow AJ, Balthazar EJ. A pattern approach to the abnormal small bowel: observations at MDCT and CT enterography. AJR Am J Roentgenol 2007;188(5):1344–55.

41. Turnage RH, Guice KS, Oldham KT. Endotoxemia and remote organ injury following intestinal reperfusion. J Surg Res 1994;56(6):571–8.

42. Balthazar EJ, Liebeskind ME, Macari M. Intestinal ischemia in patients in whom small bowel obstruction is suspected: evaluation of accuracy, limitations, and clinical implications of CT in diagnosis. Radiology 1997;205(2):519–22.

43. Frager D, Baer JW, Medwid SW, et al. Detection of intestinal ischemia in patients with acute small-bowel obstruction due to adhesions or hernia: efficacy of CT. AJR Am J Roentgenol 1996;166(1):67–71.

44. Ha HK, Kim JS, Lee MS, et al. Differentiation of simple and strangulated small-bowel obstructions: usefulness of known CT criteria. Radiology 1997;204(2):507–12.

45. Zalcman M, Sy M, Donckier V, et al. Helical CT signs in the diagnosis of intestinal ischemia in small-bowel obstruction. AJR Am J Roentgenol 2000;175(6):1601–7.

46. Bradbury MS, Kavanagh PV, Bechtold RE, et al. Mesenteric venous thrombosis: diagnosis and noninvasive imaging. Radiographics 2002;22(3):527–41.

47. Harward TR, Green D, Bergan JJ, et al. Mesenteric venous thrombosis. J Vasc Surg 1989;9(2):328–33.

48. Segatto E, Mortele KJ, Ji H, et al. Acute small bowel ischemia: CT imaging findings. Semin Ultrasound CT MR 2003;24(5):364–76.

49. Trompeter M, Brazda T, Remy CT, et al. Non-occlusive mesenteric ischemia: etiology, diagnosis, and interventional therapy. Eur Radiol 2002;12(5):1179–87.

50. Kim AY, Ha HK. Evaluation of suspected mesenteric ischemia: efficacy of radiologic studies. Radiol Clin North Am 2003;41(2):327–42.

51. Chou CK. CT manifestations of bowel ischemia. AJR Am J Roentgenol 2002;178(1):87–91.

52. Chou CK, Mak CW, Tzeng WS, et al. CT of small bowel ischemia. Abdom Imaging 2004;29(1):18–22.

Acute Infectious and Inflammatory Enterocolitides

Mark E. Baker, MD, FACR, FSAR, FSCBTMR

KEYWORDS

- Infectious • Inflammatory • Enteritis • Colitis • Ulcerative colitis • Crohn disease • Typhlitis
- Pseudomembranous colitis

KEY POINTS

- Infectious and inflammatory enterocolitides can present with an acute abdomen.
- The most common entities are ulcerative colitis, Crohn disease, and *Clostridium difficile* colitis.

This article reviews the clinical and imaging findings of patients who present acutely with infectious and inflammatory enterocolitides. The acute abdomen can be defined as the sudden onset (generally <24 hours) of severe localized or generalized abdominal pain that prompts the patient to seek immediate medical assistance; most often a visit to the emergency department.[1] In general, patients with either infectious or inflammatory enterocolitides present with a more indolent history of days or weeks and do not experience the degree of acute abdominal pain that patients with ischemia or diverticulitis experience. These 2 entities, and similar disorders, such as vasculitis and angioedema, are the subject of other reviews in this issue by Thakrar and Bodmer, and Yeh and colleagues, so they are excluded from this article.

CLINICAL PRESENTATION IN ACUTELY ILL PATIENTS WITH INFLAMMATORY BOWEL DISEASE OR INFECTION

Most patients presenting acutely with either inflammatory bowel disease (IBD) or infection involving the small bowel or colon have variable degrees of abdominal cramps and/or pain, tenesmus, diarrhea (often bloody), bloating, nausea, and vomiting.[2] The pain tends to be more generalized than from other causes of an acute abdomen. On examination, there are variable degrees of tenderness; guarding; and, if there has been a perforation, peritoneal signs.

RADIOGRAPHIC EVALUATION OF ACUTELY ILL PATIENTS WITH INFLAMMATORY BOWEL DISEASE OR INFECTION

In the past, plain radiographs were the initial radiographic examinations performed in any patient with abdominal pain. Although a kidney-ureter-bladder film alone can give important information, the combination of an upright, decubitus, or cross-table lateral film, and often a chest film (as in the acute abdominal series), is vital in identifying small amounts of free intraperitoneal gas.[3,4] However, currently, in almost all settings, computed tomography (CT) provides much more comprehensive information in patients with acute abdominal pain and this examination has almost completely replaced the plain film evaluation in these patients.[5–8]

In a large retrospective study of 874 patients from the Royal Victoria Hospital, McGill University, abdominal radiographic interpretation was normal

Disclosures: The author receives salary support as well as software and hardware from Siemens Healthcare in investigating radiation reduction in computed tomography. The author has informal consultations with Bracco about oral contrast agents for computed tomography.
Section of Abdominal Imaging, Imaging Institute, Digestive Disease Institute and Cancer Institute, Cleveland Clinic Lerner College of Medicine of Case Western Reserve University, L10, 9500 Euclid Avenue, Cleveland, OH 44195, USA
E-mail address: bakerm@ccf.org

radiologic.theclinics.com

in 34%, nonspecific in 46%, and abnormal in 19%.[9] Fifty percent of the patients underwent additional imaging: CT alone in 64% and ultrasonography alone in 22%. Of those patients whose abdominal radiography was normal, 42% had follow-up imaging. Of these, 72% of the follow-up imaging was abnormal. Of those in whom abdominal radiography was nonspecific, 52% had follow-up imaging. Of those, 78% of the follow-up imaging was abnormal. Abdominal radiography only assisted diagnosis confirmation in 2% to 8% of cases and was possibly helpful in changing patient treatment in 4% without a follow-up study.

Several other studies have shown the efficacy of CT in patients in the acute setting.[10–12] Specifically, several recent clinical studies in patients with Crohn disease have shown that CT identifies abnormalities not clinically suspected; findings that have led to management changes.[13–17] Recent investigations have shown that CT imaging in the emergency setting is efficacious in identifying important complications of Crohn disease.[15–17] However, before contemplating a CT scan, risk stratification should be performed by the ordering physician. This risk stratification should be based on history and physical findings. In one analysis, a prior history of intestinal obstruction or intra-abdominal abscess, current hematochezia, and leukocytosis (white blood cell count >12,000 μL) were all independent predictors of urgent findings on a subsequent CT (abscess, perforation, obstruction, or new or worsening non–Crohn disease findings).[17] If the patient presentation warrants immediate imaging, then a CT scan should be performed.

DOSE REDUCTION IN COMPUTED TOMOGRAPHY IN EMERGENCY DEPARTMENT/EMERGENT SETTINGS

As with all CT, efforts should be made to reduce the dose. To date, innumerable investigations have shown that efficacious scans can be obtained by reducing the dose compared with historical higher dose levels. Doses for many patients with body mass index (BMI) less than 25 to 30 kg/m^2 can be reduced to 10 to 15 mSv from historical levels of 15 to 30 mSv by altering tube voltage (peak kilovoltage or kVp) and tube current (milliamp seconds or mAs) and using noise-reducing iterative reconstruction algorithms. In a randomized controlled trial of 108 patients, low-dose CT (N = 53 patients) (2–3 mSv; 120 kVp and 64 mAs for patients with BMI<30 kg/m^2; 120 kVp and 96 mAs for patients with BMI>30 kg/m^2) was compared with abdominal radiography (N = 55 patients) (1.1 mSv).[18] A diagnosis was identified

in only 22% of the abdominal radiographs, with 51% requiring further imaging. A diagnosis was identified in 64% of the CT scans, with only 26% requiring further imaging.

OTHER IMAGING TECHNIQUES

The 2 other imaging techniques used in the emergency setting are ultrasonography and magnetic resonance (MR). Ultrasonography is generally used when the acute abdominal pain is localized to the right upper quadrant to assess for gallbladder and biliary disease, in the right lower quadrant in assessing the appendix in children and thin young adults, or in the female pelvis (these are discussed elsewhere in this issue). MR is generally not used in the setting of generalized acute abdominal pain unless the patient is pregnant.[19]

IMAGING THE ACUTE ABDOMEN IN PATIENTS WITH BOTH ULCERATIVE COLITIS AND CROHN DISEASE

Patients with ulcerative colitis and Crohn disease can both present with acute abdominal pain with severe colitis, mesenteric vein thrombi and thrombosis, and acute gastrointestinal bleeding (**Box 1**). All three entities may cause signs and symptoms that lead to imaging for diagnosis.

SEVERE COLITIS WITHOUT OR WITH MEGACOLON

A common acute entity that affects patients with either ulcerative colitis or Crohn colitis is a severe colitis, without or with megacolon. Severe colitis is common and occurs in patients with ulcerative colitis and Crohn colitis, as well as *Clostridium difficile* colitis. However, severe colitis is most common in ulcerative colitis, occurring in up to 15% of patients with ulcerative colitis.[20] The term fulminant has been defined as a critical form of severe colitis: greater than 10 bowel movements per day, daily continuous gastrointestinal bleeding

---

Box 1
Acute abdomen resulting from IBD (ulcerative colitis and Crohn disease)

- Severe colitis
  - Without megacolon
  - With megacolon
- Mesenteric venous thrombi or thrombosis
- Acute gastrointestinal hemorrhage

necessitating blood transfusions, increased erythrocyte sedimentation rate, fever, tachycardia, abdominal tenderness, distension, and colonic dilatation.[21] However, the term fulminant is now rarely used. Acute colitis with megacolon occurs in approximately 10% of patients with ulcerative colitis and 2.3% with Crohn colitis.[22] The definition of a megacolon varies between 5.5 and 8 cm depending on the author and the location of segment along the course of the colon.[23] Most clinicians consider a colonic lumen greater than 6 cm to be a megacolon when colitis is present.[24]

When radiologists describe the findings in fulminant colitis, without or with megacolon, they should not use the term toxic megacolon. Toxicity has a specific clinical definition based on findings absent on an imaging study. In 1955, Truelove and Witts[25] defined acute, severe ulcerative colitis clinically by the following: (1) stool frequency greater than or equal to 6 per day, (2) temperature greater than 37.8 C, (3) pulse rate greater than 90 beats per minute, (4) large amount of blood in stools, (5) hemoglobin level less than 10.5 g/dL, or (6) erythrocyte sedimentation rate of greater than 30 mm/h. Recent definitions of several organizations (American College of Gastroenterology, Association of Coloproctology of Great Britain and Ireland, European Crohn's and Colitis Organisation) have almost identical criteria and are based on this initial definition.[20,26,27] Jalan and colleagues'[28] initial definition of a toxic megacolon is commonly used by colorectal surgeons and includes the following, in addition to a dilated colon: (1) at least 3 of fever greater than 38 C, heart rate greater than 120 beats per minute, leukocytosis greater than 10,500/mm[3], and anemia; (2) in addition to the prior criterion, at least 1 of dehydration, altered consciousness, electrolyte disturbances, and hypotension. Note that patients may be toxic with colitis and not have a megacolon (**Fig. 1**). Patients with a severe colitis, without or with megacolon, can progress to free perforation.

Radiographic manifestations of a severe colitis are nonspecific. Further, when there is a severe pancolitis (patients with a severe colitis tend to have a pancolitis), there are no features that distinguish ulcerative colitis from Crohn colitis (unless there is obvious small bowel disease, and backwash ileitis can be confidently distinguished from Crohn ileitis). The findings of a severe colitis on plain films and cross-sectional imaging (usually CT) include nodular or asymmetric fold thickening, submucosal edema, effacement of the fold pattern with thinning of the colonic wall, pericolonic soft tissue changes and/or edema, and uncommonly free intraperitoneal gas (see **Fig. 1**; **Fig. 2**).[29–32]

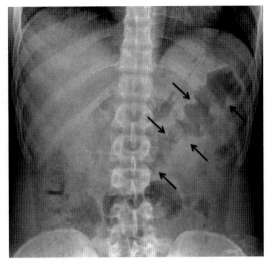

Fig. 1. Ulcerative colitis, clinically toxic without megacolon. The plain radiograph shows thick, nodular folds (*arrows*) in the distal transverse colon that is not dilated. Even so, the patient was clinically toxic and had a colectomy.

MESENTERIC VENOUS THROMBI AND THROMBOSIS

Patients with IBD, both ulcerative colitis and Crohn disease, have a propensity for thromboembolic disease. The cause of the hypercoagulable state in these patients is unknown but various factors have been postulated, including dehydration, increased coagulation factor levels, lower levels of antithrombin III, protein S and protein C deficiency caused by malnutrition, decreased endothelial protein C receptor level, thrombocytosis, and spontaneous platelet aggregation.[33–36] This complication of IBD is uncommon to rare, occurring in less than 1% of the population.[33,35] However, in patients with IBD undergoing bowel surgery, the condition seems to be more common.[37,38] In ileal pouch anal anastomosis surgery, the small bowel mesentery is completely mobilized. Further, in obese patients the ileal pouch may not reach the anal canal. In addition, if further mobilization is necessary because of the patient's body habitus, the peritoneal tissue to the right of the superior mesenteric vessels is removed with subsequent short transverse peritoneal incisions of these vessels anteriorly and posteriorly. Resecting these vessels may lead to some form of endothelial injury that can cause either shower emboli or thrombosis.[37]

Patients with IBD presenting with acute mesenteric vein thrombosis often have abdominal pain and distension. In this acute setting, the patient presentation and imaging findings depend on the

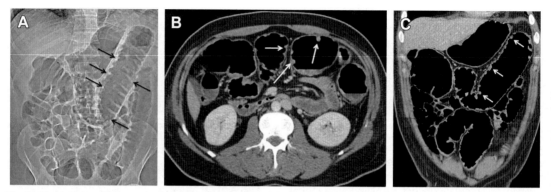

Fig. 2. Ulcerative colitis, megacolon without clinical toxicity. Scout from CT (*A*) shows a mild nodular fold pattern in a dilated transverse colon (*arrows*). Axial (*B*) and coronal (*C*) scans through the transverse colon show a thin colonic wall and small pseudopolyps (*arrows*). Despite the dilated, thin-walled colon, the patient was not toxic and was managed conservatively.

location and extent of the thrombus and whether there has been complete thrombosis of the vessel. When there has been thrombosis of a major vein, such as the superior mesenteric vein, cross-sectional imaging generally shows a long segment of symmetric small bowel wall thickening with mucosal hyperenhancement and submucosal low attenuation caused by edema. There is often adjacent mesenteric fat edema as well as ascites. If intravenous contrast has been injected, thrombus in the vein will be identified. Depending on the degree of ischemia and infarction, there may be pneumatosis and/or portal venous gas.[39–41]

Patients with IBD generally present less acutely with fever, abdominal pain, nausea and vomiting, tenderness, leukocytosis, prolonged ileus, and increased ostomy output within 1 to 3 weeks after bowel surgery. As a result, a postoperative infection and/or ileal pouch leak is suspected. In many patients, CT may only show small segmental portal vein thrombi.[38] These findings can be subtle, with thrombus present in a short segment of a small intrahepatic portal vein (**Fig. 3**), sometimes having the appearance of focal, intrahepatic biliary ductal visualization. Careful scrutiny with manual paging through the axial and coronal images can connect these small intrahepatic portal vein thrombi to the larger, more centrally located veins. Further, there is almost always some level of regional hepatic parenchymal hyperenhancement in the hepatic segment involved. This hyperenhancement is likely secondary to compensatory, increased hepatic arterial flow. If the scan is several weeks old, the regional hyperenhancement may be the only finding present, because these thrombi can resolve. In these postoperative patients, there may be thrombi or thrombosis of the larger intrahepatic portal veins, main portal vein, or superior and inferior mesenteric veins

(**Fig. 4**). However, larger vein involvement occurs in the minority of patients.[38] In almost all cases, there is no bowel wall thickening or enhancement alteration. However, most, if not all, patients have an ileus (see **Figs. 3** and **4**).

ACUTE GASTROINTESTINAL HEMORRHAGE

Although gastrointestinal bleeding is common in IBD (>50% of patients with ulcerative colitis and one-third of patients with Crohn disease), acute gastrointestinal bleeding is uncommon, accounting for less than 6% of all admissions for Crohn disease and less than 4% for ulcerative colitis.[42–44] Most patients are evaluated with endoscopy, which in many cases identifies the bleeding source. With the increasing use of multiphasic CT enterography in acute gastrointestinal bleeding, it is likely that some patients with IBD will be assessed with the technique.[45–47]

IMAGING THE ACUTE ABDOMEN IN PATIENTS WITH CROHN DISEASE

There are 2 major causes of acute abdominal pain in patients with Crohn: small bowel obstruction and penetrating disease, primarily abscess and, less commonly, free perforation (**Box 2**).

SMALL BOWEL OBSTRUCTION IN CROHN DISEASE

Of the acute presentations of Crohn disease, small bowel obstruction is one of the most common. This condition may be caused by stenotic disease without or with active inflammation or adhesive disease arising from prior surgery.[48,49] A less common cause is a complicating small bowel adenocarcinoma or neuroendocrine tumor. It is difficult to determine the causes of small bowel

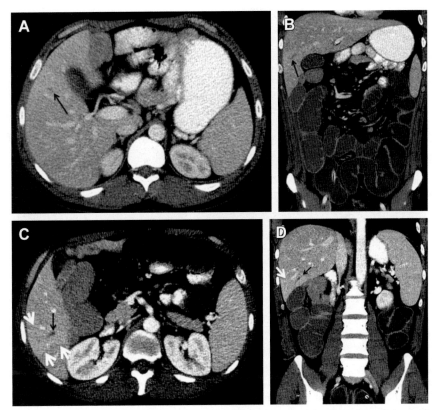

Fig. 3. Segmental portal vein thrombi after ileal pouch anal anastomosis for ulcerative colitis. Axial and coronal CT images through regions of segment V (*A*) and (*B*) and VI (*C*) and (*D*), respectively, show subtle segmental portal vein thrombi as linear hypodense areas (*black arrows*). These are associated with subtle hyperenhancing hepatic parenchyma in the affected segment (*short white arrows*). The patient had a prolonged ileus and a fever 5 days after surgery. Note the dilated fluid-filled small bowel.

obstruction in patients with Crohn, but adhesive disease is much more common than was previously realized and generally presents more acutely than in patients with stenotic disease. Imaging is very helpful in determining the cause of the small bowel obstruction, because the treatment varies depending on the cause.

When a small bowel obstruction is caused by stenotic disease, there is often concomitant acute inflammation.[48] In these cases, the bowel is dilated upstream from a short segment (<2–3 cm) of thick-walled, hyperenhancing bowel (**Fig. 5**). The hyperenhancement may be striated or homogeneous and there are dilated vasa recta.[50,51] There may be other associated mesenteric changes of edema, fluid, and penetrating disease with either fistulae or an abscess (**Fig. 6**). Pure fibrostenotic disease can cause chronic small bowel obstruction, but rarely presents acutely, unless dietary indiscretions lead to an acute obstruction at a fixed stenosis. With pure fibrostenotic disease, the bowel wall remains mildly thickened at the transition point. However, there is no hyperenhancement or vasa recta distension.

With adhesive disease without ischemia or a closed loop, the bowel wall at the transition point is normal. There is no wall thickening or hyperenhancement and the adjacent mesentery is normal as well. When there is ischemia or a closed loop obstruction, the affected segments are dilated upstream to the obstructions and there are variable degrees of wall thinning or thickening, mesenteric edema, and peritoneal fluid (**Fig. 7**).

When the bowel obstruction is caused by a complicating neoplasm, there may be an annular mass or a masslike process at the transition point, especially if it is asymmetric and nodular (**Fig. 8**).[52,53] However, many of these tumors are not detected preoperatively by imaging.

PENETRATING CROHN DISEASE

Although penetrating disease (sinus tracts, fistulae, abscess formation, and free perforation) is a hallmark of Crohn disease, and is a prime distinguishing feature from ulcerative colitis, free perforation of Crohn disease is uncommon to rare, estimated to occur in 1% to 2% of patients

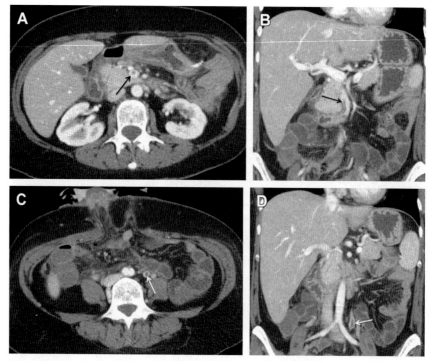

Fig. 4. Thrombi in the superior and inferior mesenteric vein, after laparoscopic subtotal colectomy for Crohn disease. Axial (*A*) and coronal (*B*) CT images show a subtle nonocclusive thrombus in the superior mesenteric vein (*black arrow*). Axial (*C*) and coronal (*D*) CT images show a near occlusive thrombus in the inferior mesenteric vein (*white arrow*). The patient had a fever and leukocytosis 7 days after surgery.

in Western countries.[22,54–57] In the largest series of 1415 patients, between 1960 and 1983, only 21 (1.5%) had free perforation.[56] These patients had a short duration of disease (mean = 3.3 years) and perforation was equally present from the small bowel and colon. In a more recent review of the Japanese literature, free perforation in Crohn disease was more common, with the incidence between 2.9% and 10.5%. Small bowel perforation was much more common than colonic perforation (88%) and most often from a solitary site (90%). Mean duration of disease was 2.1 years. In Japan, the incidence of free perforation in Crohn disease seems to be more common, occurring in between 2.9% and 10.5%.[57] As with the Western population, duration of disease in these patients is also short, with a mean of 2.1 years.

In patients presenting with free perforation, because of severe clinical manifestations, few imaging studies are performed. When performed, free intraperitoneal gas and fluid are identified. Because the bowel has decompressed, there is no bowel dilatation. The diseased bowel segments can be identified.

More commonly, penetrating disease manifests as a simple or complex fistula and/or an abscess. Patients with sinus tracts and fistulae generally do not present acutely; more often they present subacutely or with progressive symptoms. Fistulae in Crohn disease occur in 14% to 26% of patients.[58] Although perianal fistulae comprise at least 50% of these, 25% are enteroenteric, 10% to 15% are enterocutaneous or enterovesicular, and 10% are rectovaginal or anovaginal.[59] In a large

---

Box 2
Acute abdomen resulting from Crohn disease

- Small bowel obstruction
  - Mixed stenotic and active inflammatory small bowel Crohn disease
  - Adhesive disease from prior surgery
  - Small bowel tumor
    - Adenocarcinoma
    - Neuroendocrine tumor
- Penetrating disease
  - Sinus tracts/fistulae
  - Abscess
  - Free perforation

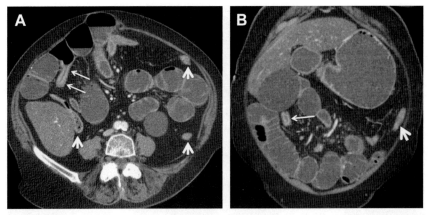

Fig. 5. Small bowel obstruction from mixed stenotic and active inflammatory small bowel Crohn disease. Axial (*A*) and coronal (*B*) CT images through the transition point show a thickened loop of small bowel with luminal occlusion and a stratified hyperenhancement pattern (*thin arrows*). Note the markedly dilated fluid-filled small bowel and the collapsed colon (*thick arrows*).

operative series from the University of Chicago, 35% of the patients had fistulae; 69% of these patients had their fistulae identified before surgery.[60] Now that CT and MR enterography are commonly performed preoperatively, most of these fistulae are now identified before surgery.[61] Investigations from Mayo have shown that fistulae are commonly identified with CT enterography in patients in whom they are clinically unsuspected.[13,14] Fistulae may be simple or complex and often are associated with small interloop abscesses. They may also be associated with a small bowel obstruction. Fistulae are identified on cross-sectional imaging as linear soft tissue attenuation strands extending from a loop of abnormal bowel toward another bowel loop, the urinary bladder, or other anatomic structure, like the psoas or iliopsoas muscle (see **Fig. 6**; **Fig. 9**). In almost all cases there is mixed disease (stenotic and active inflammatory small bowel Crohn disease).[48] The bowel wall is thickened. There is wall hyperenhancement, often with the stratified pattern. In addition, the bowel loop is often angulated or appears peaked or tethered toward the linear strand. The other bowel loops affected by the fistula are also angulated or tethered. When the urinary bladder is involved, the wall affected by the fistula is thickened and tethered. Urinary bladder gas is often absent.

Abscess formation is common in Crohn disease. In a large series from Mt Sinai, an abscess developed in 21% of patients with small bowel Crohn disease during the course of their disease.[62] In a large series from Japan studying the cumulative incidence of abscess 10 and 20 years after disease onset, 9% and 25% of patients respectively developed an abscess as a complication of Crohn disease.[63]

In almost all cases, abscesses are detected with cross-sectional imaging, usually CT, as a thick-walled collection of material with water to near-water attenuation. With the use of neutral contrast agents for CT, identification may be more difficult, but identification does not seem to be impaired by these agents.[61] There is almost always mixed active inflammatory and stenotic Crohn disease adjacent to the abscess, and a fistulous tract may also be identified extending from the abnormal bowel to the abscess (see **Fig. 9**).[64] These abscesses are often multiloculated, multiseptated, thick walled, and multiple collections, especially when the abscesses are present in the psoas or iliopsoas muscle. If accessible, and generally greater than 3 cm in diameter, these abscesses are percutaneously drained (see **Fig. 9**).

IMAGING THE ACUTE ABDOMEN IN PATIENTS WITH INFECTIONS OF THE COLON AND SMALL BOWEL

Patients with infectious enterocolitides generally do not present with symptoms severe enough to require imaging for evaluation (**Box 3**). Viruses are the most common cause of severe acute gastroenteritis leading to an emergency department visit.[65] In a large series of nearly 33,000 CT scans and 199 small bowel series performed in 1 US medical center, 446 patients had small bowel wall thickening.[66] Of these cases, approximately 25% (113 of 446) were determined to be caused by infection. Specific organisms were identified only in 30 of the 113, the most common of which were *Helicobacter pylori*, *Mycobacterium tuberculosis*, *Candida*, and *C difficile*. In general, infections can affect both the small and large bowel (**Fig. 10**). In the colon, most infections can cause a

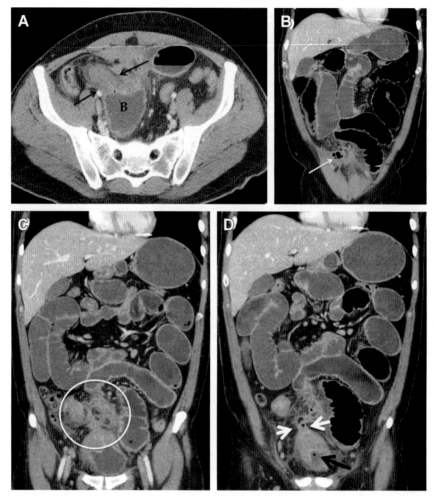

Fig. 6. Small bowel obstruction from mixed stenotic and active inflammatory small bowel Crohn disease, with penetrating disease (complex fistula and a small abscess). Axial CT image in the pelvis (*A*) through the transition point shows a very thickened loop of small bowel with luminal occlusion, subtle stratified hyperenhancement pattern (*thin black arrows*), and marked upstream dilatation (*marked by the letter B*). Anterior coronal image (*B*) in the lower abdomen shows a small abscess (*thin white arrow*). Coronal image in the pelvis (*C*) shows a complex enteroentero fistula (*contained within the white circle*). Coronal image in the pelvis more posteriorly (*D*) shows that the complex fistula (*thick white arrows*) extends inferiorly into the urinary bladder (*thick black arrow*). Note that the fistula tract is identified as a linear opacity and the wall of the superior aspect of the urinary bladder is thickened and tethered superiorly. There is also a small bubble of gas in the urinary bladder.

pancolitis.[30] Right-sided disease tends to occur in *Campylobacter*, *Salmonella*, *Yersinia*, tuberculosis, and amebiasis. Left-sided disease tends to occur in schistosomiasis, shigellosis, herpes, gonorrhea, syphilis, and lymphogranuloma venereum (**Figs. 11** and **12**). Cytomegalovirus (CMV) and *Escherichia coli* tend to be diffuse.[30,67–72] On CT, there are nonspecific findings of wall thickening and a stratified or homogeneous hyperenhancement pattern, the same as with Crohn disease. There also may be increased soft tissue attenuation stranding or edema adjacent to the affected bowel, as well as pneumatosis (**Fig. 13**).

Imaging findings cannot differentiate tuberculosis from Crohn disease. Keys to a precise diagnosis of any cause of an infectious enterocolitis lie with the history, especially if the patient is immunocompromised, and a stool culture.

CLOSTRIDIUM DIFFICILE COLITIS

As with other patients with infectious enterocolitides, patients with *C difficile* or pseudomembranous colitis generally do not require imaging because the disease is fairly self-limited and is diagnosed and treated clinically. The incidence

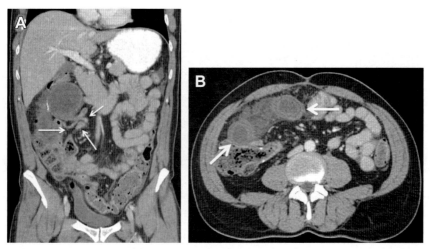

Fig. 7. Closed loop of obstruction in a patient with Crohn disease with prior surgery. Coronal CT image (*A*) in the midabdomen shows the site of the twist around the adhesive band (*thin white arrows*). Axial CT image (*B*) in the lower abdomen shows the ischemic closed loop (*thick white arrows*). The ischemic bowel has a target enhancement pattern and there is associated mesenteric fluid.

of adult, *C difficile* hospital discharge infections has increased over time, from 4.5 per 1000 in 2001 to 8.2 per 1000 in 2010.[73] In addition, severe cases of this disease are likewise increasing over time, from 7.1% in 1991 to 18.2% in 2003.[74,75] Many of these very sick patients are imaged with CT. As with colitis from IBD, patients with *C difficile* colitis can become toxic and develop a megacolon. The incidence of a toxic megacolon is up to 3% in patients with this infection.[76] The definition of toxicity for *C difficile* colitis is the same as for IBD toxic colitis. As with the other colitides, there may be a megacolon without toxicity (**Fig. 14**) and patients can be toxic without a megacolon (**Fig. 15**).

On CT, there is either focal or diffuse wall thickening associated with pericolonic soft tissue stranding and edema. In general, the wall is much more thickened than with other causes of colitis, especially Crohn colitis, but this cannot be used as a distinguishing feature. There may also be pneumatosis and/or portal venous gas, which does not imply ischemia; only loss of mucosal integrity. Some literature suggests that *C difficile* colitis can be distinguished from other forms of colitides by the presence of the so-called accordion sign.[77–79] On CT, this sign is caused by very thick haustral folds, with trapped oral contrast agent or bowel contents between the folds lined up in a parallel fashion (see **Fig. 15**; **Fig. 16**).[77] However, the

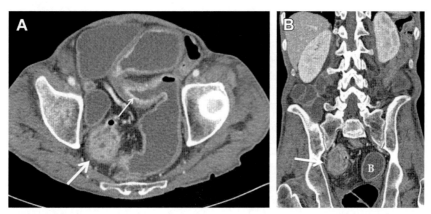

Fig. 8. Small bowel obstruction caused by a small bowel adenocarcinoma in a patient with Crohn disease. Axial (*A*) Axial CT image in the pelvis shows a mass in the distal small bowel at the transition point (*thick white arrow*). Coronal CT image of the abdomen shows the mass in the distal small bowel at the transition point (*thick white arrow*). The bowel (*marked by the letter B*) is dilated upstream to the mass. There is also mixed stenotic and active inflammatory small bowel disease upstream (*thin white arrow*).

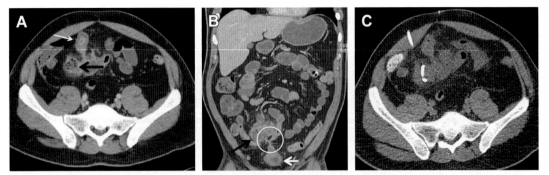

Fig. 9. Mixed stenotic and active inflammatory small bowel Crohn disease with penetrating disease (complex fistula with an abscess). Axial CT image (*A*) in the pelvis shows the mixed disease with wall thickening, luminal occlusion, and a stratified hyperenhancement pattern (*thin white arrow*). There is a mesenteric abscess (*thick black arrow*). A coronal CT image (*B*) shows a complex enterovesicular fistula (*white circle*) adjacent to the abscess (*thick black arrow*). Note the tethering of the superior aspect of the thickened urinary bladder (*thick white arrow*) and the angulation of the small bowel. The abscess was drained percutaneously (*C*).

studies suggesting that this sign is specific to the disease are largely descriptive studies specific to findings in the disease alone and do not compare the findings of *C difficile* colitis with other causes of colitis. Further, the sign is uncommon in *C difficile* colitis.[80] Although CT often detects patients with the disease, no CT finding correlates with the clinical parameters of the patient and it cannot predict surgical treatment.[81]

There are recent reports of *C difficile* affecting the small bowel. Although it is still rare, its incidence seems to be increasing and it may be associated with immunosuppression.[82] In most cases there is concomitant large and small bowel disease. The findings in the small bowel are very similar to those of any enteritis: wall thickening, mural stratification, pneumatosis, portal venous gas, adjacent mesenteric fat changes.

WHIPPLE DISEASE

Whipple disease is an infectious enteritis caused by a bacillus now called *Tropheryma whipplei*.

The disease usually occurs in white men and commonly has extraintestinal manifestations, especially migratory arthritis. On small bowel imaging there are thickened, nodular folds (**Fig. 17**).[83] CT can show low-attenuation mesenteric and retroperitoneal lymph nodes much like those seen in *Mycobacterium avium-intracellulare* and unusually in lymphoma.[84]

IMAGING THE ACUTE ABDOMEN IN PATIENTS WITH MISCELLANEOUS CAUSES OF ENTEROCOLITIDES

There are innumerable miscellaneous types of acute abdominal pain caused by other enterocolitides (**Box 4**). Only a few are highlighted here.

NEUTROPENIC COLITIS (TYPHLITIS)

Neutropenic colitis is an inflammatory process affecting the right colon, especially the cecum and terminal ileum in neutropenic patients.[30,85] The neutropenia in most cases results from chemotherapy, commonly high-dose chemotherapy used for patients after bone marrow transplant. When acutely ill with a fever and abdominal tenderness, these patients are commonly evaluated with CT. On CT, the cecum and/or right colon is thick walled and may have pneumatosis (**Fig. 18**). There is pericolonic soft tissue stranding and often pericolic gutter fluid. It is often impossible to determine whether these findings are caused by neutropenic colitis or pseudomembranous colitis because these patients are both neutropenic and *C difficile* positive (**Fig. 19**). Even so, patients are managed conservatively unless they show signs of toxicity.

Box 3
Acute abdomen resulting from infectious enterocolitides

- Miscellaneous infections
  - Viruses, *Campylobacter*, *Salmonella*, *Yersinia*, tuberculosis, amebiasis, shigellosis, herpes, gonorrhea, syphilis, lymphogranuloma, candida
- *C difficile* colitis
- Whipple disease

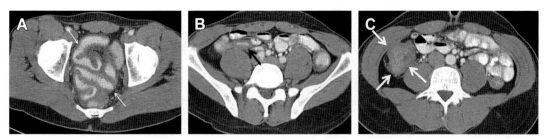

Fig. 10. *Salmonella* affecting the small bowel and colon. Axial CT images in the lower abdomen and pelvis show wall thickening in the ileum (*A*) (*thin white arrows*), terminal ileum (*B*) (*thick black arrow*), and cecum (*C*) (*thick white arrows*). The patient presented with abdominal pain and diarrhea. Stool culture was positive for *Salmonella*.

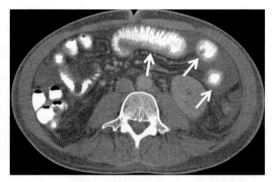

Fig. 11. *Campylobacter* affecting the small bowel. Axial CT image in the midabdomen shows small bowel wall thickening (*arrows*), ascites, and mesenteric fat edema. The patient was 7 weeks post–bone marrow transplant and presented with abdominal pain and diarrhea. Stool culture was positive for *Campylobacter*.

SMALL BOWEL DIVERTICULITIS

Small bowel diverticulitis is an uncommon to rare entity similar in presentation to large bowel diverticulitis. The disease can occur in either the jejunum or ileum and presents with acute abdominal pain, localized tenderness, fever, and leukocytosis. CT shows focal small bowel wall thickening with adjacent soft tissue stranding in the mesenteric fat and sometimes a perienteric abscess (**Fig. 20**).[86] The findings are similar to those of penetrating Crohn disease, especially if positive oral contrast medium has been administered and the distal/terminal ileum is involved. It can also mimic a foreign body perforation. The inflammatory process may obliterate the inflamed diverticulum, making the diagnosis difficult or impossible.

FOREIGN BODY PERFORATION

Detecting foreign body perforation of the small or large bowel can be challenging and is often serendipitous. However, small bones, especially from

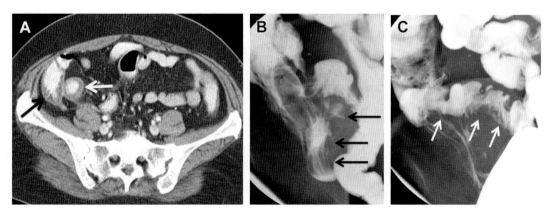

Fig. 12. *Salmonella* affecting the terminal ileum and cecum. Axial CT image (*A*) through the terminal ileum (*white arrow*) and cecum (*black arrow*) shows wall thickening. On small bowel series (*B*), the medial aspect of the cecum is narrowed and somewhat cone shaped (*black arrows*). On the same examination (*C*), the terminal ileum is mildly narrowed with nodular thickening of the folds (*white arrows*).

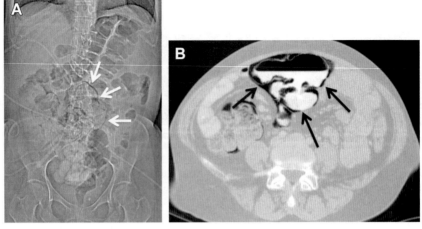

Fig. 13. CMV affecting the cecum. Scout film from a CT scan (*A*) shows pneumatosis (*white arrows*) in the wall of a mobile cecum. Axial CT image (*B*) filmed at wide windows confirms the presence of pneumatosis in the cecum (*black arrows*). The patient was 4 weeks post–bone marrow transplantation and presented with abdominal tenderness, fever, and diarrhea. Because of increasing abdominal tenderness the patient was taken to surgery and the right colon was resected. Pathology showed CMV inclusion bodies in the bowel wall.

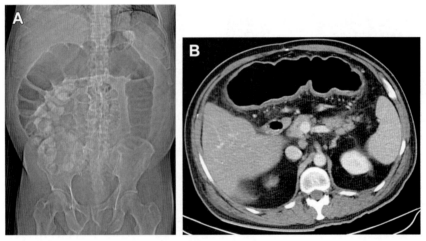

Fig. 14. *C difficile* colitis with a megacolon; patient not toxic. Scout view (*A*) and CT image (*B*) shows a dilated transverse colon with effacement of the folds. The patient was not clinically toxic.

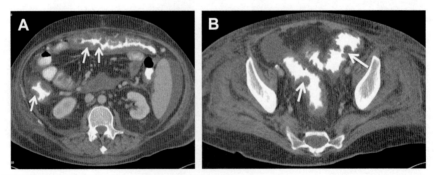

Fig. 15. *C difficile* colitis without a megacolon; patient toxic. CT images through the transverse (*A*) and sigmoid colon (*B*) show a thick-walled colon with nodular folds (*arrows*). The folds in the transverse colon trap the positive oral contrast and give an accordion sign. The colon is not dilated, but the patient was toxic and had a subsequent colectomy.

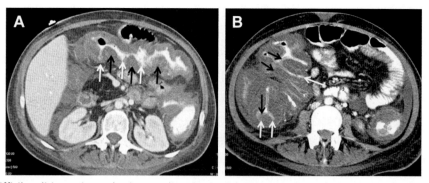

Fig. 16. *C difficile* colitis causing a classic accordion sign. Axial CT images through the transverse (*A*) and descending colon (*B*) show that the accordion sign is caused by contrast (*white arrows*) trapped between thickened, edematous folds (*black arrows*). Although there was a pancolitis without megacolon, the patient was not toxic and was treated successfully with antibiotics.

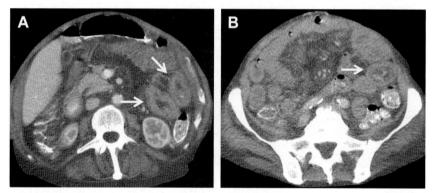

Fig. 17. Whipple disease of the small bowel. Axial CT images through the upper (*A*) and lower (*B*) abdomen show thickened small bowel (*arrows*). There was mesenteric edema, but no low-attenuation mesenteric lymph nodes.

chicken, are poorly calcified/ossified and are thus not hyperattenuating enough to be detected by plain radiographs or even CT. The problem is compounded by the ubiquitous use of scanning at 120 kVp, especially in large patients in whom the k-edge of calcium is not conducive to ideal identification. CT is sensitive in detecting these bones only after retrospective review.[87] In the area of the foreign body, the bowel wall is thickened and may contain a linear or curvilinear hyperattenuating opacity. Careful scrutiny of the bowel wall adjacent to localized soft tissue change, abscess, or soft tissue stranding facilitates identification of the foreign body.

GLUTARALDEHYDE COLITIS

Glutaraldehyde is a common germicide used for disinfecting endoscopes. The chemical is very irritating and can induce inflammation of the mucosa. If not properly removed after the endoscope

---

Box 4
Acute abdomen resulting from miscellaneous enterocolitides

- Neutropenic colitis
- Small bowel diverticulitis
- Foreign body perforation
- Glutaraldehyde colitis

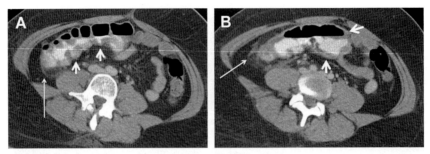

Fig. 18. Neutropenic colitis. Axial CT images through the ascending colon (*A*) and cecum (*B*) show mild colonic wall thickening (*thick white arrows*) and pericolonic soft tissue stranding (*thin white arrows*). The patient was neutropenic from high-dose chemotherapy for acute myeloid leukemia and had right lower quadrant pain and tenderness.

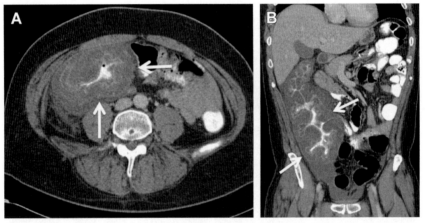

Fig. 19. Neutropenic colitis and *C difficile* colitis. Axial (*A*) and coronal (*B*) CT images through the right colon show marked colonic wall thickening (*arrows*) and an accordion sign. The colonic wall thickening was isolated to the cecum and ascending colon. The patient was neutropenic from high-dose chemotherapy for acute myeloid leukemia and had right-sided abdominal pain and tenderness. The stool was positive for *C difficile* toxin.

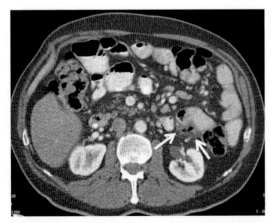

Fig. 20. Jejunal diverticulitis. Axial CT image through the jejunum shows a small amount of extraluminal gas and fluid (*arrows*) adjacent to a loop of proximal jejunum. The patient had known jejunal diverticula and presented with left mid to upper abdominal pain, tenderness, and leukocytosis. The patient was managed conservatively with antibiotics and bowel rest.

has been disinfected, it can induce a severe proctocolitis when introduced into a subsequent patient. CT shows circumferential wall thickening of the left colon.[88] There may be a stratified enhancement pattern.

DIVERSION COLITIS

Diversion colitis is a nonspecific inflammatory process that occurs in a defunctionalized colonic segment after upstream fecal diversion.[89] It is generally asymptomatic and thus its incidence is unknown, but it has been estimated to occur in up to 100% of patients. Endoscopically there is diffuse granularity, erythema, and vascular pattern blurring. Overall, the colon becomes atrophic with loss of the fold pattern.

REFERENCES

1. McNamara R, Dean AJ. Approach to acute abdominal pain. Emerg Med Clin North Am 2011; 29:159–73.

2. Fields MJ, Dean AJ. Systemic causes of abdominal pain. Emerg Med Clin North Am 2011;29:195–210.

3. Miller RE, Nelson SW. The roentgenologic demonstration of tiny amounts of free intraperitoneal gas: experimental and clinical studies. Am J Roentgenol Radium Ther Nucl Med 1971;112:574–85.

4. Miller RE, Becker GJ, Slabaugh RD. Detection of pneumoperitoneum: optimum body position and respiratory phase. AJR Am J Roentgenol 1980;135:487–90.

5. Stoker J, van Randen A, Lameris W, et al. Imaging patients with acute abdominal pain. Radiology 2009;253:31–46.

6. Panebianco NL, Jahnes K, Mills AM. Imaging and laboratory testing in acute abdominal pain. Emerg Med Clin North Am 2011;29:175–93.

7. Berdahl ED, Vermeulen MJ, Larson DB, et al. Emergency department computed tomography utilization in the United States and Canada. Ann Emerg Med 2013;62:486–94.

8. Schwartz DT. US emergency physicians order too many computed tomography scans—or do they? Ann Emerg Med 2013;62:495–7.

9. Kellow ZS, MacInnes M, Kurzencwyg D, et al. The role of abdominal radiography in the evaluation of the nontrauma emergency patient. Radiology 2008;248:887–93.

10. Ahn SH, Mayo-Smith WW, Murphy BL, et al. Acute nontraumatic abdominal pain in adult patients: abdominal radiography compared with CT evaluation. Radiology 2002;225:159–64.

11. MacKersie AB, Lane MJ, Gergardt RT, et al. Nontraumatic acute abdominal pain: unenhanced helical CT compared with three-view acute abdominal series. Radiology 2005;237:114–22.

12. Abujudeh HH, Kaewlai R, McMahon PM, et al. Abdominopelvic CT increases diagnostic certainty and guides management decisions: a prospective investigation of 584 patients in a large academic medical center. AJR Am J Roentgenol 2011;196:238–43.

13. Bruining DH, Loftus EV, Ehman EC, et al. Computed tomography enterography detects intestinal wall changes and effects of treatment in patients with Crohn's disease. Clin Gastroenterol Hepatol 2011;9:679–83.

14. Bruining DH, Siddiki HA, Fletcher JG, et al. Benefit of computed tomography enterography in Crohn's disease: effects on patient management and physician level of confidence. Inflamm Bowel Dis 2012;18:219–25.

15. Kerner C, Carey K, Mills AM, et al. Use of abdominopelvic computed tomography in emergency departments and rates of urgent diagnoses in Crohn's disease. Clin Gastroenterol Hepatol 2012;10:52–7.

16. Isreali E, Ying S, Henderson B, et al. The impact of abdominal computed tomography in a tertiary referral centre emergency department on the management of patients with inflammatory bowel disease. Aliment Pharmacol Ther 2013;38:513–21.

17. Kerner C, Carey K, Baillie C, et al. Clinical predictors of urgent findings on abdominopelvic CT in emergency patients with Crohn's disease. Inflamm Bowel Dis 2013;19:1179–85.

18. Nguyen LK, Wong DD, Fatovich DM, et al. Low-dose computed tomography versus plain abdominal radiography in the investigation of an acute abdomen. ANZ J Surg 2012;82:36–41.

19. Masselli G, Derme M, Laghi F, et al. Evaluating the Acute Abdomen in the Pregnant Patient. Radiol Clin N Am 2015, in press.

20. Brown SR, Haboubi N, Hampton J, et al. The management of acute severe colitis: ACPGBI position statement. Colrectal Dis 2008;10(Suppl 3):8–29.

21. Hanauer SB. Inflammatory bowel disease. N Engl J Med 1996;334:841–8.

22. Greenstein AJ, Sachar DB, Gibas A, et al. Outcome of toxic dilatation in ulcerative and Crohn's colitis. J Clin Gastroenterol 1985;7:137–43.

23. Autenreith DM, Baumgart DC. Toxic megacolon. Inflamm Bowel Dis 2012;18:584–91.

24. Jones JH, Chapman M. Definition of megacolon in colitis. Gut 1969;10:562–4.

25. Truelove SC, Witts LJ. Cortisone in ulcerative colitis: final report on a therapeutic trial. Br Med J 1955;2(4947):1041–8.

26. Travis SP, Stange EF, Lemman M, et al, European Crohn's and Colitis Organisation (ECCCO). European evidence based consensus on the management of ulcerative colitis. J Crohns Colitis 2008;2:24–62.

27. Kornbluth A, Sachar DB, Practice Parameters Committee of the American College of Gastroenterology. Ulcerative colitis practice guidelines in adults: American College of Gastroenterology, Practice Parameters Committee. Am J Gastroenterol 2010;105:501–24.

28. Jalan KN, Circus W, Cord WI, et al. An experience with ulcerative colitis: toxic dilation in 55 cases. Gastroenterology 1969;57:68–82.

29. Horton KM, Corl FM, Fishman EK. CT evaluation of the colon: inflammatory disease. Radiographics 2000;20:399–418.

30. Thoeni RF, Cello JP. CT imaging of colitis. Radiology 2006;240:623–38.

31. Moulin V, Dellon P, Laurent O, et al. Toxic megacolon in patients with severe acute colitis: computed tomographic features. Clin Imaging 2011;35:431–6.

32. Maddu KK, Mittal P, Shuaib W, et al. Colorectal emergencies and related complications: a comprehensive imaging review–imaging of colitis and complications. AJR Am J Roentgenol 2014;203:1205–16.

33. Hatoum OA, Spinelli KS, Abu-Hajir M, et al. Mesenteric venous thrombosis in inflammatory bowel disease. J Clin Gastroenterol 2005;39:27–31.

34. Jackson CS, Fryer J, Danese S, et al. Mesenteric vascular thromboembolism in inflammatory bowel disease: a single center experience. J Gastrointest Surg 2011;15:97–100.

35. Maconi G, Bolzacchini E, Dell'Era A, et al. Portal vein thrombosis in inflammatory bowel diseases: a single-center case series. J Crohns Colitis 2012;6:362–7.

36. Owczarek D, Cibor D, Glowacki JK, et al. Inflammatory bowel disease: epidemiology, pathology and risk factors for hypercoagulability. World J Gastroenterol 2014;20:53–63.

37. Remzi FH, Fazio VW, Oncel M, et al. Portal vein thrombi after restorative proctocolectomy. Surgery 2002;132:655–62.

38. Baker ME, Remzi F, Einstein M, et al. CT depiction of portal vein thrombi after creation of ileal-pouch-anal anastomosis. Radiology 2003;227:73–9.

39. Bradbury MS, Kavanagh PV, Bechtold RE, et al. Mesenteric venous thrombosis: diagnosis and noninvasive imaging. Radiographics 2002;22:527–41.

40. Kopylov U, Amitai MM, Lubetsky A, et al. Clinical and radiographic presentation of superior mesenteric vein thrombosis in Crohn's disease: a single center experience. J Crohns Colitis 2012;6:543–9.

41. Gore RM, Thakrar KH, Mehta UK, et al. Imaging in intestinal ischemic disorders. Clin Gastroenterol Hepatol 2008;6:849–58.

42. Cirocco WC, Reilly JC, Rusin LC. Life-threatening hemorrhage and exsanguination from Crohn's disease: report of four cases. Dis Colon Rectum 1995;38:85–95.

43. Robert JR, Sachar DB, Greenstein AJ. Severe gastrointestinal hemorrhage in Crohn's disease. Ann Surg 1991;231:207–11.

44. Pardi DS, Loftus EV, Tremaine WJ, et al. Acute major gastrointestinal hemorrhage in inflammatory bowel disease. Gastrointest Endosc 1999;49:153–7.

45. Geffroy Y, Rodallec MH, Boulay-Coletta I, et al. Multidetector CT angiography in acute gastrointestinal bleeding: why, when and how. Radiographics 2011;31:E35–47.

46. Marti M, Artigas JM, Garzon G, et al. Acute lower intestinal bleeding: feasibility and diagnostic performance of CT angiography. Radiology 2012;262:109–16.

47. Artigas JM, Marti M, Soto JA, et al. Multidetector CT angiography for acute gastrointestinal bleeding: technique and findings. Radiographics 2013;33:1453–70.

48. Baker ME, Hara AK, Platt JF, et al. CT enterography for Crohn's disease: optimal technique and imaging issues. Abdom Imaging 2015;40(5):938–52.

49. Katsanos KH, Tsianos VE, Maliouki M, et al. Obstruction and pseudo-obstruction in inflammatory bowel disease. Ann Gastroenterol 2010;23:243–56.

50. Paulson SR, Huprich JE, Fletcher JG, et al. CT enterography as a diagnostic tool in evaluating small bowel disorders: review of clinical experience with over 700 cases. Radiographics 2006;26:641–62.

51. Elsayes KM, Al-Hawary MM, Jagdish J, et al. CT enterography: principles, trends and interpretation of findings. Radiographics 2010;30:1955–74.

52. Soyer P, Hristova L, Boudghene F, et al. Small bowel adenocarcinoma in Crohn disease: CT-enterology features with pathologic correlation. Abdom Imaging 2012;37:338–49.

53. Weber NK, Fletcher JG, Fidler JL, et al. Clinical characteristics and imaging features of small bowel adenocarcinomas in Crohn's disease. Abdom Imaging 2014;40(5):1060–7.

54. Abascsal J, Diaz-Rojas F, Jorge J, et al. Free perforation of the small bowel in Crohn's disease. World J Surg 1982;6:216–20.

55. Katz S, Schulman N, Levin L. Free perforation in Crohn's disease: a report of 33 cases and review of literature. Am J Gastroenterol 1986;81:38–42.

56. Greenstein AJ, Mann D, Heimann T, et al. Spontaneous free perforation and perforated abscess in 30 patients with Crohn's disease. Ann Surg 1987;205:72–6.

57. Ikeuchi H, Yamamura T. Free perforation in Crohn's disease: review of the Japanese literature. J Gastroenterol 2002;37:1020–7.

58. Hvas CL, Dahlerup JF, Jacobsen BA, et al. Diagnosis and treatment of fistulizing Crohn's disease. Dan Med Bull 2011;58:C4338.

59. Tang L, Raswthorne P, Bernstein CN. Are perineal and luminal fistulas associated in Crohn's disease? A population-based study. Clin Gastroenterol Hepatol 2006;4:1130–4.

60. Michelassi F, Stella M, Balestracci T, et al. Incidence, diagnosis and treatment of enteric and colorectal fistulae in patients with Crohn's disease. Ann Surg 1993;218:660–6.

61. Vogel J, Moreira A, Baker ME, et al. CT enterography for Crohn's disease: accurate preoperative imaging. Dis Colon Rectum 2007;50:1761–9.

62. Ribeiro MB, Greenstein AJ, Yamazaki Y, et al. Intraabdominal abscess in regional enteritis. Ann Surg 1991;213:32–6.

63. Yamaguchi A, Matsui T, Sakurai T, et al. The clinical characteristics and outcome of intraabdominal abscess in Crohn's disease. J Gastroenterol 2004;39:441–8.

64. Booya F, Akram S, Fletcher JG, et al. CT enterography and fistulizing Crohn's disease: clinical benefit and radiographic findings. Abdom Imaging 2009;34:467–75.

65. Bresee JS, Marcus R, Venezia RA, et al. The etiology of severe acute gastroenteritis among adults visiting emergency departments in the United States. J Infect Dis 2012;205:1374–81.

66. Finkelstone L, Wolf E, Stein MW. Etiology of small bowel thickening on computed tomography. Can J Gastroenterol 2012;26:897–901.

67. Macari M, Megibow AJ, Balthazar EJ. A pattern approach to the abnormal small bowel: observations at MDCT and CT enterography. AJR Am J Roentgenol 2007;188:1344–55.

68. Katz DS, Scheirey CD, Bordia R, et al. Computed tomography of miscellaneous regional and diffuse small bowel disorders. Radiol Clin North Am 2013; 51:45–68.

69. Heller MT, Bhargava P. MDCT of acute cecal conditions. Emerg Radiol 2014;21(75):82.

70. Burrill J, Williams CJ, Bain G, et al. Tuberculosis: a radiologic review. Radiographics 2007;27:1255–73.

71. Gardiner R, Stevenson GW. The colitides. Radiol Clin North Am 1982;20:797–817.

72. Balthazar EJ, Gordon R, Hulnick D. Ileocecal tuberculosis: CT and radiologic evaluation. AJR Am J Roentgenol 1990;154:499–503.

73. Bagdasarian N, Rao K, Malani PN. Diagnosis and treatment of *Clostridium difficile* in adults: a systematic review. JAMA 2015;313:398–408.

74. Ricciardi R, Rothenberger DA, Madoff RD, et al. Increasing prevalence and severity of *Clostridium difficile* colitis in hospitalized patients in the United States. Arch Surg 2007;142:624–31.

75. Bouza E. Consequences of *Clostridium difficile* infection: understanding the healthcare burden. Clin Microbiol Infect 2012;18(Suppl 6):5–12.

76. Sayedy L, Kothari D, Richards RJ. Toxic megacolon associated *Clostridium difficile* colitis. World J Gastrointest Endosc 2010;16:293–7.

77. Fishman EK, Kavuru MK, Jones BJ, et al. Pseudomembranous colitis: CT evaluation of 26 cases. Radiology 1981;180:57–60.

78. Boland GW, Lee MJ, Cats AM, et al. Antibiotic-induced diarrhea: specificity of abdominal CT for the diagnosis of *Clostridium difficile* disease. Radiology 1994;191:103–6.

79. Boland GW, Lee JM, Cats AM, et al. *Clostridium difficile* colitis: correlation of CT findings with severity of clinical disease. Clin Radiol 1995;50:153–6.

80. Macari M, Balthazar EJ, Megibow AJ. The accordion sign at CT: a nonspecific finding in patients with colonic edema. Radiology 1999;211:743–6.

81. Ash L, Baker ME, O'Malley CM, et al. Colonic abnormalities on CT in adult hospitalized patients with *Clostridium difficile* colitis: prevalence and significance of findings. AJR Am J Roentgenol 2006;186:1393–400.

82. Wee B, Poels JA, McCafferty IJ, et al. A description of CT features of *Clostridium difficile* infection of the small bowel in four patients and a review of the literature. Br J Radiol 2009;82:890–5.

83. Philips R, Carson HC. The roentgenographic and clinical findings in Whipple's disease: a review of 8 patients. AJR Am J Roentgenol 1975;123:268–73.

84. Davis SJ, Patel A. Case report: distinctive echogenic lymphadenopathy in Whipple's disease. Clin Radiol 1990;42:60–2.

85. Schmit M, Bethge W, Beck R, et al. CT of gastrointestinal complications associated with hematopoietic stem cell transplantation. AJR Am J Roentgenol 2008;190:712–9.

86. Macari M, Balthazar EJ, Krinsky G, et al. CT diagnosis of ileal diverticulitis. Clin Imaging 1998;22(4): 243–5.

87. Goh BK, Tan YM, Lin SE, et al. CT in the preoperative diagnosis of fish bone perforation of the gastrointestinal tract. AJR Am J Roentgenol 2006;187:710–4.

88. Birnbaum BA, Gordon RB, Jacobs JE. Glutaraldehyde colitis: radiologic findings. Radiology 1995; 195:131–4.

89. Kabir SI, Kabir SA, Richards R, et al. Pathophysiology, clinical presentation and management of diversion colitis; a review of the current literature. Int J Surg 2014;12:1088–92.

Acute Urinary Tract Disorders

Rakhee H. Goel, MD[a], Raman Unnikrishnan, MD[b], Erick M. Remer, MD[c],*

KEYWORDS

• Flank pain • Urolithiasis • Hemorrhage • Pyelonephritis • Urinary obstruction

KEY POINTS

• Flank pain is a nondiscriminatory symptom due to the autonomic innervation of multiple organ systems, including the urinary tract.
• Low-dose computed tomography (CT) is the recommended test for patients who have an initial presentation with flank pain from presumed urinary colic.
• Most patients with pyelonephritis do not require imaging unless they fail to respond to antibiotics within 72 hours.
• Patients who present with pyelonephritis and any of the following conditions should be imaged at presentation: patients who are pregnant, diabetic, elderly, or immunocompromised or have a history of stone disease or congenital genitourinary (GU) abnormalities.
• The most common cause of renal infarction is an embolus from a cardiac source, whereas the most common cause of nontumoral renal vein thrombosis (RVT) is coagulopathy, such as in nephrotic syndrome.

INTRODUCTION

Acute urinary tract disorders often manifest as flank pain and are a common complaint of patients who present to the emergency department (ED). The pain is often a vague, poorly localized sensation that can have a variety of causes. Laboratory and clinical findings, such as hematuria, are neither sensitive nor specific for determining the cause of the flank pain. Accordingly, imaging is an important tool in determining a diagnosis and management plan. Patients with acute urinary tract disorders who present with pain include those with calculi, as well as renal infection, vascular disorders, and hemorrhage.

ANATOMY

The flank is the region between the posterior costal margin and the top of the iliac crest. The referred pain to the flank is due to both the dermatomal pattern of autonomic innervation and the common embryologic origin of various organs. The renal capsule and collecting system are innervated by sympathetic fibers from the T12 dermatome. In addition to the kidneys and ureters, these fibers also innervate gastrointestinal organs, resulting in poor pain localization. Pain from mid to lower ureteral distention radiates into the testes or labia, given the common embryologic origin from the urogenital ridge. Stimulation of the sympathetic fibers by either visceral organ distention or inflammation causes both pain and autonomic symptoms such as nausea and vomiting.[1]

IMAGING TECHNIQUE

The American Urological Association[2] and the American College of Radiology (ACR)[3] recommend low-dose (for body mass index [BMI] <30)

[a] Imaging Institute, Cleveland Clinic, 9500 Euclid Avenue, L10, Cleveland, OH 44195, USA; [b] Glickman Urological and Kidney Institute, Cleveland Clinic, 9500 Euclid Avenue, Q10, Cleveland, OH 44195, USA; [c] Imaging Institute, Glickman Urological and Kidney Institute, Cleveland Clinic, 9500 Euclid Avenue, A21, Cleveland, OH 44195, USA
* Corresponding author.
E-mail address: remere1@ccf.org

Radiol Clin N Am 53 (2015) 1273–1292
http://dx.doi.org/10.1016/j.rcl.2015.06.011
0033-8389/15/$ – see front matter © 2015 Elsevier Inc. All rights reserved.

noncontrast CT for the initial presentation of flank pain (**Table 1**). Noncontrast CT is a fast, readily available technique that provides a broad overview of the abdomen and pelvis, which is especially useful in the setting of vague symptoms. In addition, CT also provides important information for the management of renal calculi, such as stone burden and precise calculus location.

Miller and colleagues[4] performed a study to evaluate the utility of intravenous (IV) contrast in patients with flank pain and found that of the 708 patients who received IV contrast only 43 (6%) had actionable findings that required IV contrast, including 32 patients who had pyelonephritis, for which imaging is not initially indicated unless the patient has complicating factors.[5] Of the 8 patients, 6 with renal cell carcinoma had masses large enough to be distinguished without IV contrast.[4] Specific indications for IV contrast in patients who present with flank pain include unilateral renal stranding/enlargement with risk factors for renal infarct or vein thrombosis (ie, patients with dysrhythmia, thromboembolic disease history, or elevated levels of lactate dehydrogenase), perirenal fluid collection, renal mass/complicated cyst, or unexplained hematuria.[6]

During the past decade, there has been an emphasis on reducing the radiation dose of CT scans performed for flank pain given the young age and frequency of imaging within the affected patient population. Poletti and colleagues[7] demonstrated 100% sensitivity for calculi greater than 3 mm and nonurinary tract disorders for low-dose CT (30 mAs, 1.6–2.1 mSv) in patients with BMI less than 30. Ciaschini and colleagues[8] reconstructed raw CT data at 100%, 50%, and 25% of the original tube current using simulation software and demonstrated sensitivities of 91.7%, 83.3%, and 67.1%, respectively, for each reconstruction level. Although the sensitivity for stone detection is high, stone size measurements can vary on low-dose CT by 20% compared with standard-dose CT.[7]

Methods for dose reduction include the use of automated tube current modulation, increased slice thickness, and decreased tube current and/or voltage. Automatic tube current modulation maintains constant image quality by altering tube current based on patient size and allows for a reduction in effective dose of up to 66%, without any difference in stone conspicuity[9] and is routinely used. Memarsadeghi and colleagues[10] demonstrated that, although fewer stones are detected at a 5-mm section thickness, all missed stones measured less than 3 mm (in the range in which most pass spontaneously). By reducing tube voltage to 100 kV (dose reduction of 35%), there is an increase in noise of 30%. However,

Table 1
Sensitivity and specificity for detecting stones

Modality	Sensitivity	Accuracy	Key Points
XR	58%–62% (renal or ureteral)[3,12] 45%–58% for ureteral calculus[12,13]	61%[21]	• Main utility: surgical planning SWL, stent placement, follow up calculus • No information concerning hydronephrosis
XR + US	79%[21]	71%[21]	• Can be used in young women and patients with prior history of stones
IVU	85%[19]	92%[21]	• Requires IV contrast
CT	95%–96%[3]	98%[3]	• Low-dose (for BMI <30) NCCT study of choice for acute flank pain new presentation
US	24%–57% (renal/ureteral calculus)[3,20] 73%–86% (secondary signs of obstruction)	69%[21]	• Useful in the following population: young women, pregnant women, prior history of calculus
MR imaging	50%–60% (renal/ureteral calculus) 100% (secondary signs of obstruction)[26,27]	—	• Examination of choice for hydronephrosis in the first trimester • T1 postcontrast can increase specificity for a calculus, but gadolinium not allowed in pregnancy

Abbreviations: IV, intravenous; IVU, intravenous urography; NCCT, noncontrast computed tomography; SWL, shockwave lithotripsy; US, ultrasonography; XR, radiography.

by using adaptive iterative reconstruction (IR), which improves the signal to noise ratio while preserving image contrast (unlike filtered back projection), use of lower voltage is possible with maintained imaging quality. Given the dramatic advancement in computational power during the past 2 decades, IR can now be used in the clinical setting.[11]

Multiple studies have demonstrated the limited utility of the plain abdominal radiography (kidneys, ureters, and bladder [KUB]) in the workup for new-onset acute flank pain, with a sensitivity of 45% to 58% and a specificity of 70% to 80% for ureteral calculi.[12,13] The main value of KUB is in surgical planning for patients undergoing shock wave lithotripsy, visualization of stent positioning, and follow-up of known calculi. About 50% of ureteral calculi (particularly ureteral calculi that are >4 mm, in the upper ureter, and have Hounsfield units (HU) >100[14]) are seen on the CT scout and can be subsequently followed up with KUB. Although not seen on the initial CT scout image, an additional 10% of calculi is seen on a KUB because of the lower peak kilovoltage used.[15] A recent study also suggests that a baseline KUB improves the clinician's ability to interpret follow-up KUBs.[16]

Compared with plain radiography, intravenous urography (IVU) provides more physiologic information, including the degree of the delayed nephrogram, which is associated with the severity of the obstruction[17] (**Fig. 1**). However, given that IVU has a dose similar to that of low-dose noncontrast CT (3.63 mSv),[18] requires IV contrast, can

take several hours to complete in the setting of obstruction, and still misses 31% to 48% of stones, CT is the preferred imaging modality.[19]

Ultrasonography (US) can assess for dilation of the renal and ureteral collecting system without the use of ionizing radiation. The sensitivity of US for a renal/ureteral calculus is 24% to 57% (worse in the left kidney), with poor visualization of stones less than 5 mm.[3,20] When also incorporating secondary signs of obstruction (such as hydronephrosis), the sensitivity improves to 73% to 86%. However, hydronephrosis can take several hours to develop after acute obstruction and varies with the level of patient hydration. Absence of an ipsilateral ureteral jet in the bladder can support the presence of obstruction; however, the patient needs to be well hydrated, and a jet may still be present with partial obstruction[17,21] (**Fig. 2**).

A prospective study comparing CT with the KUB/US combination revealed that all stones not detected by KUB/US passed spontaneously.[22] Smith-Bindman and colleagues[23] also demonstrated that utilization of US in the initial ED flank evaluation does not increase the rate of serious adverse events or return ED visits/hospitalizations. However, between 27% and 41% of patients who initially had US required a subsequent CT during the same ED visit.

US is the recommended initial imaging modality for flank pain in pregnant and young women because of the lack of ionizing radiation. Young women (<45 years) have a much lower rate of stone detection (24.1%) than do men (61.6%), related to

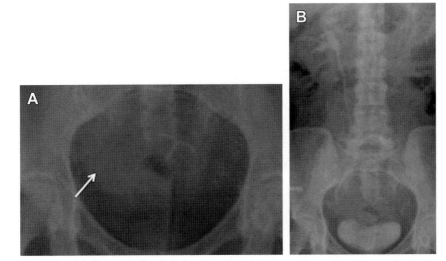

Fig. 1. Distal right ureteral calculus. (A) Pelvis plain radiograph demonstrates a faint radiopaque density in the right pelvis, could represent a ureteral calculus or phlebolith (*arrow*). Intrauterine device in place. (B) Intravenous urogram shows a mildly dilated right renal collecting system and ureter to the level of an obstructing calculus.

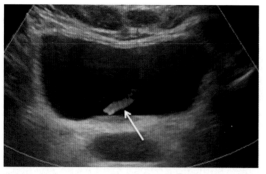

Fig. 2. Right ureteral jet. Color Doppler ultrasound image shows a right ureteral jet (*arrow*), which excludes complete right ureteral obstruction.

the high rate of gynecologic causes for pain (such as ovarian cysts).[24] In addition, the organ dose for women is higher because of the positioning of the ovaries. Given that 83% of women with stones greater than 4 mm had hydronephrosis Patatas and colleagues[24] recommended that KUB/US be the initial imaging modality for the young female population.

In pregnant patients, physiologic right hydroureteronephrosis is a confounding phenomenon seen in the second trimester. It occurs secondary to obstruction of the right distal ureter by the gravid uterus. ACR appropriateness criteria recommend the use of MR imaging in the first trimester during organogenesis and CT in the second trimester given its higher sensitivity for calculi (100% CT vs 69% MR imaging)[3] (**Table 2**).

Although MR imaging is 100% sensitive for diagnosing GU obstruction, its value in acute flank pain evaluation is limited by inherent lower spatial resolution and the low signal intensity of calculi.[25] In particular, calculi less than 1 cm are not well visualized on T2 sequences, with a sensitivity of 50% to 60% for ureteral calculi.[26,27] T1 postcontrast urogram images have a higher sensitivity for calculus detection and can exclude an enhancing tumor at the site of obstruction.[27] However, contrast cannot be administered in pregnancy. Phleboliths are not visualized on MR imaging, also decreasing diagnostic utility.

URINARY TRACT CALCULUS IMAGING

An obstructing renal or ureteral calculus is the most frequent cause of flank pain and is seen in 35% to 55% of patients who undergo imaging for pain.[28] Obstructing proximal ureteral stones typically cause symptoms of flank discomfort radiating to the ipsilateral groin, often with coexistent nausea and vomiting. Distal ureteral calculi often present with ipsilateral groin and scrotal or labial pain in addition to irritative voiding symptoms of urinary frequency and urgency.

The lifetime risk for a urinary calculus disease is 12% for men and 6% for women.[29] Risk factors include a personal or family history of stones, urinary tract anatomic abnormality, obesity, and metabolic disorders. The incidence for stone disease is highest in warm regions and during the summer months because of an increased rate of dehydration.[30]

There are multiple types of calculi, with the most common type being calcium based (75%), followed by struvite (15%), uric acid (UA) (8%), and cysteine (3%).[31] Struvite stones are associated with infections from urease splitting organisms resulting in

Table 2			
Imaging recommendations for acute flank pain by patient population			
Presentation		**Study**	**Comments**
Acute flank pain	Concern for stone disease	Noncontrast CT	Most rapid and accurate
	Recurrent stone disease	Noncontrast CT	Ultralow dose recommended due to repeat imaging
		KUB/US	History of stones visible on KUB
	Pregnant	MR imaging or US	First trimester
		CT	Second and third trimesters
Flank pain with fever	Simple infection	No imaging recommended	CT with contrast if symptoms >72 h despite antibiotics
	Complicated infection	CT with contrast	Assess for complications and underlying anatomic abnormalities
		US	When there is concern for pyonephrosis

Data from Coursey CA, Casalino DD, Remer EM, et al. ACR appropriateness criteria: acute onset flank pain—suspicion of stone disease. In: ACR Criteria. 2011. Available at: http://www.acr.org/~/media/ACR/Documents/AppCriteria/Diagnostic/AcuteOnsetFlankPainSuspicionStoneDisease.pdf. Accessed January 15, 2015.

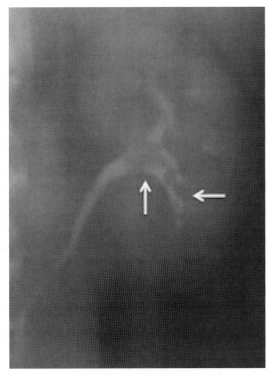

Fig. 3. Left renal collecting system uric acid stone. IVU demonstrates 3 radiolucent round filling defects (*arrows*) in the left renal collecting system.

alkaline urine. UA calculi are seen with a low urinary pH, are radiolucent on plain radiographs, and have attenuation values on CT imaging typically of less than 400 HU (**Fig. 3**). The rare matrix stone and calculi related to protease inhibitor treatment are low attenuation on CT[32] (**Fig. 4**).

On CT, a calculus is a high attenuation focus within the renal collecting system, ureteral lumen, bladder, or urethra (**Fig. 5**). Calculi often become lodged at the 3 narrowest segments of the ureter: (1) the ureteropelvic junction, (2) the crossing of the iliac vessels, and (3) the ureterovesical junction. The main differential diagnosis for a calculus is a phlebolith within a gonadal or pelvic vein. Characteristics that distinguish a ureteral calculus from a phlebolith within a pelvic vein include the following:

- Comet tail sign, tapering soft tissue that corresponds to the noncalcified portion of the vein
- Tissue rim, edematous ureter that surrounds the ureteral stone

Kawashima and colleagues[33] demonstrated that, although the tissue rim is specific for ureterolithiasis, its absence does not rule out a calculus. If uncertainty remains, CT urogram with IV contrast can be performed.

On US, a renal calculus is an echogenic focus with posterior shadowing, which is best visualized when the calculus is greater than 5 mm. Although the twinkle artifact is a useful color Doppler artifact to distinguish between small stones less than 5 mm and vascular calcifications, it can have a high false-positive rate.[34] Color comet tail artifact is another color Doppler artifact, immediately deep to the calculus, which can aid in diagnosis (**Fig. 6**).

Imaging findings for GU obstruction include ipsilateral hydronephrosis (69%–80%), hydroureter

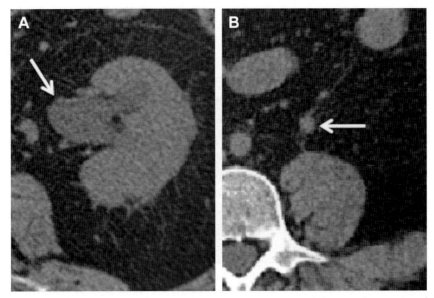

Fig. 4. Obstructive distal right ureteral idinavir calculus. Noncontrast axial CT images demonstrate (*A*) mild right hydronephrosis (*arrow*), (*B*) with a soft-tissue attenuation filling defect in the mid/distal right ureter (*arrow*).

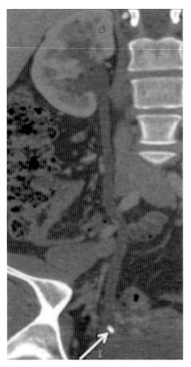

Fig. 5. Right ureterovesical junction calculus. Coronal CT noncontrast image demonstrates a calculus at the right ureterovesical junction (*arrow*) causing upstream dilation.

(64%–90%), unilateral renal enlargement (36%–71%), and perinephric edema (36%–82%).[35,36] Assessment for hydronephrosis should be based on dilation of the upper and lower pole calyces because of the frequent presence of an extrarenal pelvis. Although multiple early studies demonstrated the severity of perinephric edema as a reflection of the degree of functional obstruction,[37]

the most important factors in stone management are stone location, attenuation, size, and duration of symptoms.[38]

Chemical composition of a calculus is also important for management decision making, given that UA stones are treated with alkalization of the urine, struvite stones require antibiotics, and cysteine, brushite, or calcium oxalate stones can be resistant to shockwave lithotripsy (SWL). Therefore, dual-energy CT (DECT), which evaluates the change in attenuation in a material at high versus low kilovoltage peak, is being explored to quantify stone composition.[39] A case series demonstrated that DECT is 2 times more accurate for determining stone composition (UA vs non-UA) than Hounsfield unit criteria.[40] Pitfalls for DECT include calculi less than 3 mm and morbidly obese patients.

Frequently, nonobstructive calyceal calculi are encountered on CT imaging. Several prior retrospective studies suggest that a subset of these stones can cause a chronic, dull, vague pain over the kidney, rather than the acute episodic pain of renal colic, with resolution of symptoms after stone management.[41,42] A retrospective review of association between calculus location and symptoms demonstrated that 17% of calyceal stones were associated with pain/symptoms.[43]

Passage of a ureteral calculus depends on size and location, with a spontaneous passage rate of 48% for proximal versus 75% for distal ureteral calculi and 76%, 60%, 48%, and 25% for 2 to 4, 5 to 7, 7 to 9, and greater than 9 mm diameter, respectively.[29,44]

α-Blocker therapy (most commonly tamsulosin) has been shown to improve passage rates by 25%.[45] Therefore, for patients with ureteral calculi less than 8 mm with well-controlled symptoms,

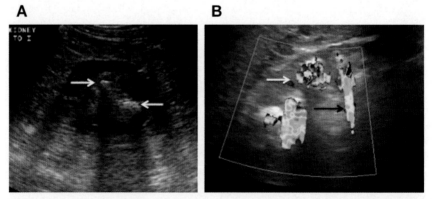

Fig. 6. Nonobstructive renal calculi. (*A*) Sagittal gray-scale ultrasound image demonstrates echogenic foci with posterior acoustic shadowing, consistent with calculi (*arrows*). (*B*) Sagittal color Doppler shows twinkle artifact (*white arrow*), related to reflection from a coarse surface, and comet tail artifact (*black arrow*), a form of reverberation artifact, both of which are associated with renal calculi.

normal renal function, and no concerns for urinary sepsis, observation with medical expulsive therapy in the form of tamsulosin is typically offered initially. Evidence suggests that spontaneous passage occurs within 4 to 6 weeks.[46] Most ureteral calculi greater than 10 mm do not pass spontaneously, and surgical treatment is typically offered.

If the patient is not a candidate for observation, there are 3 treatment modalities for ureteral and renal calculi: extracorporeal SWL, ureteroscopy with laser lithotripsy, and percutaneous nephrolithotomy (PCNL). SWL, performed under conscious sedation, involves shocking the calculus with sound waves to cause fragmentation. The calculus must be radiopaque on plain film, as fluoroscopy is needed to target the calculus. For morbidly obese patients, a skin to stone distance (measured on an axial CT from the stone to the overlying flank) should be less than 10 cm; otherwise the stone cannot be positioned in the focal zone of the shock wave. Stone-free rates vary depending on stone location, size, and attenuation. Significantly lower stone-free rates are seen with lower pole calculi (55%) than for mid or upper pole stones (71.8% and 76.5%, respectively).[47,48]

Stones with an attenuation value greater than 1000 HU also do not respond significantly to extracorporeal SWL.[49,50] Ureteroscopy, performed under spinal or general anesthesia, involves passage of a semirigid or flexible ureteroscope up the ureter with laser fragmentation of the stone. In general, it yields greater stone-free rates than SWL except for proximal ureteral stones less than 10 mm. PCNL, performed under general anesthesia, involves percutaneous access to the renal collecting system through the flank, with antegrade removal of the stone. It is typically reserved for renal stones greater than 20 mm[47] (**Box 1**).

Other causes for hydronephrosis that may present with acute flank pain include external obstruction due to a pelvic mass/inflammatory process, internal filling defect (such as a sloughed papilla or blood clot), or a ureteral wall abnormality (such as a ureteral transitional cell carcinoma or stricture). Renal leaks, which are related to disruption of the calices is usually due to trauma; however, occasionally a high level of backpressure can cause calyceal rupture with an associated perirenal urinoma (**Fig. 7**).[51]

RENAL INFECTION IMAGING

In patients who present with fever in addition to flank pain, nausea, and vomiting, GU infection should be considered. Additional signs of infection include dysuria and costovertebral angle

---

Box 1
Stone disease, what does the referring physician want to know?

Size of the renal or ureteral calculus

  Is the stone greater than 8 mm?

Location of the calculus

  Renal calculus—upper or lower pole

  Ureteral calculus—upper or lower

  Bladder—ureterovesical junction versus in the bladder

Stone attenuation

  Is the stone less than 400 HU?

  Homogenous versus heterogeneous

Stone burden

  How many stones are there?

Secondary signs of obstruction

  Degree of perinephric stranding

  Severity of hydronephrosis

Skin to stone distance

Adapted from Kambadakone AR, Eisner BH, Catalano OA, et al. New and evolving concepts in the imaging and management of urolithiasis: urologist's perspective. Radiographics 2010;30:603–23.

---

tenderness. Pyelonephritis is a common diagnosis, with an incidence of 120 to 130 cases annually per 100,000 women and 30 to 40 cases per 100,000 men.[52] Most cases are related to gram-negative enteric bacteria (such as *Escherichia coli*), which use special virulence factors such as endotoxins that inhibit ureteral peristalsis and adhesion fimbria to ascend from the lower urinary tract to the kidney.[53,54] Urinalysis and urine culture are used to confirm the diagnosis.

Imaging is not necessary to diagnose simple pyelonephritis. As suggested by the ACR appropriateness criteria, imaging is generally only necessary in the 5% of patients who do not demonstrate clinical improvement within 72 hours of initiating antibiotic therapy.[5] In addition, imaging should be used in specific patient groups who have an increased rate of disease progression, including patients who are pregnant, diabetic, elderly, or immunocompromised or have a history of stone disease and congenital GU abnormalities.[54] Clinical findings that are of concern for progression of infection include urine pH greater than 7.0 and renal insufficiency (glomerular filtration rate <40 mL/min/1.73 m^2).[55] The purpose of imaging is to assess for an obstructing stone, identify

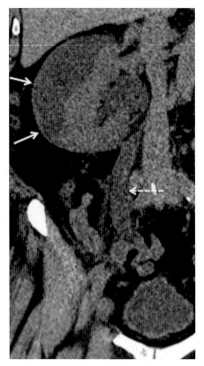

Fig. 7. Perinephric urinoma. Coronal noncontrast CT image demonstrates moderate right hydroureteronephrosis (*dashed white arrow*) due to a prostate cancer extending into the bladder (not shown). Forniceal rupture with associated subcapsular urinoma (*white arrow*) is a rare complication of hydronephrosis.

rare causes for pyelonephritis (such as anatomic abnormalities), and rule out complications (such as abscess) (**Table 3**).

The recommended CT protocol for complicated GU infection is a noncontrast examination (to assess for stone disease) followed by an enhanced phase at 90 to 120 seconds when there is uniform nephrographic phase enhancement of the renal parenchyma.[5,45] CT findings of pyelonephritis include a persistent and/or striated nephrogram, thickening and mucosal enhancement of the urothelium, renal enlargement, and inflammatory changes in

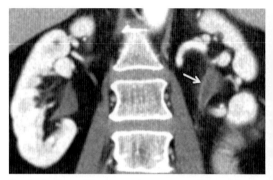

Fig. 8. Left pyelitis. Coronal contrast-enhanced image shows enhancement of the left renal collecting system urothelium with adjacent fat stranding (*arrow*), related to acute inflammation. Normal enhancement of the left renal parenchyma (not shown).

Gerota fascia and/or the renal sinus[56,57] (**Figs. 8 and 9**). In addition, perinephric fluid collections/effusions can form after pyelonephritis, which may need aspiration to rule out infection. Variant forms of pyelonephritis include the following[58]:

- Hemorrhagic bacterial nephritis: wedge-shaped area of increased attenuation related to an intraparenchymal hemorrhage
- Focal pyelonephritis: focal ill-defined infection with a masslike appearance that can mimic a neoplasm (**Fig. 10**)
- Hematogenous seeding: multiple, bilateral peripheral round low-attenuation lesions in the setting of systemic staphylococcal or streptococcal infection (**Fig. 11**).
- Emphysematous pyelonephritis: gas within the renal parenchyma

The differential diagnosis for the imaging findings of pyelonephritis includes other causes for striated nephrogram (CT contrast toxicity and renal infarcts) (**Fig. 12**) or a renal infiltrative process (leukemia, lymphoma, and transitional cell carcinoma [TCC]).[57]

Table 3 When to image for pyelonephritis		
Clinical Risk Factors[3,54]	**Concerning Symptoms**[54]	**Abnormal Laboratory Results**[55]
Diabetes	Symptoms >72 h, despite antibiotics	Urine pH >7.0
Immunocompromised	Acute renal colic	GFR <40
Elderly	Unstable patient (AMS, low BP)	50% decline in renal function
History of stone disease	Recurrent symptoms after completion of antibiotics	—

Abbreviations: AMS, altered mental status; BP, blood pressure; GFR, glomerular filtration rate.

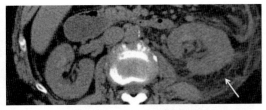

Fig. 9. Left pyelonephritis. Axial noncontrast CT shows edematous enlargement of the left kidney with surrounding perinephric fat stranding (*arrow*).

US findings are usually normal in the setting of pyelonephritis, and is, therefore, only useful to exclude obstruction as a cause for the infection. Endotoxins, released by the bacteria, inhibit ureteral peristalsis and can cause mild dilation of the collecting system. Nonspecific findings of pyelonephritis on US include focal hypoechoic region with decreased vascular flow, renal enlargement, and loss of the sinus fat and/or corticomedullary differentiation.[57,58] Both gas and calculi have decreased T2 signal intensity, limiting the utility of MR imaging in infection. Specific applications for diffusion-weighted imaging include differentiating between pyonephrosis/hydronephrosis and a fluid collection or abscess and increasing the

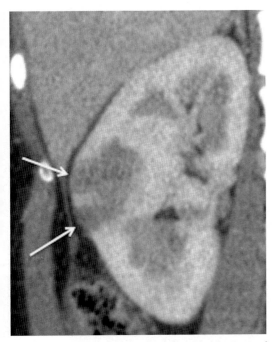

Fig. 10. Right interpolar focal pyelonephritis. Coronal contrast-enhanced CT image shows focal region of decreased enhancement (*arrows*) in the lateral interpolar kidney with a striated appearance. Mild adjacent fat stranding/fascial thickening.

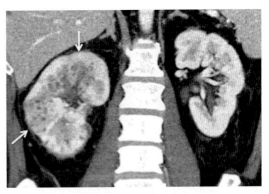

Fig. 11. Methicillin-resistant *Staphylococcus aureus*–related hematogenous pyelonephritis. Coronal contrast-enhanced CT demonstrates ill-defined regions of heterogeneous enhancement (*arrows*), which involve both the cortex and medulla. There is surrounding fat stranding.

sensitivity for detecting simple pyelonephritis[59] (**Fig. 13**).

When both infection and obstruction are present, pyonephrosis may result. Pyonephrosis (aka pus under pressure) requires urgent decompression of the urinary tract, via either a nephrostomy tube or a ureteral stent, to avoid rapid destruction of the renal parenchyma and deterioration in clinical status.[57] US is 90% sensitive and 97% specific for pyonephrosis and demonstrates debris or a fluid-fluid level within a dilated collecting system.[60] CT findings of pyonephrosis include thickening (>2 mm) and enhancement of the renal pelvis, dilation, and layering of debris within the collecting system. Fluid attenuation measurements within the renal pelvis are not reliable for assessment for pyonephrosis unless a layering debris level is seen. Similar findings are seen on MR imaging.[54,61]

When infection causes liquefactive necrosis of the renal parenchyma, microabscesses coalesce and a renal abscess forms (**Fig. 14**). About 75%

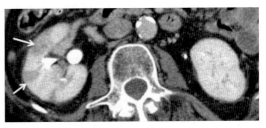

Fig. 12. Acute renal infarcts. Axial contrast-enhanced CT demonstrates wedge-shaped regions of decreased enhancement in the right kidney (*arrows*) with mild surrounding fat stranding.

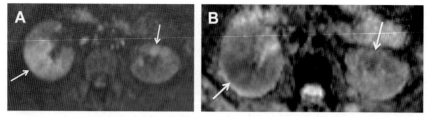

Fig. 13. Acute pyelonephritis. Diffusion-weighted MR imaging demonstrates bilateral wedge-shaped regions of restricted diffusion. (*A*) Diffusion-weighted imaging (*arrows*); (*B*) apparent diffusion coefficient image (*arrows*).

of renal abscesses occur in diabetic patients and can have an insidious presentation because of a lack of flank pain related to diabetic neuropathy. In addition, 15% to 20% of patients with a renal abscess have negative results on urine culture.[54] On CT, a renal abscess is seen as a low-attenuation collection with a thick wall (pseudocapsule) that has diminished enhancement compared with normal renal parenchyma during the corticomedullary phase that retains contrast on delayed imaging. CT can also assess for extension into the perinephric fat and other adjacent structures (**Fig. 15**). US can be useful to assess for a fluid component within the complex mass but is limited for assessing perinephric extension.[62]

Emphysematous pyelonephritis and pyelitis are also diagnoses seen primarily in diabetic patients. About 90% of patients with emphysematous pyelonephritis have diabetes and present with costovertebral tenderness, fever, and rarely crepitus in the flank region or scrotum. The most common causative organism is *E coli*, followed by *Klebsiella pneumoniae*. About 50% of patients have bacteremia.[63,64] CT, the imaging study of choice for emphysematous pyelonephritis, demonstrates gas within the renal parenchyma, asymmetric renal enhancement with delayed contrast excretion, and focal regions of necrosis or abscess. Wan and colleagues[65] delineated a

classification system based on the presence of fluid collections (type I no collections, type II with collections). Type II has a significantly better prognosis with respect to mortality (18% vs 69%), because the presence of fluid collections indicates an immune response (**Fig. 16**). Treatment is generally emergent nephrectomy, but conservative treatment with resuscitation, antibiotics, and in some cases percutaneous drainage, has been advocated for those who are clinically stable and have gas only in the collecting system or as initial management in those with perinephric collections.[66]

Gas in the bladder lumen may be from a gas-forming urinary tract infection (typically *E coli*), a bowel-bladder fistula, or recent instrumentation. Emphysematous cystitis involves gas within the bladder wall and is most commonly seen in middle-aged diabetic women (**Fig. 17**). In contrast to the high mortality rate and surgical management of emphysematous pyelonephritis, 90% of patients are treated with medical management, and the mortality rate is only 7%.[67]

Renal Arterial Infarct

Nonspecific acute-onset flank pain, often with nausea and vomiting, is the most common presentation of renal vascular events. In addition, patients

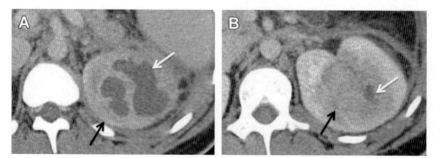

Fig. 14. Left renal abscess. Axial contrast-enhanced CT images demonstrate (*A*) a central fluid attenuation lesion (*white arrow*) with a thin enhancing rim and a thicker hypoenhancing rind (*black arrow*). More superiorly (*B*), there is a hypoenhancing region (*black arrow*), consistent with infected parenchyma, with a small central necrotic focus (*white arrow*).

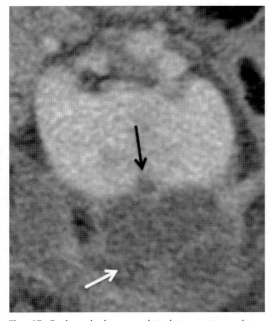

Fig. 15. Perirenal abscess related to acute pyelonephritis. Axial CT image demonstrates a posterior pararenal abscess (*white arrow*) with an enhancing rim and septations, which communicates with a ruptured calyx (*black arrow*).

can have a mild leukocytosis and fever for 1 to 2 days after a renal infarct, further complicating the diagnostic process.[68]

In the setting of relevant risk factors (myocardial infarction, malignancy, aortic aneurysm, and cardiac valvular disease), CT imaging with contrast should be performed when there is an enlarged kidney with surrounding perinephric edema of unknown cause on an initial unenhanced CT.[4] The most common cause for renal infarction is thromboembolism from a cardiac source. Although nonspecific, markedly elevated serum lactate dehydrogenase levels, a serum marker for cell necrosis, is helpful in suggesting the diagnosis.[69]

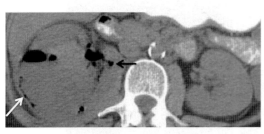

Fig. 16. Emphysematous pyelonephritis with fluid collection. Axial noncontrast CT image demonstrates a fluid collection replacing the renal parenchyma that contains gas (*white arrow*), with extension of gas into the adjacent psoas muscle (*black arrow*).

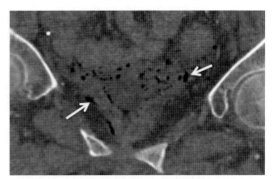

Fig. 17. Emphysematous cystitis. Coronal noncontrast CT image demonstrates gas within the bladder wall (*white arrows*).

CT protocol includes both the corticomedullary (to assess for patency of the renal vasculature) and nephrographic phases. CT findings for renal artery infarction include an occluded renal vessel and wedge-shaped region of decreased parenchymal attenuation (**Fig. 18**). The cortical rim sign, seen in 20% of global renal infarcts, related to capsular artery enhancement, is often not seen for at least 8 hours after infarct.[70,71] Given the appearance of medullary striations due to intrarenal collaterals vessels, pyelonephritis is the leading diagnostic differential consideration in the subacute period. In contrast to a renal infarct, acute pyelonephritis would demonstrate urothelial enhancement and perinephric inflammatory change. Additional differential diagnostic considerations include vasculitis and renal trauma. The MR imaging appearance of an acute infarct is a focal T1 and T2 hypointense region without internal enhancement.[72]

Acute cortical necrosis is a rare variant (2% of acute renal failure) of global ischemia related to either diffuse vasospasm or injury to the distal arcuate arteries (acute tubular necrosis) in which there is a relative decrease in peripheral cortical enhancement, with sparing of the medulla (**Fig. 19**). More than 50% of cases are associated with obstetric-related hemorrhage, most commonly placental abruption. There is bilateral kidney damage due to the systemic causes, resulting in high mortality (>50%).[73]

Renal vein thrombosis
The clinical and radiologic signs associated with RVT vary with the acuity of onset and amount of thrombus within the renal vein. Typical symptoms and signs include flank pain, microscopic hematuria, and deterioration of renal function. The most common causes for RVT are extension of renal tumor, trauma, or a hypercoagulable state as seen in nephrotic syndrome (ie, membranous

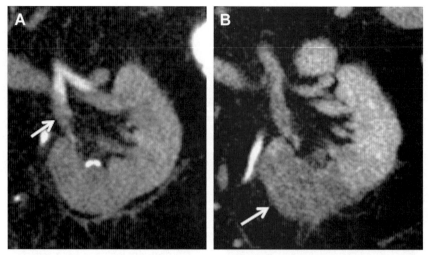

Fig. 18. Acute left lower pole renal infarct. Multiphase contrast-enhanced coronal CT images demonstrate (*A*) a filling defect (*arrow*) within an inferior pole renal artery on the arterial phase, (*B*) with an associated wedge-shaped region of decreased enhancement (*arrow*) in the inferior pole on the renal parenchymal phase.

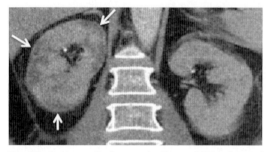

Fig. 19. Acute cortical necrosis. Coronal CT enhanced image demonstrates patchy decreased enhancement of the right renal cortex (*arrows*) with surrounding fat stranding and fascial thickening.

glomerulonephritis), systemic lupus erythematosus, or an inherited syndrome.[74] Renal vein thrombus occurs in 20% of patients with nephrotic syndrome.[75]

RVT is more common on the left, because of the longer course of the left vein. CT imaging findings include filling defect in the renal vein (**Fig. 20**), enlarged kidney with extension of edema into the sinus and perinephric fat, and coarse striations. In contrast to bland thrombus, tumor-related thrombus heterogeneously enhances and distends the vein.[76] US gray-scale findings include enlarged, hypoechoic kidneys with loss of the

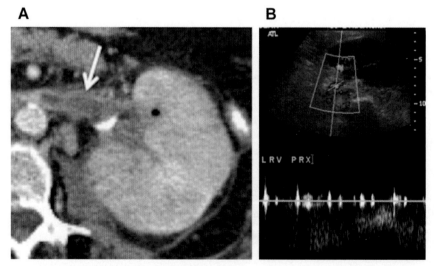

Fig. 20. Renal vein thrombus. (*A*) Axial contrast-enhanced image demonstrates filling defect in the left renal vein (*arrow*), with associated decreased enhancement of the left renal parenchyma and surrounding fat stranding. Focus of gas within the left renal collecting system is related to recently inserted ureteral stent. (*B*) Color Doppler image with spectral waveform demonstrates flow within the left renal vein, a false-negative finding.

normal corticomedullary differentiation. Spectral Doppler findings, both arterial and venous, are neither sensitive nor specific for RVT[77]; color Doppler venous flow can still be seen in RVT. MR imaging, which demonstrates high contrast between flowing blood and vascular walls, is useful for determining the superior extent of thrombus extension, given the mixing of nonopacified blood that occurs in the suprarenal IVC on CT.[74]

Renal hemorrhage

When an acute drop in hemoglobin is noted during initial flank pain evaluation, the primary diagnostic consideration is spontaneous perirenal hemorrhage, the Wunderlich syndrome. The most common underlying cause is a renal mass (both benign and malignant) (62%). However, other considerations include vascular diseases (inflammatory and aneurysm) (17%), infection (3%), anticoagulation, and idiopathic causes (13%).[78]

Multiphasic CT, the study of choice for perirenal hematoma, has a sensitivity of approximately 57% for determining the cause of hemorrhage at the time of presentation.[78,79] The unenhanced phase is used to identify the hemorrhage, which is high attenuation (HU 40–70) in the acute phase. Active contrast extravasation may be recognized on the arterial phase, which is also useful for ruling out aneurysms and other vascular causes.[80] Underlying masses are best visualized on the nephrographic phase. Short-term follow-up CT at 2 to 3 months should be done to assess for an underlying mass. If no mass is visualized, MR imaging with contrast and subtraction imaging or angiography should be performed.

MR imaging, with its superior contrast resolution, is a secondary option when the source of bleeding is not apparent on CT. Acute hemorrhage is T1 hyperintense, and subacute hemorrhage is heterogeneously both T1 and T2 hyperintense. Gadolinium-enhanced images with subtraction

postprocessing can be used to identify an underlying renal mass. After assessment with both CT and MR imaging, the source of bleeding is still not identified in 20% of cases. Then, selective renal arteriography can be used to identify subtle causes for bleeding such as vasculitis, small masses, and aneurysms.[80,81] US has poor sensitivity of identification of an underlying renal lesion, given that the echogenicity of the hemorrhage matches an adjacent lesion.[79]

The most common cause of a perirenal hemorrhage is a renal mass. Although less than 1% of renal cell carcinomas bleed, clear cell carcinoma is most prone to hemorrhage given its hypervascularity[82] (**Fig. 21**). Angiomyolipoma (AML), the most common benign renal tumor, is composed of smooth muscle, adipose tissue, and perivascular epithelial cells that form elastin-poor aneurysmal vessels (**Fig. 22**). This benign tumor is more prevalent in women (2.5:1), with a mean age of 41 years. Most patients with a small AML can undergo interval surveillance to assess for growth. In one series of 130 patients, 79% were found incidentally.[83] When an AML is greater than 4 cm, 82% to 94% are symptomatic and 50% to 60% bleed spontaneously.[84] Aneurysmal vessels within an AML that are greater than 5 mm was the most important factor linked to AML hemorrhage in a multivariate analysis[85] (**Fig. 23**). Selective embolization is the treatment of choice in patients with large AMLs, with a majority (94%) of patients not requiring surgical intervention at 5 years.[86]

Polyarteritis nodosa (PAN), a necrotizing small-medium vessel vasculitis, is the most common cause of bilateral renal hemorrhage.[79] PAN is antineutrophil cytoplasmic antibody negative and more common in patients with hepatitis B infection.[87] About 60% of patients with PAN have renal involvement, with intrarenal microaneurysms due to fibrinoid necrosis. CT findings include enlarged kidneys with decreased attenuation, segmental

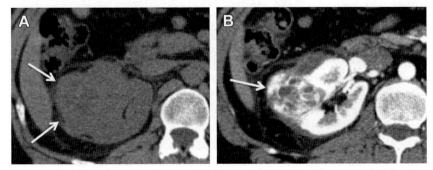

Fig. 21. Renal cell carcinoma with hemorrhage. Multiphase axial CT images demonstrate (*A*) subcapsular hyperdense region (*arrows*) with surrounding fat stranding concerning for hemorrhage on this noncontrast image; (*B*) contrast-enhanced image shows a central enhancing mass (*arrow*) with mild adjacent hemorrhage.

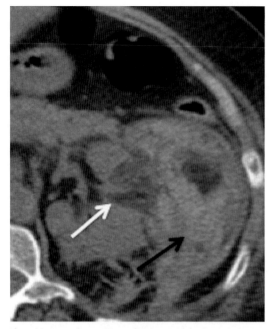

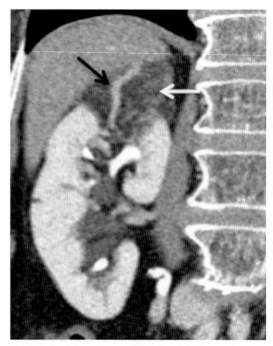

Fig. 22. Renal angiomyolipoma with hemorrhage. Axial noncontrast CT image demonstrates a fat-containing lesion (*white arrow*) that arises from the anterior interpolar kidney with acute perinephric hemorrhage (*black arrow*).

Fig. 23. Renal angiomyolipoma with internal aneurysmal vessel. Coronal contrast-enhanced CT image demonstrates a fat-containing lesion (*white arrow*) in the superior pole with an aneurysmal central enhancing vessel (*black arrow*).

infarcts, and multiple microaneurysms.[88] Because of the risk of hemorrhage with biopsy, diagnosis is usually confirmed with angiography to demonstrate the aneurysms.[80] Other causes for renal artery aneurysms include congenital, fibromuscular dysplasia, atherosclerosis, and prior trauma/instrumentation (including 1% of patients with prior partial nephrectomy) (**Fig. 24**).[89]

Additional subtypes of GU hemorrhage include the following:

- Adrenal hemorrhage: most often due to trauma but can also be associated with stress, bleeding diatheses, or tumor. Acute adrenal insufficiency is rare, even in the setting of bilateral hemorrhage; therefore, this is most commonly an incidental finding[90] (**Fig. 25**).

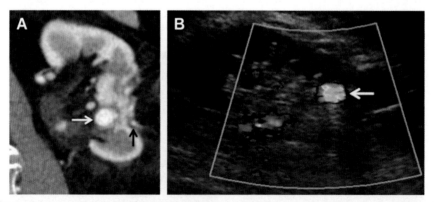

Fig. 24. Lobar renal artery pseudoaneurysm due to partial nephrectomy. (*A*) Axial contrast-enhanced CT image demonstrates a round enhancing focus (*white arrow*) with attenuation, which matches the vessels adjacent to a partial nephrectomy defect (*black arrow*), (*B*) Color Doppler image demonstrates yin-yang flow within the pseudoaneurysm (*arrow*).

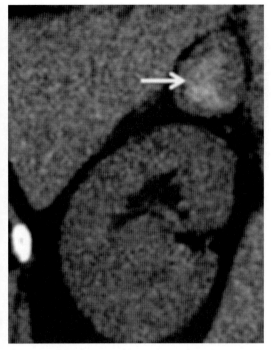

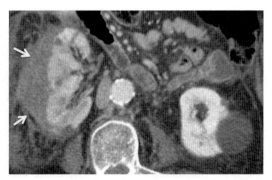

Fig. 26. Subcapsular hematoma. Axial contrast-enhanced CT image demonstrates a right subcapsular hematoma (*arrows*) causing mass effect on the right kidney and persistent corticomedullary phase nephrogram compared with nephrographic phase on left.

Fig. 25. Adrenal hemorrhage. Coronal noncontrast CT demonstrates high attenuation (*arrow*) and enlargement of right adrenal.

- Antopol-Goldman lesion: subepithelial pelvic hematoma, of unknown cause, which can mimic a urothelial neoplasm. Patients present with flank pain and gross hematuria. CT findings include a high-attenuation renal pelvis mass that does not enhance.[91]
- Subcapsular hematoma causing a Page kidney: renal compression by a subcapsular

hematoma compromises renal vascular inflow, activating the renin-angiotensin system and causing hypertension. Subcapsular hematomas are most common after trauma or intervention, such as percutaneous biopsy[92] (Fig. 26).
- Hemorrhage into a cyst: most commonly seen in patients with autosomal dominant polycystic kidney disease (ADPKD) or acquired renal cystic disease. About 80% of patients with ADPKD have acute pain at least once in their lives. Hemorrhagic cysts are CT high attenuation and MR imaging T1 hyperintense[93] (Fig. 27).

Alternative diagnoses
One reason that noncontrast CT is the study of choice for acute flank pain is its ability to

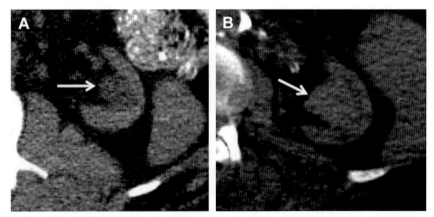

Fig. 27. Hemorrhage into a renal cyst. (*A*) Noncontrast CT examination in 2013 demonstrates a left interpolar parapelvic cyst (*arrow*). (*B*) Noncontrast CT examination in 2014 demonstrates enlargement of the cyst with new internal high attenuation material (*arrow*) in a patient presenting with acute left flank pain.

A   **B**

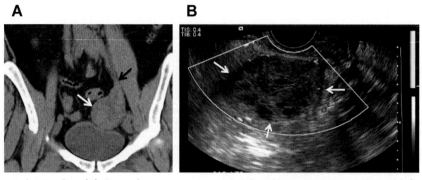

Fig. 28. Left ovarian torsion. (*A*) Coronal noncontrast examination demonstrates an enlarged left ovary (*white arrow*) with cephalad tapered extension representing a twisted pedicle (*black arrow*). (*B*) Color Doppler ultrasound image demonstrates absent flow within an enlarged left ovary (*arrows*).

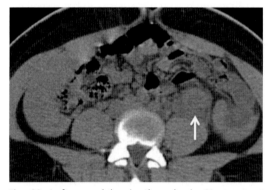

Fig. 29. Left gonadal vein thrombosis. Noncontrast axial CT image demonstrates the left gonadal vein distended with thrombus (*arrow*) with surrounding fat stranding and soft-tissue thickening.

diagnose non-GU causes for pain. Prior research indicates that a calculus is present on a CT obtained for indication of flank pain in 35% to 55% of patients and approximately 10% of patients have an alternative non-GU diagnosis. In women, gynecologic conditions, in particular adnexal cysts, account for 30% to 50% of the alternative diagnoses (**Figs. 28** and **29**). Additional less common alternative diagnoses include appendicitis/diverticulitis (10% of alternative diagnoses) (**Fig. 30**), acute cholecystitis/choledocolithiasis, vascular conditions (such as abdominal aortic aneurysm), musculoskeletal pain, and intraperitoneal fat infarction (omental infarction or epiploic appendagitis).[28,94]

A   **B**

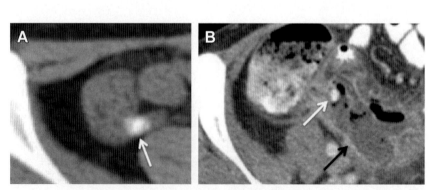

Fig. 30. Acute appendicitis. (*A*) Axial noncontrast CT image shows an appendicolith (*arrow*) at the base of the appendix with normal appendix. Subsequent contrast-enhanced image 5 days later when patient returned with persistent pain, (*B*) demonstrates a perforated appendix (*white arrow*) with an adjacent periappendiceal abscess (*black arrow*).

SUMMARY

Acute flank pain is a nonspecific presenting symptom with a variety of causes, including GU, gastrointestinal, and musculoskeletal causes. Low-dose noncontrast CT is the study of choice because of its ability to provide a broad survey of the abdomen in an efficient manner. For select patient groups, including young women, pregnant women, and patients with frequent stones, KUB/US is an alternative option. Radiologists play a key role in the diagnostic process by providing a diagnosis and key information for management decisions.

REFERENCES

1. Bueschen AJ. Flank pain. Chapter 182. In: Walker HK, Hall WD, Hurst JW, editors. Clinical methods: the history, physical, and laboratory examinations. 3rd edition. Boston (MA): Butterworths; 1990. p. 845–6.

2. Fulgham PF, Assimos DG, Pearle MS, et al. Clinical effectiveness protocols for imaging in the management of ureteral calculus disease: AUA technology assessment. J Urol 2013;189:1203–13.

3. Coursey CA, Casalino DD, Remer EM, et al. ACR appropriateness criteria: acute onset flank pain–suspicion of stone disease. In: ACR Criteria. 2011. Available at: http://www.acr.org/~/media/ACR/Documents/AppCriteria/Diagnostic/AcuteOnsetFlankPainSuspicionStoneDisease.pdf. Accessed January 15, 2015.

4. Miller FH, Kraemer E, Dalal K, et al. Unexplained renal colic: what is the utility of IV contrast? Clin Imaging 2005;29:331–6.

5. Nikolaidis P, Casalino DD, Remer EM, et al. ACR appropriateness criteria–acute pyelonephritis. In: ACR Criteria. 2012. Available at: https://acsearch.acr.org/docs/69489/Narrative/. Accessed January 15, 2015.

6. Akpinar E, Turkbey B, Eldem G, et al. When do we need contrast-enhanced CT in patients with vague urinary system findings on un-enhanced CT? Emerg Radiol 2009;16:97–103.

7. Poletti PA, Platon A, Rutschmann OT, et al. Low-dose versus standard-dose CT protocol in patients with clinically suspected renal colic. AJR Am J Roentgenol 2007;188:927–33.

8. Ciaschini MW, Remer EM, Baker ME, et al. Urinary calculi: radiation dose reduction of 50% and 75% at CT–effect on sensitivity. Radiology 2009;251:105–11.

9. Mulkens TH, Daineffe S, De Wijngaert R, et al. Urinary stone disease: comparison of standard-dose and low-dose with 4D MDCT tube current modulation. AJR Am J Roentgenol 2007;188:553–62.

10. Memarsadeghi M, Heinz-Peer G, Helbich TH, et al. Unenhanced multi-detector row CT in patients suspected of having urinary stone disease: effect of section width on diagnosis. Radiology 2005;235:530–6.

11. Kulkarni NM, Uppot RN, Eisner BH, et al. Radiation dose reduction at multidector CT with adaptive statistical iterative reconstruction for evaluation or urolithiasis: how low can we go? Radiology 2012;265:158–66.

12. Mutgi A, Williams JW, Nettleman M. Renal colic. Utility of the plain abdominal roentgenogram. Arch Intern Med 1991;151:1589–92.

13. Levine JA, Neitlich J, Verga M, et al. Ureteral calculi in patients with flank pain: correlation of plain radiography with unenhanced helical CT. Radiology 1997;204:27–31.

14. Yap WW, Belfield JC, Bhatnagar P, et al. Evaluation of the sensitivity of scout radiographs on unenhanced helical CT in identifying ureteral calculi: a large UK tertiary referral centre experience. Br J Radiol 2012;85:800–6.

15. Johnston R, Lin A, Du J, et al. Comparison of kidney-ureter-bladder abdominal radiography and computed tomography scout films for identifying renal calculi. BJU Int 2009;104:670.

16. Foell K, Ordon M, Ghiculete D, et al. Does baseline radiography of the kidneys, ureters, and bladder facilitate stone management in patients presenting to the emergency department with renal colic? J Endourol 2013;271:425–30.

17. Reddy S. State of the art trends in imaging of renal colic. Emerg Radiol 2008;15:217–25.

18. Eikefjord EN, Thorsen F, Rorvik J. Comparison of effective radiation dose in patients undergoing unenhanced MDCT and excretory urography for acute flank pain. AJR Am J Roentgenol 2007;188:934–9.

19. Pfister SA, Deckart A, Laschke S, et al. Unenhanced helical computed tomography versus intravenous urography in patients with acute flank pain: accuracy and economic impact in a randomized prospective trial. Eur Radiol 2003;13:2513–20.

20. Fowler KA, Locken JA, Duchesne JH, et al. US for detecting renal calculi with nonenhanced CT as the reference standard. Radiology 2002;222:109–13.

21. Svedstrom E, Alanen A, Nurmi M. Radiologic diagnosis of renal colic: the role of plain films, excretory urography, and sonography. Eur J Radiol 1990;11:180–3.

22. Ripolles T, Agramunt M, Errando J, et al. Suspected ureteral colic: plain film and sonography versus unenhanced helical CT. A prospective study in 66 patients. Eur Radiol 2004;14:129–36.

23. Smith-Bindman R, Aubin C, Bailitz J, et al. Ultrasonography versus computed tomography for suspected nephrolithiasis. N Engl J Med 2014;371:1100–10.

24. Patatas K, Panditaratne N, Wah TM, et al. Emergency department imaging protocol for suspected

renal colic: re-evaluating our service. Br J Radiol 2012;85:1118–22.

25. Regan F, Bohlman ME, Khazan R, et al. MR urography using HASTE imaging in the assessment of ureteric obstruction. AJR Am J Roentgenol 1996; 167:1115–20.

26. Kalb B, Sharma P, Salman K, et al. Acute abdominal pain: is there a potential role for MRI in the setting of the emergency department in a patient with renal calculi? J Magn Reson Imaging 2010;32:1012–23.

27. Sudah M, Vanninen R, Partanen K, et al. MR urography in evaluation of acute flank pain: T2-weighted sequences and gadolinium-enhanced three-dimensional FLASH compared with urography. Fast low-angle shot. AJR Am J Roentgenol 2001;176:105–12.

28. Rucker CM, Menias CO, Bhalla S. Mimics of renal colic: alternative diagnoses at unenhanced helical CT. Radiographics 2004;24:S11–33.

29. Bultitude M, Rees J. Management of renal colic. BMJ 2012;345:1–8.

30. Curhan GC. Epidemiology of stone disease. Urol Clin North Am 2007;34:287–93.

31. Cheng PM, Moin P, Dunn MD, et al. What the radiologist needs to know about urolithiasis: part 1–pathogenesis, types, assessment, and variant anatomy. AJR Am J Roentgenol 2012;198:W540–7.

32. Pearle MS, Lotan Y. Urinary lithiasis. Chapter 45. In: Wein AJ, Kavoussi LR, Novick AC, et al, editors. Campbell-Walsh urology. 10th edition. Philadelphia: Saunders; 2012. p. 1257–86.

33. Kawashima A, Sandler CM, Boridy IC, et al. Unenhanced helical CT of ureterolithiasis: value of the tissue rim sign. AJR Am J Roentgenol 1997;168: 997–1000.

34. Dillman JR, Kappil M, Weadock WJ, et al. Sonographic twinkling artifact for renal calculus detection: correlation with CT. Radiology 2011;259:911–6.

35. Ege G, Akman H, Kuzucu K, et al. Acute ureterolithiasis: incidence of secondary signs on unenhanced helical CT and influence on patient management. Clin Radiol 2003;58:990–4.

36. Smith RC, Verga M, Dalrymple N, et al. Acute ureteral obstruction: value of secondary signs of helical unenhanced CT. AJR Am J Roentgenol 1996;167: 1109–13.

37. Boridy IC, Kawahima A, Goldman SM, et al. Acute ureterolithiasis: nonenhanced helical CT findings of perinephric edema for prediction of degree of ureteral obstruction. Radiology 1999;213:663–7.

38. Taourel P, Thuret R, Hoquet MD, et al. Computed tomography in the nontraumatic renal causes of acute flank pain. Semin Ultrasound CT MR 2008; 29:341–52.

39. Jepperson MA, Cernigliaro JG, Sella D, et al. Dual-energy CT for the evaluation of urinary calculi: image interpretation, pitfalls, and stone mimics. Clin Radiol 2013;68:707–14.

40. Jepperson MA, Ibrahim EH, Taylor A, et al. Accuracy and efficiency of determining urinary calculi composition using dual-energy computed tomography compared with Hounsfield unit measurements for practicing physicians. Urology 2014;84:561–4.

41. Furlan A, Federle MP, Yealy DM, et al. Nonobstructing renal stones on unenhanced CT: a real cause for renal colic? AJR Am J Roentgenol 2008;190:W125–7.

42. Coury TA, Sonda LP, Lingeman JE, et al. Treatment of painful caliceal stones. Urology 1988;32:119–23.

43. Lallas CD, Liu XS, Chiura AN, et al. Urolithiasis location and size and the association with microhematuria and stone-related symptoms. J Endourol 2011; 25:1909–13.

44. Coll DM, Varanelli MJ, Smith RC. Relationship of spontaneous passage of ureteral calculus to stone size and location as revealed by unenhanced helical CT. AJR Am J Roentgenol 2002;178:101–3.

45. Pearle MS, Goldfarb DS, Assimos DG, et al. Medical management of kidney stones. In: AUA guideline. 2014. Available at: https://www.auanet.org/education/guidelines/management-kidney-stones.cfm. Accessed January 15, 2015.

46. Miller OF, Kane CJ. Time to stone passage for observed ureteral calculi: a guide for patient education. J Urol 1999;162:688.

47. Kambadakone AR, Eisner BH, Catalano OA, et al. New and evolving concepts in the imaging and management of urolithiasis: urologist's perspective. Radiographics 2010;30:603–23.

48. Weld KJ, Montiglio C, Morris MS, et al. Shock wave lithotripsy success for renal stones based on patient and stone computed tomography characteristics. Urology 2007;70:1043–6.

49. Joseph P, Mandal AK, Singh SK, et al. Computerized tomography attenuation value of renal calculus: can it predict successful fragmentation of the calculus by extracorporeal shock wave lithotripsy? J Urol 2002;167:1968–71.

50. Gupta NP, Ansari MS, Kesarvani P, et al. Role of computed tomography with no contrast medium enhancement in predicting outcome of extracorporeal shock wave lithotripsy for urinary calculi. BJU Int 2005;95:1285–8.

51. Titton RL, Gervais DA, Hahn PF, et al. Urine leaks and urinomas: diagnosis and management. Radiographics 2003;23:1133–47.

52. Czaja CA, Scholes D, Hooton TM, et al. Population-based epidemiologic analysis of acute pyelonephritis. Clin Infect Dis 2007;45:273–80.

53. Schaeffer AJ, Schaeffer EM. Infections of the urinary tract. Chapter 10. In: Wein AJ, Kavoussi LR, Novick AC, et al, editors. Campbell-Walsh urology. 10th edition. Philadelphia: Saunders; 2012. p. 257–326.

54. Craig WM, Wagner BJ, Travis MD. From the archives of the AFIP: pyelonephritis: radiologic-pathologic review. Radiographics 2008;28:255–76.

55. van Nieuwkoop C, Hoppe BPC, Bonten TN, et al. Predicting the need for radiologic imaging in adults with febrile urinary tract infection. Clin Infect Dis 2010;51:1266–72.

56. Kawashima A, Sandler C, Goldman S, et al. CT of renal inflammatory disease. Radiographics 1997; 17:851–66.

57. Demertzis J, Menias CO. State of the art: imaging of renal infections. Emerg Radiol 2007;14:13–22.

58. Hammond NA, Nikolaidis P, Miller FH. Infectious and inflammatory diseases of the kidney. Radiol Clin North Am 2012;50:259–70.

59. Chan JH, Tsui EY, Luk SH, et al. Diffusion-weighted imaging of the kidney: differentiation between hydronephrosis and pyonephrosis. Clin Imaging 2001;25: 110–3.

60. Subramanyam BR, Raghavendra BN, Bosniak MA, et al. Sonography of pyonephrosis: a prospective study. AJR Am J Roentgenol 1983;140:991–3.

61. Fultz PJ, Hampton WR, Totterman SM. Computed tomography of pyonephrosis. Abdom Imaging 1993; 18:82–7.

62. Ifergan J, Pommier R, Brown MC, et al. Imaging in upper urinary tract infections. Diagn Interv Imaging 2012;93:509–19.

63. Ubee SS, McGlynn L, Fordham M. Emphysematous pyelonephritis. BJU Int 2010;107:1474–8.

64. Grayson DE, Abbott RM, Levy AD, et al. Emphysematous infections of the abdomen and pelvis: a pictorial review. Radiographics 2002;22:543–61.

65. Wan YL, Lee TY, Bullard MJ, et al. Acute gas-producing bacterial renal infection: correlation between imaging findings and clinical outcome. Radiology 1996;198:433–8.

66. Weintrob AC, Sexton DJ. Emphysematous urinary tract infections. Boston (MA): UpToDate; 2013.

67. Thomas AA, Lane BR, Thomas AZ, et al. Emphysematous cystitis: a review of 135 cases. BJU Int 2007;100:17–20.

68. Robinson S, Nichols D, MacLoed A, et al. Acute renal artery embolism: a case report and brief review of the literature. Ann Vasc Surg 2008;22: 145–7.

69. Antopolsky M, Simanovsky N, Stalnikowicz R, et al. Renal infarction in the ED: 10 year experience and review of the literature. Am J Emerg Med 2012;30: 1055–60.

70. Kamel IR, Berkowitz JF. Assessment of the cortical rim sign in posttraumatic renal infarction. J Comput Assist Tomogr 1996;20:803–6.

71. Suzer O, Shirkhoda A, Jafri SZ, et al. CT features of renal infarction. Eur J Radiol 2002;44:59–64.

72. Sidhu R, Lockhart ME. Imaging of renovascular disease. Semin Ultrasound CT MR 2009;30:271–88.

73. Matlin RA, Gary NE. Acute cortical necrosis: case report and review of the literature. Am J Med 1974; 56:110–8.

74. Kawashima A, Sandler CM, Ernst RD, et al. CT evaluation of renovascular disease. Radiographics 2000;20:1321–40.

75. Llach F, Papper S, Massry SG. The clinical spectrum of renal vein thrombosis: acute and chronic. Am J Med 1980;69:819–27.

76. Glazer GM, Frances IR, Gross BH, et al. Computed tomography of renal vein thrombosis. J Comput Assist Tomogr 1984;8:288–93.

77. Platt JF, Ellis JH, Rubin JM. Intrarenal arterial Doppler sonography in the detection of renal vein thrombosis of the native kidney. AJR Am J Roentgenol 1994;162:1367–70.

78. Zhang JQ, Fielding JR, Zou KH. Etiology of spontaneous renal hemorrhage. J Urol 2002;167:1593–6.

79. Diaz JR, Agriantonis DJ, Aguila J, et al. Spontaneous perirenal hemorrhage: what radiologists need to know. Emerg Radiol 2011;18:329–34.

80. Katabathina VS, Katre R, Prasad SR, et al. Wunderlich syndrome: cross-sectional imaging review. J Comput Assist Tomogr 2011;35:425–33.

81. Belville JS, Morgentaler A, Loughlin KR, et al. Spontaneous perinephric and subcapsular renal hemorrhage: evaluation with CT, US, and angiography. Radiology 1989;172:733–8.

82. Mydlo JH, Kaplan J, Thelmo W, et al. Spontaneous renal hemorrhage associated with renal tumors. Clin Imaging 1997;21:287–9.

83. Ouzaid I, Autorino R, Fatica R, et al. Active surveillance for renal angiomyolipoma: outcomes and factors predictive of delayed intervention. BJU Int 2014; 114:412–7.

84. Soulen MC, Faykus MH, Shlansky-Goldberg RD, et al. Elective embolization for prevention of hemorrhage from renal angiomyolipmas. J Vasc Interv Radiol 1994;5:587–91.

85. Yamakado K, Tanaka N, Nakagawa T, et al. Renal angiomyolipoma: relationships between size, aneurysm formation, and rupture. Radiology 2002;225: 78–82.

86. Ramon J, Rimon U, Garniek A, et al. Renal angiomyolipoma: long-term results following selective arterial embolization. Eur Urol 2009;55:1155–62.

87. Nadwani GM, Musker MP, Chaplin BJ, et al. Spontaneous perirenal hemorrhage in polyarteritis nodosa. J Coll Physicians Surg Pak 2013;23:445–7.

88. Ozaki K, Miyayama S, Ushiogi Y, et al. Renal involvement of polyarteritis nodosa: CT and MR findings. Abdom Imaging 2009;34:265–70.

89. Jain S, Nyirenda T, Yates J, et al. Incidence of renal artery pseudoaneurysm following a minimally invasive partial nephrectomy: a systematic review and comparative analysis. J Urol 2013;189:1643–8.

90. Lattin GE, Sturgill ED, Tujo CA, et al. From the radiology pathology archives: adrenal tumors and tumor-like conditions in the adult: radiologic-pathologic correlation. Radiographics 2014;34:805–29.

91. Cardin AL, Marshall J, Bhatt S, et al. Antopol-Goldman lesion of the kidney diagnosed by radiology: a case report of observation. Acta Radiol 2008;6:715–7.

92. Heffernan E, Zwirewich C, Harris A, et al. Page kidney after renal allograpft biopsy: sonographic findings. J Clin Ultrasound 2009;37:226–9.

93. Tonolini M, Rigiroli F, Villa F, et al. Complications of sporadic, hereditary, and acquired renal cysts: cross-sectional imaging findings. Curr Probl Diagn Radiol 2014;43:80–90.

94. Moore CL, Daniels B, Singh D, et al. Prevalence and clinical importance of alternative causes of symptoms using a renal colic computed tomography protocol in patient with flank or back pain and absence of pyuria. Acad Emerg Med 2013;20:470–8.

FURTHER READING

Bove P, Kaplan D, Dalrymple N, et al. Reexamining the value of hematuria testing in patients with acute flank pain. J Urol 1999;162:685–7.

Wang LJ, Wong YC, Chuang CK, et al. Predictions of outcomes of renal stones after extracorporeal shock wave lithotripsy from stone characteristics determined by unenhanced helical computed tomography: a multivariate analysis. Eur Radiol 2005;14:665.

Acute Gynecologic Disorders

Carolyn K. Donaldson, MD

KEYWORDS

- Ultrasound ● Acute pelvic pain ● Pregnancy ● Acute management

KEY POINTS

- Ultrasound is the preferred imaging modality of choice when a gynecologic source of actue pain is suspected. CT is more useful when GI or urinary tract pathology is more likely.
- Ectopic pregnancy is one of the most serious causes of acute pelvic pain. It should be always considered in patients with a positive pregnancy test and no IUP.
- A hemorrhagic physiologic cyst is the most common adnexal lesion and frequently the cause of acute pelvic pain. Bleeding is often limited but irritates the peritoneum.
- Dermoids are the most common benign ovarian neoplasm. They have characteristic appearances on ultrasound allowing for specific diagnosis. Dermoids pose a risk for torsion and can rupture resulting in acute pain.
- Gynecologic malignancies can present with acute symptoms in the emergency department. The most specific feature of malignancy in an adnexal lesion is solid elements with internal vascularity.

INTRODUCTION

Premenopausal women with acute pelvic pain comprise a significant percentage of patients who present to the emergency room. Etiologies can be gynecologic, urologic, gastrointestinal, or vascular. Signs and symptoms are often nonspecific and overlapping. The choice of imaging modality is determined by the clinically suspected differential diagnosis. Ultrasound (US) is the preferred imaging modality for suspected obstetric or gynecologic disorders. CT is more useful when gastrointestinal or urinary tract pathology is likely.[1] MR imaging is rarely used in the emergent setting, except to exclude appendicitis in pregnant women. This article presents a comprehensive review of imaging of acute gynecologic disorders.

ECTOPIC PREGNANCY

Ectopic pregnancy (EP) is one of the most serious causes of acute pelvic pain. Patients who present with pain and bleeding in the first trimester of pregnancy often undergo pelvic US to exclude an EP.

EP typically present near 6 weeks gestation. Atypical locations of EP, including interstitial EP and abdominal pregnancy (**Fig. 1**), can present later. Premenopausal women with pelvic pain usually undergo pregnancy testing regardless of menstrual history.

Imaging findings are variable in the setting of EP. The gestational sac of an EP is often not identifiable on US. The more common US findings are the result of tubal rupture and include an adnexal mass and complex free fluid (hemoperitoneum). Hemoperitoneum, although life threatening, can be very subtle on US. It is an extremely important finding to recognize because hemoperitoneum is very specific finding for ruptured EP with a reported sensitivity of 93%.[2]

On US, hemoperitoneum appears as complex fluid, usually with low- to medium-level echoes (**Fig. 2**). Acute hemorrhage can mimic a solid adnexal mass as well as obscure visualization of an ovary. In the setting of hemoperitoneum, scanning should include the right upper quadrant. Morrison's pouch is the most dependent portion of the peritoneum and may indicate a larger volume

Department of Radiology, NorthShore University HealthSystem, 2650 Ridge Avenue, Evanston, IL 60201, USA
E-mail address: cdonaldson2@northshore.org

Radiol Clin N Am 53 (2015) 1293–1307
http://dx.doi.org/10.1016/j.rcl.2015.06.012
0033-8389/15/$ – see front matter © 2015 Elsevier Inc. All rights reserved.

radiologic.theclinics.com

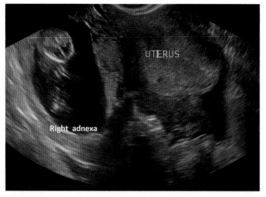

Fig. 1. Abdominal ectopic pregnancy. Transvaginal ultrasound of the pelvis reveals an empty uterus, complex-free fluid in the pelvis, and an obvious extrauterine pregnancy in the right adnexal region. A biparietal diameter could even be measured.

hemorrhage. The finding of hemoperitoneum should be reported immediately because intraperitoneal bleeding can be life threatening. On CT, blood manifests as hyperdense fluid (**Fig. 3**).

HETEROTOPIC PREGNANCY

Heterotopic pregnancy (HP) is the simultaneous occurrence of 2 implantation sites (**Fig. 4**). It is most often manifested as an intrauterine pregnancy and EP. HP is a rare entity that is most frequently seen in fertility patients. The incidence of HP is 1 in 7000 fertility patients and occurs spontaneously 1 in 30,000 pregnancies.[3] The incidence of HP has increased owing to assisted reproduction and the increasing incidence of pelvic inflammatory disease (PID). Risk factors for HP are the same for EP. Treatment of HP is usually surgical (laparoscopy). Nonsurgical management

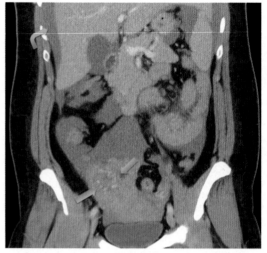

Fig. 3. Ruptured ectopic pregnancy: CT findings. Coronal reformatted CT reveals high-density free fluid in the pelvis with even higher density pooling in the right adnexal region (*straight arrows*). At surgery, active bleeding from a ruptured ectopic pregnancy was found. Note the free fluid surrounding the liver (*curved arrow*), spleen, and gallbladder.

with US-guided injection of potassium chloride may be used in a nonviable and nonruptured EP. The β-human chorionic gonadotropin levels are often misleading in the setting of EP and therefore falsely reassuring in the setting of HP. The β-human chorionic gonadotropin is often within the normal range owing to the coexisting intrauterine pregnancy.[4]

HEMORRHAGIC OVARIAN CYST

Rupture of an ovarian cyst can cause acute pain secondary to irritation of the peritoneum from

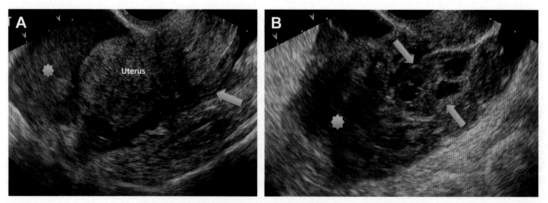

Fig. 2. Hemoperitoneum associated with ectopic pregnancy. (*A*) Sagittal pelvic sonogram shows complex fluid (blood) surrounding the uterus. A large amount of blood is present in the anterior cul de sac (*asterisk*) and surrounding the uterine fundus. More echogenic, even solid appearing, blood is present in the posterior cul de sac (*arrow*). (*B*) The hemoperitoneum obscures the ovary. Sagittal pelvic sonogram depicts the ovary (*arrows*) surrounded by blood (*asterisk*). Follicles allow for identification of the ovary.

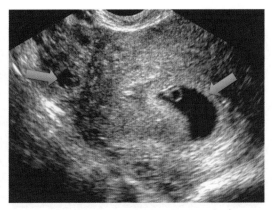

Fig. 4. Heterotopic pregnancy. Transvaginal sonogram demonstrates a well-formed intrauterine gestational sac with a yolk sac (*right arrow*). A subtle right adnexal gestational sac also contains a yolk sac (*left arrow*).

blood. Bleeding is often very limited, but can be sufficiently extensive to require surgery. These patients often present mid cycle with rupture owing to ovulation. The bleeding is usually limited, but rarely can result in significant hemoperitoneum and pain prompting surgery. Hemorrhagic cysts are the most common cause of complex cystic ovarian lesions. They are usually the result of hemorrhage into a corpus luteum.

The ultrasonographic features of hemorrhagic cysts are variable. The 1 consistent feature of hemorrhagic cysts is the lack of internal vascularity. Fine, lacelike reticulations are often present. Acute hemorrhage can be echogenic, mimicking a solid component (**Fig. 5**). Retracting blood clots may be present demonstrating concave margins.

CORPUS LUTEUM

A corpus luteum develops within a dominant follicle after rupture (ovulation). A corpus luteum often undergoes hemorrhage and causes pain. This diagnostic abnormality should be considered in the setting of ipsilateral pain. The ultrasonographic hallmark finding of a corpus luteum is the intense peripheral vascularity on color Doppler (**Fig. 6**). The spectral Doppler waveform demonstrates low-resistance flow typical of a metabolically active structure.

A corpus luteum is a common incidental finding on CT. The intense peripheral vascularity of a corpus luteum is confirmed with a dense peripheral rind on a postcontrast CT of the pelvis (**Fig. 7**). On PET scanning, a corpus luteum demonstrates increased activity owing to its metabolic activity and increased uptake of fluorodeoxyglucose.

OVARIAN TORSION

Ovarian torsion can be a difficult diagnosis even in the hands of an experienced imager. Often it is the clinical picture of acute, severe pain that leads to surgical intervention. Although usually acute, torsion can be subacute or chronic. It usually occurs in the setting of an ovarian lesion. Occasionally, a paraovarian lesion, usually a peritubal cyst, can undergo torsion. The clinical presentation is similar to that of ovarian torsion, which presents with similar clinical features.

The most consistent finding of ovarian torsion (**Fig. 8**) is an enlarged ovary with or without a mass. Doppler findings are variable and can be misleading. Lack of internal vascularity allows for a fairly confident diagnosis. However, the presence of either arterial or venous flow does not entirely exclude the diagnosis. Diminished or absent venous flow is more common then absent arterial flow.[5] In 2004, the ultrasonographic "whirlpool" sign was described as an extraovarian mass of a twisted vascular pedicle.[6]

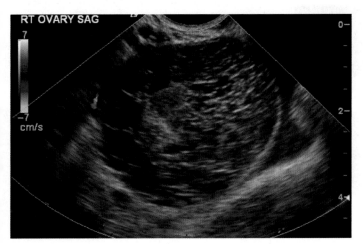

Fig. 5. Hemorrhagic ovarian cyst. Acute blood can mimic a solid lesion as shown in this hemorrhagic cyst. Note the lack of internal vascularity on color Doppler ultrasound. Lacelike reticulations or fish net appearance are seen in the periphery of this lesion.

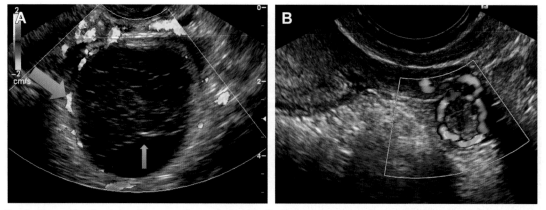

Fig. 6. Hemorrhagic corpus luteum: ultrasonographic findings. (*A*) Note the fine, lacelike reticulations and retracting clot (*thin arrows*) consistent with a hemorrhagic lesion. The intense peripheral vascularity is typical of a corpus luteum (*thick arrow*). (*B*) Color Doppler ultrasonography demonstrating the peripheral flow characteristic of a corpus luteum. An isoechoic corpus luteum can be identified with color Doppler in this image.

The "classic" ultrasonographic appearance is an enlarged ovary with heterogeneous central stroma and small peripheral follicles (**Fig. 9**). The "follicular ring sign" describes the echogenic rim surrounding the peripheral follicles.[7] Often, the appearance of the torsed ovary reflects the appearance of the underlying lesion. The most common lesions associated with ovarian torsion is a dermoid. On MR (**Fig. 10**), the torsed ovary is hyperintense on T2-weighted images secondary to edema. Subacute hemorrhage can be seen as a rim of hyperintense signal on fat-saturated T1 weighted images (**Fig. 11**).[8]

PELVIC INFLAMMATORY DISEASE–TUBOOVARIAN ABSCESS

PID is a spectrum of infection beginning with a localized endometritis progressing to tuboovarian abscesses and potentially to a diffuse bacterial peritonitis. The infectious agents most frequently cultured are *Chlamydia trachomatis* and *Neisseria gonorrhea*. The fallopian tubes provide a route for extension of the inflammatory process to the adnexae and peritoneal cavity.

Clinical signs and symptoms of PID can be nonspecific and include pain, fever, nausea, and vomiting. Purulent vaginal discharge and cervical motion tenderness are more specific for PID. Elevated white blood cell count is often present. Although the diagnosis of PID can be made clinically, patients who present to the emergency room with PID often undergo imaging before seeing a gynecologist. Often, the blood test results are not yet available while imaging is performed. Pelvic US and CT are routinely performed in suspected cases of PID.

Imaging findings are a spectrum ranging from normal to extensive abnormalities and reflect the stage of disease (**Fig. 12**). Early in the course of the disease, pelvic US may be normal. Infiltration of the pelvic fat can be seen with CT. The US correlate of this finding is echogenic pelvic fat. As the infection spreads, occlusion of the fallopian tubes can occur with resultant pyosalpinx. Pyosalpinx has several appearances, including an oval or pearshaped and fluid filled, containing low-level echoes.[8] With inflammation of the fallopian tube, the walls become nodular and have been described as having a "cogwheel appearance" (**Fig. 13**). When the tube folds over on itself, it creates the appearance of a partial septation allowing for more confident diagnosis.

As infection spreads to the ovary, the ovary becomes enlarged with increased number of follicles owing to oophoritis.[9] The inflamed ovary and tube

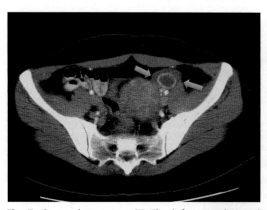

Fig. 7. Corpus luteum on CT. The left ovary (*arrows*) contains a peripherally enhancing lesion consistent with a corpus luteum.

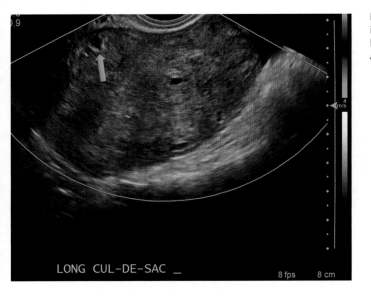

Fig. 8. Ovarian torsion. Color Doppler image revealing an enlarged, feature-less ovary. Several peripheral follicles are identified (*arrow*).

become adherent to one another and form the so-called tuboovarian complex.[8] PID can progress to complete breakdown of the ovary and tube resulting in a tuboovarian abscess. US findings at this stage include thick walled complex cystic lesions containing debris. Flow is often visible in the periphery of the abscesses. Complex free fluid may be present.

On CT, these complex cystic adnexal lesions have a nonspecific appearance. It is the extensive surrounding inflammatory changes in the pelvis that allow for the CT diagnosis of PID. Tuboovarian abscesses can be unilateral or bilateral.

Pelvic free fluid is usually present in the setting of PID. In the early stages, this fluid is usually simple. With progression of disease, the fluid becomes complex.

INTRAUTERINE DEVICE IN PREGNANCY

A patient with a history of prior IUD placement and a positive pregnancy test should be assumed to have an extrauterine pregnancy until proven otherwise (**Fig. 14**). The most likely scenario is the IUD has fallen out allowing pregnancy to occur; however, extrauterine pregnancy is a risk for patients with IUDs.

Management of pregnant patients with an IUD varies depending on gestational age and location of the IUD. The difficulty and risks of removal increase with increasing gestational age. There are multiple adverse outcomes in pregnancy complicated by an IUD. These include spontaneous abortion (40%–50%), premature labor, chorioamnionitis, and low birth weight. These risks are

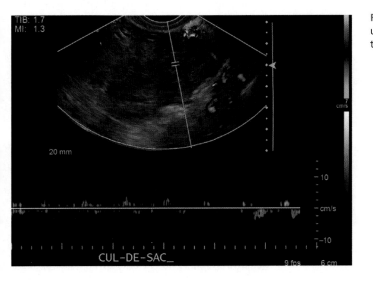

Fig. 9. Ovarian torsion. Color Doppler ultrasonographic tracing with questionable ovarian flow.

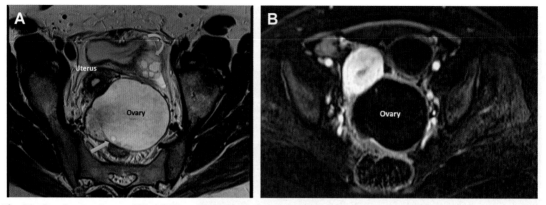

Fig. 10. Ovarian torsion on MR. (*A*) T2 weighted MR of the pelvis demonstrating an enlarged right ovary with few peripheral follicles (*thin arrow*). Note the normal left ovary (*curved arrow*). (*B*) Post contrast MR reveals complete lack of enhancement of the right ovary. Note how the uterus is deviated to the side of the torsed ovary.

reduced with removal of the IUD in early pregnancy.[10] Three-dimensional US is helpful in evaluating the position of an IUD because it provides a bird's eye view of the endometrial cavity.

INTRAUTERINE DEVICE COMPLICATIONS

Uterine perforation occurs in 1 in 1000 IUDs placed.[10] It usually occurs during placement of an IUD and can go unnoticed. Perforation ranges from an arm of an IUD embedded in the myometrium to migration into the peritoneal cavity. US may not adequately define extrauterine extension of an IUD. The bowel gas and pelvic fat surrounding the uterus obscure visualization of extrauterine extension of an IUD. IUDs that perforate but are partially contained in the uterus can be retrieved hysteroscopically. Symptoms of perforation are varied. Patients can be asymptomatic, have pain, or experience abnormal bleeding.

Missing IUDs pose potential complications. It is not uncommon for a patient to give a history of prior IUD placement but no IUD is seen during

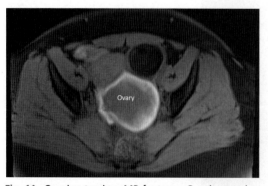

Fig. 11. Ovarian torsion: MR features. Ovarian torsion with resultant hemorrhage seen as increased signal on a fat-suppressed, T1 weighted image.

pelvic US scanning. In these situations, an abdominal radiograph should be performed to evaluate for an extrauterine location of the IUD. If an IUD is seen on an abdominal radiographic (**Fig. 15**), but not in the uterus on pelvic US, patients should be further evaluated with CT to determine location of the IUD (**Fig. 16**). Surgery is usually performed to prevent bowel perforation or other injuries that can be caused by an IUD freely moving in the peritoneal cavity.

The more common explanation for lack of visualization of an IUD on pelvic US is that the IUD was expelled spontaneously. Surprisingly, this can occur without women realizing that the device has been expelled or experiencing symptoms during its passage.

ACUTE APPENDICITIS

Pelvic US is often used in premenopausal women with right lower quadrant pain. The clinical diagnosis of acute appendicitis is difficult in women during the reproductive years because the clinical presentation of acute appendicitis overlaps with gynecologic disorders. Clinical mimickers of appendicitis include physiologic processes such as a ruptured ovarian cyst and pathologic conditions, particularly PID.[11,12]

The appendix, particularly an abnormal appendix, may be visible with transvaginal US imaging of the pelvis. Caspi and colleagues[13] studied 28 women with confirmed acute appendicitis and found that 66% of the patients had an abnormal appendix seen on transvaginal US. Ultrasonographic features of acute appendicitis include a dilated (>6 mm), fluid-filled, blind-ending tubular structure. Hyperemia may be demonstrated with color or power Doppler. An appendicolith may be visible (**Fig. 17**). Inflamed periappendiceal fat becomes hyperechogenic. Echogenic fat is seen with inflammation.

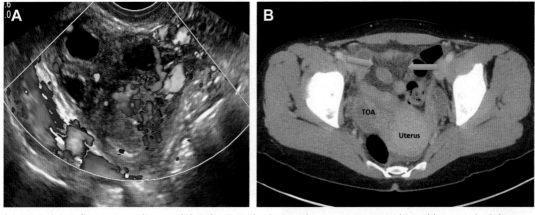

Fig. 12. Pelvic inflammatory disease. (*A*) Color Doppler image demonstrates an enlarged hyperemic right ovary with multiple cystic structures with surrounding flow. (*B*) CT image from the same patient demonstrates a nonspecific right adnexal lesion. The extensive inflammatory changes seen in the pelvis anteriorly (*arrows*) allow for the diagnosis of pelvic inflammatory disease in the proper clinical setting.

The CT correlate (**Fig. 18**) of this finding is edema or infiltration of periappendiceal fat. A ruptured or gangrenous appendix will have an atypical appearance and may be difficult to diagnose on US.

Patients will be tender when scanning near an abnormal appendix, allowing for a more specific diagnosis. Free fluid in the pelvis is usually present with acute appendicitis. CT is more sensitive than US for the detection of acute appendicitis particularly in the setting of a retrocecal appendix.

ADNEXAL MASSES

Both benign and malignant ovarian lesions can present with acute pain and are not infrequently diagnosed emergently in the ED. Occasionally, advanced ovarian cancer can present in the emergent setting with pelvic masses, ascites and

obvious metastatic disease. It is much more common to see benign ovarian lesions in the setting of acute pain. These lesions include ovarian cysts (usually a dominant follicle), a corpus luteum, hemorrhagic cysts, endometriomas, and dermoid cysts. Adnexal lesions pose a risk for torsion. Dermoids can leak and cause peritoneal symptoms. It is possible to diagnosis these common, benign ovarian lesions with their characteristic ultrasonographic features.[14] These common, benign lesions are described elsewhere in this article.

OVARIAN CYSTS

Acute pain can result from an ovarian cyst, particularly a large cyst. These cysts are usually follicles but occasionally become quite large and symptomatic. They are usually simple with

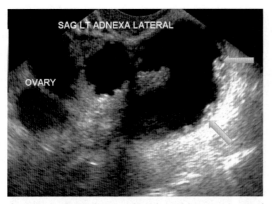

Fig. 13. Hydrosaplinx with salpingitis. Transvaginal image of the fallopian tube en face (*asterisk*) and on end (*arrows*). Note the cogwheel appearance that results from inflammation of the tube. SAG LT, sagittal left.

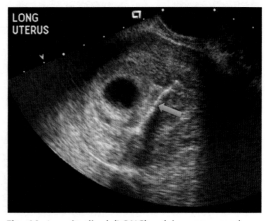

Fig. 14. Longitudinal (LONG) pelvic sonogram shows an early intrauterine gestational sac adjacent to an intrauterine device (*arrow*).

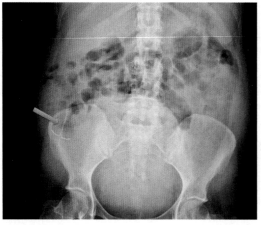

Fig. 15. Extrauterine intrauterine device. On this abdominal plain radiograph an intrauterine device (*arrow*) is located in the right iliac fossa laterally.

ultrasonographic features typical of cysts seen elsewhere in the body. Cysts can be ovarian or paraovarian and both cause increased incidence of torsion. The incidence of malignancy in simple cysts less than 7.5 cm is virtually nil.[15]

ENDOMETRIOMAS

Endometriosis is a well-known cause of chronic pelvic pain, but these patients can present with acute episodes of pain resulting in emergent imaging. Symptomatic endometriosis is usually the result of endometrial implants that are not usually visible on US. These implants, however, can often be seen with MR imaging. Endometriomas, also know as "chocolate cysts" because of their appearance at surgery, result from endometrial implants in the ovaries. Endometriomas can be seen

in patients with known endometriosis or can be an incidental finding in asymptomatic patients.[16]

Endometriomas are among the more common adnexal lesions identified with pelvic US. Ultrasonographic features of endometriomas include homogeneous low-level echoes often referred to as ground glass echoes. The homogeneous low-level echoes within the lesion result from cyclical bleeding. The diagnosis of a classic endometrioma can be made with ultrasonography. Often, a short-term follow-up is recommended to confirm the diagnosis and exclude a hemorrhagic cyst, which resolves on follow-up examination. Endometriomas cause acoustic enhancement owing to their cystic nature (**Fig. 19**). They are avascular and should not demonstrate flow with color Doppler imaging. Ultrasonographic evaluation of a suspected endometrioma requires careful evaluation with color Doppler US to exclude internal vascularity.[17]

Endometriomas can be complex. A recently describe feature of endometriomas are punctate echogenic foci in the periphery of these lesions. This ultrasonographic feature allows for increased diagnostic specificity.[18] Endometriomas can be even more complex with larger peripheral nodules or coalescent debris. These complex endometriomas can demonstrate ultrasonographic features, which overlap with malignancy. MR imaging plays an important role in distinguishing atypical endometriomas from malignancy.

Classic endometriomas are often treated conservatively without surgery. Approximately 1% of endometriomas are believed to undergo malignant transformation. Most malignancies occur in large lesions (>9 cm) and in older women (>45 years old).

A   **B**

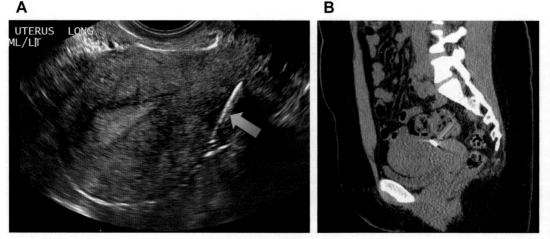

Fig. 16. Intrauterine device (IUD) perforation: imaging findings. (*A*) Sagittal sonogram of the uterus with the IUD perforating the posterior lower uterine segment (*arrow*). (*B*) Sagittal CT image confirms IUD perforation into the lower uterine segment.

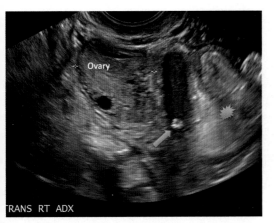

Fig. 17. Appendicitis on transvaginal ultrasound. A dilated, fluid-filled appendix with an appendicolith (*arrow*) is seen medial to the right ovary. Note the hyperechoic fat medial to the appendix (*asterisk*).

DERMOIDS

Mature cystic teratomas, often referred to as dermoids, are the most common benign ovarian neoplasm and the most common neoplasm responsible for ovarian torsion. They frequently present with acute pain owing to rupture or torsion. If free fluid is present in the setting of a dermoid and acute pain, rupture should be considered. Pain results from a chemical peritonitis secondary to leaking of the oily material of dermoids.[19]

Because they have classic ultrasonographic features (**Fig. 20**), most dermoids can be accurately characterized by US.[20] The classic ultrasonographic features of dermoids on gray scale US include hyperechoic line and dots (hair en face or on end), focal or diffuse hyperechoic component (fat or oil), calcifications with dense shadowing, and no internal flow with color or spectral Doppler. Rare but pathognomic features include floating echogenic spherules in a cystic mass and a fluid–fluid level.

"Tip of the iceberg" is a term used to describe the ultrasonographic findings of a dermoid.[21] Dermoids can contain large fatty components that absorb the sound beam, preventing adequate evaluation of the lesion. Therefore, only the anterior margin of a lesion may be imaged with US. The posterior margin is obscured. Thus, large lesions are often undermeasured. The same lesion on CT is much larger (**Fig. 21**).

Dermoids do not contain internal vascularity. This is an important feature that distinguishes dermoids from malignant lesions. Dermoids are usually benign. Malignant transformation in up to 2% occurs in older women (>50 years) and in large dermoids (>10 cm). Dermoids are usually removed because of the risk of rupture, or torsion. They can grow slowly and destroy ovary. They are bilateral in 12% to 20% of cases. Dermoids may elude detection by US, but are subsequently seen on CT.[22]

MALIGNANT ADNEXAL LESIONS

Gynecologic malignancies are not uncommonly diagnosed through the emergency department. Patients present with nonspecific symptoms of abdominal distension and pain. Ascites, peritoneal masses, and adnexal lesions are highly specific for gynecologic malignancy. Evaluation of an isolated adnexal lesion for malignancy requires careful ultrasonographic technique. The most specific feature for malignancy is solid elements with internal vascularity (**Fig. 22**). Mural nodules or nodular septations are also suspicious for malignancy.[23]

Occasionally, ovarian masses are secondary to metastatic disease. The most common primary malignancies include colon, breast, and lung primaries. A rare example are the Krukenberg tumors, which are an adenocarcinoma of the ovary

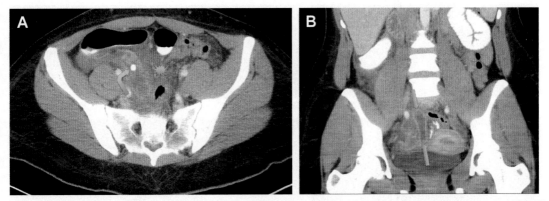

Fig. 18. Appendicitis: CT features. Axial (*A*) and coronal (*B*) reformatted images of the same patient as **Fig. 17** confirm the diagnosis of acute appendicitis. Curved arrow denotes the appendicolith. *Asterisk* denotes edematous fat. A fluid filled enhancing appendix is situated between the straight arrows on coronal reformatted image (*B*).

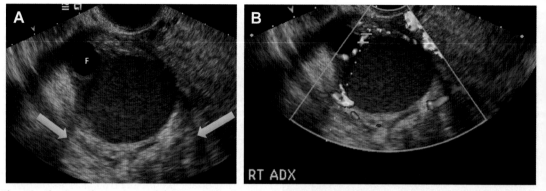

Fig. 19. Classic endometrioma. (*A*) Gray scale ultrasound image of the pelvis shows well-circumscribed lesions with low-level internal echoes. Acoustic enhancement is present distal to the lesion (*arrows*). (*B*) Color Doppler ultrasonography shows no internal vascularity.

with signet ring cells. They represent only 1% to 2% of ovarian cancers and are most commonly metastatic gastric carcinoma (70%). Signet ring cell adenocarcinomas of solid organs metastasize to the ovaries more commonly than other malignancies from the same organs. Spread is felt to be lymphatic. They are usually bilateral (80%).[24] They are complex but predominantly solid and can be very large.

Krukenberg tumors (**Fig. 23**) present in younger women than ovarian cancer. The average age at presentation is 45 years. The primary tumor can be occult and in these instances, the prognosis is very poor. In general, Krukenberg tumors have a very low survival rate, namely, 15% at 2 years. The diagnosis of Krukenberg tumors is usually made at surgery.[24,25]

HYDROSALPINX

Patients with hydrosalpinx can be asymptomatic or have significant symptoms such as PID. Hydrosalpinx, or dilation of the fallopian tubes, can be unilateral or bilateral. The contents of the tube can be simple or complex. The tube itself can exhibit thin walls or be thickened owing to inflammation. In advanced inflammation such as in the setting of a tuboovarian abscess, the tubes can be so abnormal so as not to be recognized.

The imaging features of hydrosalpinx are quite characteristic (**Fig. 24**). As a fluid-filled structure folds on itself, it creates a partial septation. As the tube becomes inflamed, it develops nodular thickening and can result in a "beads on a string" appearance or a "cogwheel" appearance of the tube in cross-section (see **Fig. 19**). This is the

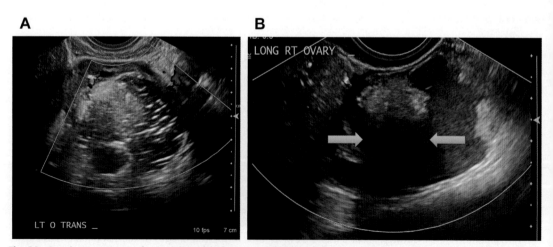

Fig. 20. Ovarian teratoma: ultrasonographic features. (*A*) Echogenic lines and dots are characteristic of dermoids. (*B*). Fat nodules diagnostic of dermoid will cause dirty shadowing (*arrows*).

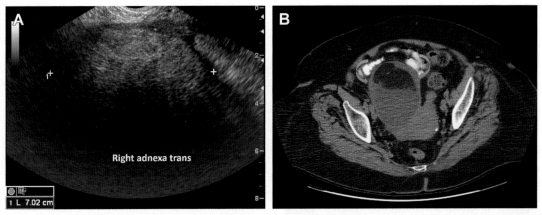

Fig. 21. Ovarian teratoma: imaging features. (A) This large dermoid resulted in complete absorption of the ultrasound beam allowing for only visualization of the front of the lesion ("tip of the iceberg") on this transverse pelvic sonogram. (B) CT provides complete depiction of this lesion. Note the fat fluid layer (curved arrows).

result of thickening of the endosalpingeal folds and such nodular thickening creates small nodules (<3 mm). Cine clips or 3-dimensional imaging may be helpful in establishing the diagnosis.[26] Visualization of the ipsilateral ovary is imperative when diagnosing hydrosalpinx. Classic findings of hydrosalpinx do not need further imaging or follow-up to establish the diagnosis. Recommendations for follow-up should be based on patient age and clinic symptoms.

A rare mimicker of hydrosalpinx is mucocele of the appendix (mucus accumulation in the appendix). Most mucoceles are benign and caused by mucinous cystadenomas.[27] Recognition (Fig. 25) and surgical resection of appendiceal mucoceles are important because some of these lesions are

malignant adenocarcinomas that can rupture leading to psuedomyxoma peritonei.[28] Nodular enhancing lesions in the wall of a mucocele are a finding suggestive of a malignant cause of mucocele.[29]

HEMATOCOLPOS

Hematocolpos (blood in the vagina) and hematometrocolpos (blood in the uterus and vagina) can cause acute pain and develops in adolescent girls; it is usually owing to an imperforate hymen. With an imperforate hymen, the obstruction is at the level of the introitus and patients may present with bulging of the perineum. The vagina is more distensible than the muscular uterus. Blood is not

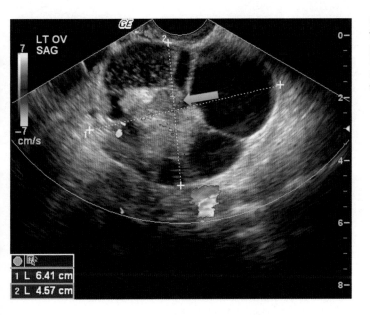

Fig. 22. Mucinous cystadenoma of the ovary. Sagittal sonogram of the pelvis shows a complex left ovarian lesion with cystic and solid elements. Color Doppler demonstrates internal vascularity (arrow).

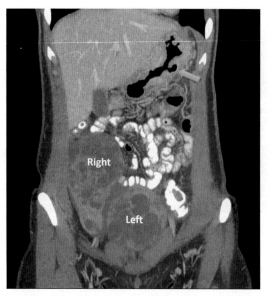

Fig. 23. Krukenberg tumors: CT features. Large, bilateral ovarian masses with an ulcerating gastric mass (*arrow*) consistent with Krukenberg tumors are seen on this coronal reformatted CT scan of the abdomen and pelvis. Left, left ovary; Right, right ovary.

usually retained within the endometrial cavity (**Fig. 26**A). The vagina can become very large, containing blood from recurring menses (see **Fig. 26**B).[30]

The ultrasonographic appearance of hemotocolpos is similar to an endometrioma. Both result from cyclical bleeding accumulating in a contained space. With US imaging, a low pelvic midline cystic mass with homogeneous low level internal echoes and no internal vascularity allow for diagnosis. MR may be helpful to distinguish the point and cause of obstruction thereby facilitating surgical planning. The blood-filled vaginal demonstrates signal characteristics of blood and T2 shading similar to an endometrioma.[31]

Imperforate hymen is the most common anomaly of the vagina. It is not an anomaly of Mullerian duct origin and therefore it is not associated with other congenital anomalies. Treatment is surgical.

RETAINED PRODUCTS OF CONCEPTION

Post partum patients may present to the ED with persistent or increased bleeding. US imaging is usually performed in attempt to evaluate for

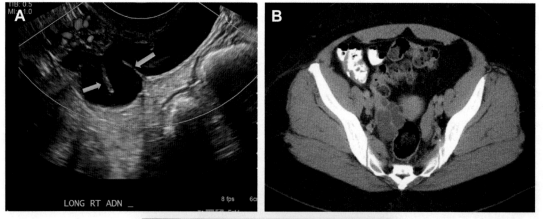

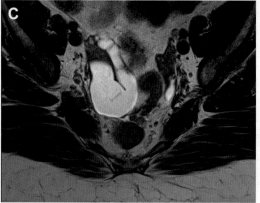

Fig. 24. Hydrosalpinx: imaging findings. (*A*) Longitudinal pelvic ultrasound shows a tubular structure with septations (*arrows*) owing to folding upon itself. (*B*) Axial CT of the pelvis shows cystic lesions in the adnexa. CT is not as specific as MR or ultrasonography for the diagnosis of hydrosalpinx. (*C*) Axial T2 weighted MR imaging of the pelvis demonstrating simple fluid within a dilated right fallopian tube (*arrow*).

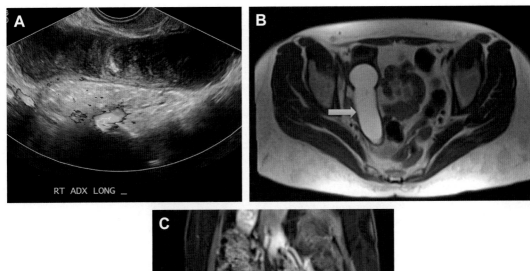

Fig. 25. Mucocele of the appendix: imaging features. (*A*) Longitudinal pelvic sonogram shows an avascular tubular structure containing heterogeneous material representing layers of inspissated mucus. This dilated appendix (*arrow*) contains high signal material on T2 weighted axial images (*B*) and low signal on T1 weighted sagittal (*C*) MR images.

retained products of conception (RPOC). RPOC usually is placental tissue (chorionic villi). Because of its very vascular connection to the uterus, it results in continued bleeding. The incidence of

RPOC is greatest after second trimester delivery or termination of pregnancy.[32]

The most sensitive finding of RPOC is a thickened endometrial echo complex. Thickened is

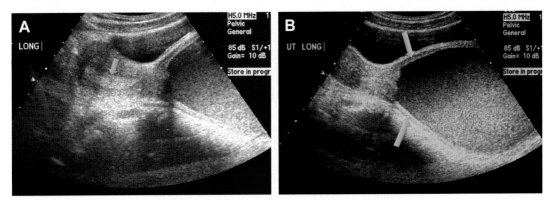

Fig. 26. Hemotocolpos. (*A*) Longitudinal sonogram shows that the vagina is dilated but the endometrium (*arrow*) is not. The muscular uterus prevents distension of the endometrial cavity. (*B*) The vagina is markedly distended and contains low-level echoes resulting from cyclical bleeding in a contained space. The walls of the vagina are splayed anteriorly and posteriorly (*arrows*).

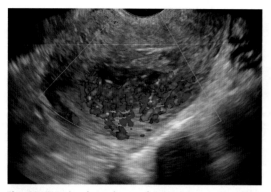

Fig. 27. Retained products of conception: ultrasonographic features. Thickened, heterogeneous endometrium demonstrating internal vascularity. Note the hypervascularity in the adjacent myometrium.

defined as greater than 1 cm. Vascularity in a thickened endometrial echo complex or endometrial mass is likely to be RPOC. Blood clots in the endometrium are avascular. An additional finding recently described with RPOC is hyperemia of the adjacent myometrium.[32,33] With color Doppler imaging, geographic areas of hyperemia are present in the myometrium (**Fig. 27**). This can be a very helpful finding, because the diagnosis of RPOC can be difficult to make given the presence of normal postpartum lochia. Dilation and curettage is sometimes needed with equivocal US findings. Preexisting endometrial polyps and submucosal myomas can mimic RPOC.

REFERENCES

1. Andreotti RF, Lee SI, Choy G, et al. ACR appropriateness criteria on acute pelvic pain in the reproductive age group. J Am Coll Radiol 2009;6:235–41.
2. Mazzariol FS, Roberts J, Oh SK, et al. Pearls and pitfalls in first-trimester obstetric sonography. Clin Imaging 2015;39:176–85.
3. Barrenetxea G, Barinaga-Remeteria L, Lopez de Larruzea A, et al. Heterotopic pregnancy: two cases and a comparative review. Fertil Steril 2007;87:9–15.
4. Avitabile NC, Kaban NL, Siadecki SD, et al. Two cases of heterotopic pregnancy: review of the literature and sonographic diagnosis in the emergency department. J Ultrasound Med 2015;34(3):527–30.
5. Gerscovich EO, Corwin MT, Sekhon S, et al. Sonographic appearance of adnexal torsion, correlation with other imaging modalities, and clinical history. Ultrasound Q 2014;30:49–55.
6. Wilkinson C, Sanderson A. Adnexal torsion-a multimodality imaging review. Clin Radiol 2012;67(5):476–83.
7. Sibal M. Follicular ring sign: a simple sonographic sign for early diagnosis of ovarian torsion. J Ultrasound Med 2012;31:1803–9.
8. Allison SO, Lev-Toaff AS. Acute pelvic pain, what we have learned from the ER. Ultrasound Q 2010;26:211–8.
9. Cacciatore B, Leminen A, Ingman-Griberg S, et al. Transvaginal sonographic findings in ambulatory patients with suspect pelvic inflammatory disease. Obstet Gynecol 1992;80:912–6.
10. Boortz HE, Margolis DJ, Ragavendra N. Migration of Intrauterine devices: radiologic findings and implications for patient care. RadioGraphics 2012;32:335–52.
11. Khandelwal A, Fasih N, Kielar A. Imaging of acute abdomen in pregnancy. Radiol Clin North Am 2013;51(6):1005–22.
12. Leeson K, Leeson B. Pediatric ultrasound: applications in the emergency department. Emerg Med Clin North Am 2013;31(3):809–29.
13. Caspi B, Zbar AP, Mavor E. The contribution of transvaginal ultrasound in the diagnosis of acute appendicitis: an observational study. Ultrasound Obstet Gynecol 2003;21(3):273–6.
14. Levine DI, Brown DL, Andreotti RF, et al. Management of Asymptomatic ovarian and other adnexal cysts imaged at US: Society of Radiologist in US consensus conference Statement. Radiology 2010;256(3):943–54.
15. Brown D. A practical approach to the ultrasound characterization of adnexal masses. Ultrasound Q 2007;23:87–105.
16. Exacoustos C, Manganaro L, Zupi E. Imaging for the evaluation of endometriosis and adenomyosis. Best Pract Res Clin Obstet Gynaecol 2014;28(5):655–81.
17. Gui B, Valentini AL, Ninivaggi V, et al. Deep pelvic endometriosis: don't forget round ligaments. Review of anatomy, clinical characteristics, and MR imaging features. Abdom Imaging 2014;39:622–32.
18. Asch E, Levine D. Variations in the appearance of endometriomas. J Ultrasound Med 2007;26:993–1002.
19. Marret H, Cayrol M. Sonographic diagnosis of presumed benign ovarian tumors. J Gynecol Obstet Biol Reprod 2013;42(8):730–43 [in French].
20. Saba L, Guerriero S, Sulcis R, et al. Mature and immature ovarian teratomas: CT, US and MR imaging characteristics. Eur J Radiol 2009;72(3):454–63.
21. Laing FC, Allison SJ. Ultrasound of the ovary and adnexa: to worry or not to worry? Radiographics 2012;32:1621–39.
22. Choudhary S, Fasih N, Mc Innes M, et al. Imaging of ovarian teratomas: appearances and complications. J Med Imaging Radiat Oncol 2009;53(5):480–8.
23. Chu LC, Coquia SF, Hamper UM. Ultrasonography evaluation of pelvic masses. Radiol Clin North Am 2014;52(6):1237–52.
24. Valentin L, Ameye L, Testa A, et al. Ultrasound characteristics of different types of adnexal malignancies. Gynecol Oncol 2006;102(1):41–8.

25. Smorgick N, Maymon R. Assessment of adnexal masses using ultrasound: a practical review. Int J Womens Health 2014;23(6):857–63.
26. Kim MY, Rha SE, Oh SN, et al. MR imaging findings of hydrosalpinx: a comprehensive review. Radiographics 2009;29(2):495–507.
27. Wang H, Chen YQ, Wei R, et al. Appendiceal mucocele: a diagnostic dilemma in differentiating malignant from benign lesions with CT. AJR Am J Roentgenol 2013;201(4):W590–5.
28. Spyropoulos C, Rentis A, Alexaki E, et al. Appendiceal mucocele and pseudomyxoma peritonei; the clinical boundaries of a subtle disease. Am J Case Rep 2014;15:355–60.
29. Malya FU, Hasbahceci M, Serter A, et al. Appendiceal mucocele: clinical and imaging features of 14 cases. Chirurgia (Bucur) 2014; 109(6):788–93.
30. Chirop R. A case of retention of urine and haematocolpometra. Eur J Emerg Med 2003;10(3):244–5.
31. Salvat J, Slamani L. Hematocolpos. J Gynecol Obstet Biol Reprod (Paris) 1998;27(4):396–402.
32. Sellmyer MA, Desser TS, Maturen KE, et al. Physiologic, histologic, and imaging features of retained products of conception. Radiographics 2013;33(3): 781–96.
33. Laifer-Narin SL, Kwak E, Kim H, et al. Multimodality imaging of the postpartum or posttermination uterus: evaluation using ultrasound, computed tomography, and magnetic resonance imaging. Curr Probl Diagn Radiol 2014;43(6):374–85.

Evaluating the Acute Abdomen in the Pregnant Patient

Gabriele Masselli, MD[a],*, Martina Derme, MD[b],
Francesca Laghi, MD[a], Marialuisa Framarino-dei-Malatesta, MD[b],
Gianfranco Gualdi, MD[a]

KEYWORDS

- Acute abdominal pain • Pregnancy • Ultrasound • Computed tomography • MR imaging

KEY POINTS

- US and MR imaging are the preferred investigations for acute abdominal pain during pregnancy.
- US remains the primary imaging investigation because of availability and portability.
- MR imaging helps differentiate causes of acute abdominal pain when US is inconclusive.

INTRODUCTION

The management of acute abdominal pain in pregnancy is challenging for a variety of reasons. Complications and conditions that are associated with or unrelated to pregnancy (urinary tract disorders, gastrointestinal and vascular diseases) may cause abdominal pain or the acute abdomen.[1] The diagnosis of acute abdominal pain in pregnant women is particularly difficult because of multiple confounding factors related to normal pregnancy: nonspecific leukocytosis, displacement of abdominal and pelvic structures from their normal locations by the gravid uterus, difficult abdominal examination, and nonspecific nausea and vomiting.[2] Prompt diagnosis and treatment are crucial for the well-being of the mother and the fetus, and imaging is often required to clarify the clinical picture. Because of exposure of the fetus to ionizing radiation, computed tomography (CT) or plain abdominal radiographs are not the imaging modalities of choice in these patients. Ultrasound

(US) and MR imaging are the preferred primary imaging investigations of pregnancy, because of the lack of ionizing radiation.

US is widely used as the initial diagnostic imaging technique during pregnancy because of its availability, portability, and lack of ionizing radiation. US can elucidate the cause of abdominal pain, particularly if pain is caused by an obstetric and gynecologic abnormality. However, evaluation of the bowel, pancreas, ureters, and mesenteric vasculature may be limited on US because of patient body habitus, a small field of view, and the presence of overlying structures. Air within the bowel can particularly limit evaluation of the mesenteric vessels, pancreas, and bowel.

MR imaging is often used when US is inconclusive. CT is used more sparingly in pregnancy because of its level of ionizing radiation. It is the investigation of choice when there is a life-threatening situation and in case of traumatic injuries when a rapid diagnosis is required.[3] This article explains the role of the different imaging

Authors have no conflict of interest to declare.
[a] Radiology Department, Umberto I Hospital, Sapienza University, Viale del Policlinico 155, Rome 00161, Italy;
[b] Department of Gynecological, Obstetrical and Urological Sciences, Sapienza University, Viale del Policlinico 155, Rome 00161, Italy
* Corresponding author.
E-mail address: g.masselli@policlinicoumberto1.it

techniques for the diagnosis and the management of the most common causes of acute abdominal pain during pregnancy.

IMAGING TECHNIQUE AND SAFETY

US is the first-line diagnostic test in pregnant women with acute abdominal pain, because of the universal availability, the low cost, and the lack of ionizing radiation. Limitations of US include operator dependency, altered body habitus, small field of view, and presence of interfering overlying structures. There are no documented adverse fetal effects of diagnostic US. The US Food and Drug Administration proposed an upper limit of 720 mW/cm^2 for spatial-peak temporal average intensity. Doppler US should be limited to the minimum necessary for clinical diagnosis and its use is discouraged in the first trimester.[4]

The American College of Radiology states that MR imaging is a useful problem-solving tool in the evaluation of abdominal and pelvic pain during pregnancy.[5] It is the preferred investigation when US is inconclusive. The potential advantages of MR imaging are multiplanar imaging capabilities and the ability to detect and distinguish blood from other fluid collections. A comprehensive multiplanar imaging protocol is used to evaluate the most common causes of acute abdominal pain. The protocol includes breath-hold multiplanar T2-weighted sequences based on the half-Fourier reconstruction technique (half-Fourier RARE or single-shot fast spin echo) and balanced gradient echo sequences (FIESTA, true FISP), axial and sagittal T1-weighted gradient-recalled echo sequences, and axial and sagittal diffusion sequences. The time required for this MR protocol is 20 minutes (Table 1).[3]

The detection of acute inflammatory changes is a critical component in the imaging of acute abdominal pain, and MR imaging is sensitive for depiction of inflammation by demonstration of elevated T2 signal within, or adjacent to, the affected tissues. The elevated abnormal T2 signal related to inflammatory disease processes has the potential to be obscured by the inherent high signal of intraperitoneal and retroperitoneal fat. Thus, the acquisition of an additional T2 single-shot sequence that is combined with reliable, high-quality fat suppression is an important component of any abdominopelvic MR imaging. Fat suppression using a spectral adiabatic inversion-recovery technique has been found to produce improved suppression of lipid signal over conventional inversion recovery or spectral saturation techniques. This spectral adiabatic inversion-recovery technique allows the fat-suppressed T2-weighted images to serve as a sensitive marker sequence for edema and inflammatory changes. Compared with CT, the detection of edema with fat-suppressed T2 single-shot MR imaging sequences provides higher levels of contrast and therefore higher sensitivity and specificity for inflammatory changes in the affected tissues and in the surrounding retroperitoneal and mesenteric fat.

Table 1
MR imaging parameters

Parameter	Balanced Gradient Echo Sequence (FIESTA, True FISP, BSSFP) Axial	Coronal/ Sagittal	T2 Half-Fourier Sequence (HASTE) Axial/ Axial Fat Sat	Coronal/ Sagittal	T1 Three-Dimensional Sequence Gradient Echo Sequence Axial/Sagittal	Diffusion-Weighted Image Axial, Coronal
Repetition time/echo time (ms)	4.3/2.2	4.3/2.2	1000/90	1000/90	4.1/1.1	3200/75
Flip angle (degrees)	50	50	150	150	10	10
Field of view (mm)	320–400	320–400	320–400	320–400	320–400	320–400
Matrix	256 × 224	256 × 224	256 × 224	256 × 224	256 × 224	256 × 192
Parallel imaging factor	2	2	2	2	3	2
Section thickness (mm)	5	5	4	4	2.5	10
Intersection gap (mm)	0	0	0	0	0	0
NEX	1	1	1	1	1	6
Receiver bandwidth	125	125	62.50	62.50	62.50	1930

Despite the lack of any evidence of adverse fetal effects after MR imaging studies, gadolinium-based contrast agents are classified as category C drugs by the Food and Drug Administration and should only be administered to a pregnant patient "if the potential benefit justifies the potential risk to the fetus and using the smallest dose of the most stable gadolinium agent."[6]

Examinations using ionizing radiation, in particular CT, can also accurately diagnose many causes of abdominal pain during pregnancy. A risk-benefit analysis is particularly warranted before performing an examination involving ionizing radiation on a pregnant or potentially pregnant patient. However, most diagnostic imaging studies using ionizing radiation do not expose the fetus to a radiation dose high enough to result in developmental or neurologic deficits. Therefore, ionizing radiation examinations can still be offered to pregnant women when the study is in the best health interest of the mother and the patient understands the minimal and unknown risks to the fetus.

This dose is below the recommended 50-mGy (5-rad) maternal dose limit for avoiding deterministic radiation effects (ie, effects that have a radiation threshold below which they should not occur), such as fetal teratogenesis. There is no known maternal radiation limit for fetal stochastic effects (ie, effects that can occur regardless of radiation dose), such as carcinogenesis; therefore, radiation levels should be kept as low as reasonably achievable for all ionizing radiation studies.

CT is used more sparingly in pregnancy because of its higher level of ionizing radiation. It is the investigation of choice when there is a life-threatening situation, such as hypovolemic blunt or penetrating trauma or severe sepsis, and a rapid diagnosis is required. When CT is used in pregnant patients, it is important to use automatic exposure control to reduce the radiation exposure. Protocols should minimize the use of multiphase studies and should optimize settings to reduce the dose as much as possible without losing image quality. It is common practice to wrap areas adjacent to those being scanned with shielding. Indeed, this may provide a psychological benefit to the patient and her physicians.[7] European society of urogenital radiology (ESUR) guidelines recommend that intravascular iodinated contrast medium should be administered only if absolutely necessary and after an informed consent has been obtained.[8]

OBSTETRIC CAUSES
Ectopic Pregnancy

An ectopic pregnancy (EP) is the implantation of a fertilized ovum outside the endometrial lining of the uterus. The incidence of EP is 1% to 2% of all reported pregnancies and it remains the main cause of maternal death during the first trimester. Potential risk factors are previous EP, prior pelvic inflammatory disease, previous tubal surgery, abdominal surgery, tubal blockage, advanced maternal age, cigarette smoking, intrauterine device, prior abortions, and a history of subfertility.[9]

EP is usually tubal (95%); more rarely, it is ovarian (1%–3%), interstitial (2%–4%), abdominal (1.4%), and cervical (<1%).[10] Signs and symptoms are nonspecific and include acute abdominal pain, vaginal bleeding, and an adnexal mass. Early diagnosis and treatment of EP are crucial to reduce maternal mortality and preserve future fertility. The initial evaluation includes a quantitative measurement of serum human chorionic gonadotropin (hCG) and transvaginal US. If hCG levels increase by less than 50% during a 48-hour period, the pregnancy is almost always nonviable.[11] Transvaginal US demonstrates a gestational sac (GS) when hCG levels are greater than 2000 mIU/mL,[12] with a sensitivity of 69% to 99% and a specificity of 84% to 99.9%.[13] Sometimes US provides a definitive diagnosis showing an extrauterine GS with a yolk sac or embryo; more frequently, it is only suggestive of an EP showing the presence of an adnexal mass (the most common sonographic finding in EP) and pelvic free fluid.[14–16] The adnexal mass usually appears as a saclike ring, solid or complex (**Fig. 1**).

MR imaging is an excellent problem-solving modality to confirm or better define suspected EP, especially when transvaginal US fails to demonstrate focus of EP or to distinguish from incomplete abortion. MR imaging can help to diagnose the rare or complicated form of EP.[17] However, its use may be limited in hemodynamically unstable patients, especially because of ruptured EP. Reported MR imaging findings of EP include GS-like structure that typically appears as a cystic saclike structure, an adnexal or abdominal hematoma, tubal dilatation caused by hemosalpinx, and tubal wall enhancement.[13,17,18] MR imaging is also important to make an accurate differential diagnosis between GS and corpus luteum cyst. On transvaginal US, a corpus luteum appears as a cystic structure with the ring of fire on color Doppler imaging, which resembles the feature of EP. On MR imaging, the distinction may be facilitated by focusing on the signal intensity of the peripheral area, location (intraovarian or extraovarian), and enhancement pattern.[13]

MR imaging is superior to US in detecting hemoperitoneum and in differentiating it from ascites.

Expectant management is a possible option for clinically stable asymptomatic women with a US

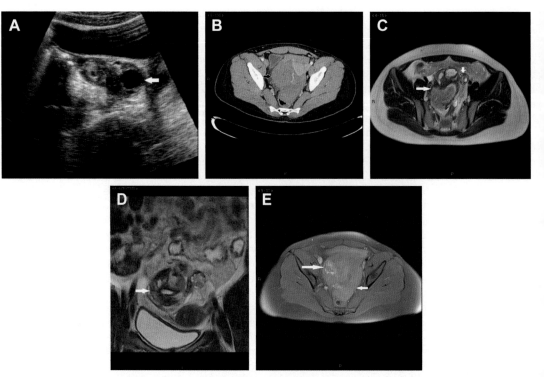

Fig. 1. A 32-year-old woman presenting with acute pelvic pain. Transvaginal US (*A*) shows the presence of a right complex saclike ring (*arrow*). Axial CT scan (*B*) confirms the presence of a right voluminous adnexal mass (*arrow*). Axial (*C*) and coronal (*D*) T2-weighted images of the pelvis show a right heterogeneous adnexal mass (*long arrow*) with fallopian tube hematoma. Note the normal right ovary (*short arrow*) in *C*. Precontrast T1-weighted fat-saturated image (*E*) shows the presence of fallopian tube hematoma (*long arrow*) and hemoperitoneum (*short arrow*).

diagnosis of EP and a decreasing serum hCG value, initially less than 1000 mIU/mL. Medical therapy, using methotrexate, should be offered to women with a serum hCG value less than 3000 mIU/mL, and minimal symptoms. Surgery is usually needed when EP causes severe symptoms, bleeding, or high hCG levels are present. Laparoscopic surgery is typically used. For a ruptured EP, emergency laparotomy is needed.

Placental Abruption

Placental abruption (PA), the premature separation of a normally implanted placenta from the uterine wall before delivery of the fetus, complicates about 1% of all pregnancies and it is an important cause of maternal and neonatal morbidity and mortality.[19] Evidence suggests that hypertensive disorders, advanced maternal age, grand-multiparity, thrombopenia, cigarette smoking, illicit drug use, and external abdominal trauma are associated with an increased risk of PA.[20]

The main clinical features of PA are vaginal bleeding associated with abdominal pain, uterine contractions or uterine tenderness, and signs of fetal distress. The most important US criteria for PA (sensitivity, 80%; specificity, 92%) are the detection of preplacental/retroplacental collections, evidence of marginal subchorionic or intra-amniotic hematomas, increased placental thickness (>5 cm), and jelly-like movements of the chorionic plate.[21,22] However, 25% to 50% of hematomas, mostly retroplacental in location, remain undetected by US[21–23] because the echo texture of recent hemorrhage is similar to that of the placenta[24] or because of the small dimensions of the bleed. Moreover clots resulting from chronic abruption may drain through the cervix.

MR imaging is superior to US in the evaluation of placenta hemorrhage, because it improves soft tissue contrast and has a wider field of view.[25] The diffusion- and T1-weighted sequences (sensitivity, 100% and 94%, respectively; diagnostic accuracy, 100% and 97%, respectively) are more accurate than the T2-weighted half-Fourier RARE (sensitivity, 94%; diagnostic accuracy, 87%) and true FISP sequences (sensitivity, 79%; diagnostic, accuracy 90%) in the detection of PA (**Fig. 2**).[25,26]

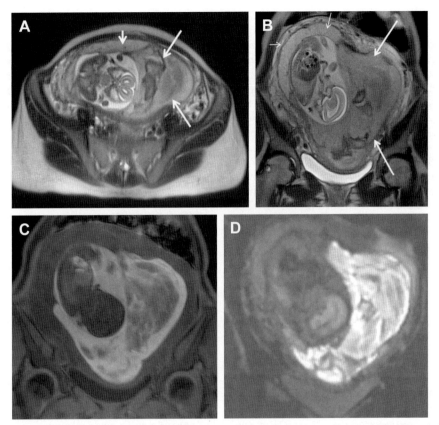

Fig. 2. A 29-year-old woman at 30 weeks' gestation with acute pelvic pain and vaginal bleeding. Axial (*A*) and coronal (*B*) T2-weighted images show the intrauterine clot with mixed hypointense and hyperintense areas placed along the left side of the uterine cavity and extended inferiorly to cover the uterine ostium. Coronal T1-weighted fat-saturated gradient echo (*C*) and diffusion-weighted (*D*) images show heterogeneous signal of the hematoma, indicating the coexistent acute and subacute hemorrhage. Note the normal placenta located on the right (*short arrow*).

Additionally, MR imaging is able to date hemorrhage based on the paramagnetic effects of methemoglobin and to classify intrauterine hematomas as hyperacute (first few hours, intracellular oxyhemoglobin), acute (1–3 days, intracellular deoxyhemoglobin), early subacute (3–7 days, intracellular methemoglobin), late subacute (≥14 days, extracellular methemoglobin), and chronic (>4 weeks, intracellular hemosiderin and ferritin).[27]

Because abruption may rapidly worsen, requiring rapid surgical delivery to prevent adverse maternal and fetal outcomes, an accurate diagnosis of PA and, possibly, the prediction of its worsening are extremely important when considering conservative treatment. The presence of a hematoma with hyperacute or acute MR signal intensity characteristics might correlate with progression of the abruption to higher grades. Because of the possible rapid and unpredictable worsening of abruption, it is important to avoid

any delay in performing MR imaging. Moreover, when taking a pregnant patient with a potentially unstable condition to an MR unit, continuous monitoring and emergency preparedness are mandatory. MR imaging is an extremely accurate investigation that identifies, with an excellent interobserver agreement, the origin of second- and third-trimester uterine bleeding.

MR imaging is an extremely accurate modality able to identify PA, even in cases with negative US findings. Signs of acute or recent bleeding within a hematoma indicate a potentially unstable abruption, whereas hematomas with late, subacute bleeding are stable.

Placental Adhesive Disorders

Placental adhesive disorders (PAD) include placenta accreta (placental villi attached to the myometrium), placenta increta (placental villi invading the myometrium), and placenta percreta (placental villi penetrating up to the uterine serosa). The incidence of PAD is 1 in 2000 pregnancies, with a rapid increase reflecting the rising number of cesarean sections and other uterine surgery.[28] The presence of acute abdominal pain is generally related to placenta percreta. US is the first imaging modality used to diagnose PAD. Sonographic features are loss of the normal hypoechoic retroplacental myometrium zone; thinning or disruption of the hyperechoic uterine serosa-bladder interface; presence of focal exophytic masses; and the presence of lacunae in the placenta, which is the most predictive sonographic sign showing a sensitivity of 79% and a positive predictive value of 92%.[29] Color Doppler can add information and, when three dimensions are available, can often distinguish placenta accreta from placenta percreta, highlighting areas of increased vascularity with dilated blood vessels that cross the placenta and uterine wall.[30]

MR imaging is not used as the first imaging modality to diagnose PAD but can provide additional information in equivocal cases, especially in patients with posterior placenta and previous myomectomy.[30–32] Lim and colleagues[33] found that the volume of dark placental bands was the most predictive finding in detecting PAD. Derman and colleagues[34] confirmed that the most reliable sign is the larger dark band on T2 HASTE series. They added an additional finding: vessels of 6 mm or greater (which presumably correspond to lacunae). When the placenta is percreta, MR imaging is able to detect infiltration of adjacent organs by evaluating tenting of the bladder, interruption of the myometrial line, and direct infiltration of pelvic organs (**Fig. 3**).[30]

If US findings suggest possible percreta or are inconclusive or negative in an at-risk woman, MR imaging can be useful. Invasion of adjacent organs is better depicted with MR imaging than on US. Situations in which MR imaging may also contribute additional information include women with placenta previa with a posterior or lateral implantation, a posterior scar from a myomectomy, a history of difficult placental removal in the past with a posterior or lateral placenta in the present pregnancy, or a history of endometrial ablation.[30] The correct and prompt diagnosis of placenta percreta is important because this condition may cause uterine rupture, requiring an emergency cesarean section.

Uterine Rupture

Uterine rupture is an obstetric complication characterized by a breach in the uterine wall and the overlying serosa. It often occurs during labor or third trimester of pregnancy. Two main categories are distinguished: rupture in a scarred uterus and rupture in an intact uterus. The term "scarred uterus" indicates a uterus subjected to previous surgery, in particular cesarean section, which constitutes the principal cause of overall uterine ruptures. According to the literature, incidence of spontaneous uterine rupture in a previously intact uterus is approximately 1 in 15,000.[35]

The diagnosis of uterine rupture on US relies on nonspecific and secondary signs, such as the presence of free fluid or hematoma formation. In comparison with US, MR imaging is less operator-dependent and provides a more comprehensive study with a larger field of view. MR imaging allows a better evaluation of soft tissues than US and CT. Finally, MR imaging allows clear visualization of the uterine wall; therefore, it helps to diagnose antepartum uterine rupture when US is indeterminate, showing the tear itself. Moreover MR imaging is more accurate than US in differentiating uterine

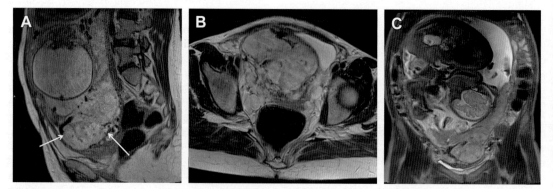

Fig. 3. A 25-year-old woman at 28 weeks' gestation with acute pelvic pain. Sagittal (*A*), axial (*B*), and coronal (*C*) T2-weighted HASTE images show multiple irregular areas of the placenta bulging into the myometrium with invasion of the right parametrium (*arrows*). These findings indicate placenta percreta. A hysterectomy was performed at delivery, which confirmed the presence of placenta percreta.

rupture from other uterine wall defects including uterine dehiscence and uterine sacculation.[36,37]

A correct differential diagnosis between complete uterine rupture and uterine dehiscence is important to choose the most appropriate management. In fact, when a diagnosis of complete uterine rupture is established, the immediate stabilization of the mother and the surgical delivery of the fetus are imperative, although expectant management can be used after the diagnosis of uterine dehiscence.

GYNECOLOGIC CAUSES
Adnexal Masses

The incidence of adnexal masses during pregnancy is about 1%.[38] Common adnexal lesions include simple cysts, hemorrhagic cysts, and hyperstimulated ovaries in patients who have undergone fertility assistance therapy. Lower abdominal pain is the most common symptom. Although ovarian cyst torsion or rupture is uncommon in pregnancy, some women may require emergency surgery for these complications. US is the study of choice for primary evaluation of adnexal masses but it is less accurate for complex or indeterminate lesions, even when combined with color Doppler imaging. MR imaging has been shown to be more specific and accurate than US and Doppler assessment in the diagnosis and characterization of adnexal masses, with an accuracy ranging from 83% to 89%, compared with 63% of ultrasonography.[39] Using frequency-selective fat saturation pulse sequences, MR imaging can determine whether a mass contains fat, which can be useful in the diagnosis of a teratoma. MR imaging can distinguish benign ovarian cysts from ovarian neoplasms because of the presence of papillary projections and nodular septa in neoplasms (Fig. 4).[40]

Most ovarian masses diagnosed in pregnancy are benign and resolve spontaneously. Surgical management is warranted when masses are suspicious for malignancy, at risk for torsion, or clinically symptomatic. With increasing numbers of successful laparoscopic procedures reported in pregnancy, laparoscopy seems to be a safe option with trained and experienced providers.

Ovarian Torsion

Ovarian torsion during pregnancy is a rare event, with a reported incidence of 1 to 10 per 10,000 spontaneous pregnancies. The highest risk of ovarian torsion exists in the first trimester of gestation.[41] Many cases of ovarian torsion are associated with the presence of an ovarian mass. Risk factors for ovarian torsion are mass size of 5 cm or greater, presence of a benign mass, ovarian hyperstimulation, and the pregnancy.[41] The clinical signs and symptoms are often confused with those of other abdominal conditions, and the imaging features are sometimes nonspecific.

US is typically the first imaging modality used to diagnose ovarian torsion in pregnancy. US findings include an enlarged ovary with multiple peripherally located follicles, a twisted vascular pedicle (the "whirlpool sign"), and free pelvic fluid. Normal Doppler flow can be observed in 45% to 61% of all ovarian torsion cases.[42,43] MR imaging should be performed after inconclusive US. Asymmetric enlargement of the ovary and stromal edema are well demonstrated by MR imaging, especially using T2-weighted sequences (Fig. 5). A twisted vascular pedicle can also be observed by MR imaging. Ovarian hemorrhage, a frequent sequela of torsion, can be identified on MR imaging, especially using T1-weighted images where blood products are hyperintense.[42] Chiou and colleagues[43] found that the presence on MR imaging of pelvic fat infiltration, hematoma formation, and the lack of enhancement sign were highly associated with necrosis of the involved adnexa, requiring rapid surgical intervention.

In some cases it may be necessary to perform a CT in emergency situations, such as when there is a massive hemoperitoneum in the unstable patient.

A missed diagnosis of ovarian torsion may lead not only to ovarian necrosis and sepsis, but also threaten the pregnancy. Early diagnosis and subsequent laparoscopic management are needed to optimize maternal and fetal outcomes.

Uterine Leiomyoma

Leiomyomas (fibroids or myomas) have prevalence during pregnancy of up to 20%, with higher frequency in women of advancing maternal age. They have been associated with a variety of different obstetric complications including spontaneous abortion, fetal malpresentation, intrauterine growth restriction, placenta previa, labor dystocia, PA, retained placenta, preterm labor, premature rupture of membranes, postpartum hemorrhage, and an increased frequency of cesarean sections.[44]

Leiomyomas are often asymptomatic during pregnancy. Abdominal pain and uterine contractions can result from their degeneration and necrosis. The Muram criteria have been widely used to evaluate the presence of a leiomyoma by US. The original criteria included visualization of a spherical mass with diameter greater than or equal to 3 cm; distortion of the adjacent myometrium by the mass; and a distinctive echogenicity,

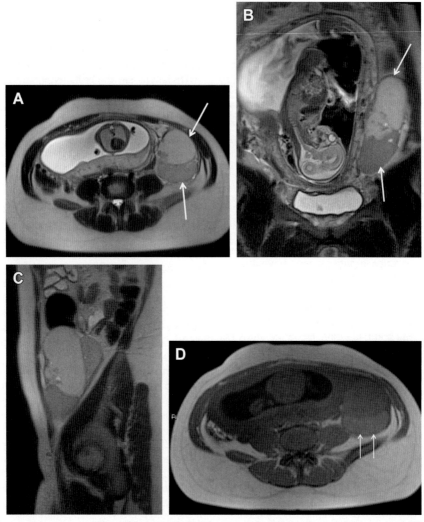

Fig. 4. A 35-year-old woman at 25 weeks' gestation with acute left-sided pain. Axial (*A*), coronal (*B*), and sagittal (*C*) T2-weighted HASTE MR images show a complex mass, with fluid and solid components in the left ovary. High-intensity areas are seen on axial T1-weighted sequence (*D*). Borderline mucinous cystadenoma was confirmed at surgery.

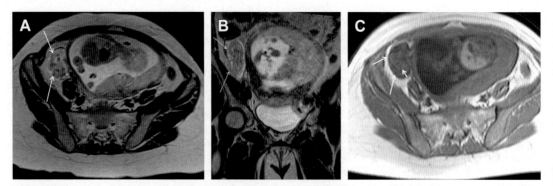

Fig. 5. Ovarian torsion in a 38-year-old woman at gestational week 26 with acute pelvic pain. Axial (*A*) and coronal (*B*) T2-weighted HASTE images show an enlarged, edematous right ovary (*arrows*). Axial T1-weighted sequence (*C*) shows areas of increased signal intensity (*short arrow*) within the right ovary indicating hemorrhagic infarction.

differentiating the mass from myometrium.[45] In acute hemorrhagic infarction (red degeneration), US shows heterogeneous or hyperechoic lesions and later anechoic components resulting from cystic necrosis.[3] MR imaging is the most accurate imaging technique for detection and localization of leiomyomas. On T2-weighted images, nondegenerated leiomyomas appear as well-circumscribed masses of decreased signal intensity. Leiomyomas with hemorrhagic degeneration often exhibit diffuse or peripheral high signal intensity on T1-weighted imaging and variable signal intensity on T2-weighted imaging.[46,47]

There is no consensus regarding the best approach to the treatment of symptomatic leiomyomas during pregnancy. Conservative therapy is the first option to be considered. Myomectomy may be performed in selected patients, with low perioperative and postoperative morbidity, presenting symptomatic, subserosal, or pedunculated leiomyomas with signs of degeneration, after the failure of a conservative treatment.

NONOBSTETRIC AND NONGYNECOLOGIC CAUSES
Urolithiasis

Renal colic is the most frequent nonobstetric and nongynecologic cause for abdominal pain and subsequent hospitalization during pregnancy. Symptomatic nephrolithiasis complicates 1 in 3300 pregnancies with an incidence ranging from 1 in 200 to 1 in 1500.[48] Renal colic has been associated with several pregnancy complications, such as preterm labor and delivery, recurrent abortions, hypertensive disorders, gestational diabetes, and cesarean sections.[49] US is the first investigation when there is a suspicion of stone disease during pregnancy. US is operator dependent and its sensitivity for detecting nephrolithiasis during pregnancy ranges from 34% to 92.5%.

Renal sonographic findings may be nonspecific and may be unable to differentiate between ureteral obstruction secondary to calculi and physiologic hydronephrosis. Transvaginal US is helpful to evaluate distal ureter and distinguish obstruction from physiologic hydronephrosis, which can occur in up to 90% of pregnant patients. Doppler-assisted measurement of the resistive index (RI) (peak systolic velocity of intrarenal blood flow minus the end-diastolic velocity divided by the peak systolic velocity) has shown some promise in pregnancy. The RI does not seem to be affected by the physiologic hydronephrosis during pregnancy. Normal pregnancy does not usually affect the intrarenal RI, and an elevated RI (>0.70) should not therefore be attributed to pregnancy.

Color Doppler US can also be used to detect the passage of urine at the ureterovesical junction by visualizing a normal ureteral jet. In the nonpregnant abdomen, absence of this sign on the symptomatic side has a very high sensitivity and specificity for obstruction. However, its diagnostic value is hampered because ureteral jets may be absent in 15% of asymptomatic pregnant women. Possible false-positive results are decreased by imaging patients in the contralateral decubitus position; this maneuver reduces the degree of physiologic dilatation. The value of intravenous urography in pregnancy is limited because of the confounding physiologic hydroureter and superimposed gravid uterus. The fetal osseous structures can obscure visualization of ureteral calculi. Moreover, the radiation dose is not significantly lower than that from the renal stone CT protocol.[50,51]

MR urography without contrast is a safe, effective, and accurate procedure in differentiating obstructive from physiologic hydronephrosis. The presence of a standing column of urine below the level of the pelvic brim, in addition to proximal ureteral dilation, is suggestive of an obstructing distal ureteral calculus ("double kink sign"). Other MR imaging features that suggest pathologic rather than physiologic hydronephrosis include an "unusual" site of obstruction (such as the pelvoureteral junction or vesicoureteral junction), an abrupt ending of the ureter (rather than a smooth taper at the level of the pelvic brim), and perinephric or periureteral edema (**Fig. 6**).[48,51] MR imaging is helpful in demonstrating complications, such as pyelonephritis that manifests as an enlarged edematous kidney. Areas of focal pyelonephritis have lower signal intensity on T2-weighted and restricted proton diffusion on diffusion-weighted images.

Urinary tract calculi appear as signal voids overlying the high signal of urine within a dilated ureter. The degree of sensitivity for diagnosing renal stones increases with larger stone size. The use of high-resolution T2 fast spin echo sequence with thin section (3 mm) is mandatory to increase the accuracy in detecting small stones. In unresolved cases, CT remains a reliable technique for depicting obstructing urinary tract calculi in pregnant women.

A conservative approach is usually taken in the initial management in all pregnant patients with symptomatic ureteric stones. Conservative treatment, which requires close communication between the urologist and obstetrician, includes hydration (oral or intravenous), analgesia, antibiotics (if infection is present), antiemetics, rest, and routine sieving of urine. If the conservative approach fails, ureteral stenting may be performed as an initial procedure in patients who have fever

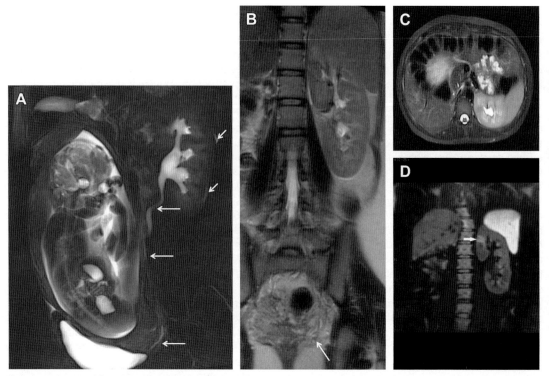

Fig. 6. A 33-year-old woman at 32-gestational week was admitted with fever and acute left-side pain. MR urography image (*A*) shows the standing column sign indicating obstructive hydronephrosis (*arrows*). Coronal T2-weighted HASTE MR image (*B*) demonstrates a 4-mm low-signal-intensity (*arrow*) calculus within the distal left ureter. Axial T2-weighted fat-saturated image (*C*) through the kidney showing swelling on the left with slight parenchymal edema and reduction in corticomedullary differentiation. Coronal diffusion-weighted image (b value = 800) (*D*) shows an area of restricted proton diffusion (*arrow*) indicating focal pyelonephritis at the level of the upper left kidney.

and/or proximal ureteric stones. Percutaneous nephrostomy should be reserved for patients with urosepsis or pyonephrosis if a stent cannot be placed. Ureteroscopy with laser therapy has become the procedure of choice in pregnancy for symptomatic stones less than 1 cm and in those patients without evidence of sepsis or a history of transplanted kidney.

Anti-inflammatory agents and intravenous antibiotics are required in the treatment of pyelonephritis. Rarely, rapid spread of infection may result in a perinephric abscess. This may occur because of a delay in diagnosis, inappropriate treatment, diabetes mellitus, or an immunocompromised state. Aggressive treatment with intravenous antibiotics and surgical or percutaneous drainage of the abscess are indicated.

Gastrointestinal Causes

Acute appendicitis
Acute appendicitis occurs in 1 in 2000 pregnancies and it is the most common nonobstetric

surgical emergency. Fetal mortality of 37% if the maternal appendix perforates and surgical delay of greater than 24 hours results in a 66% increase in the rate of appendiceal perforation. Thus, early and accurate diagnosis of appendicitis in pregnant patients is critical to prevent adverse outcomes to mother and fetus.

Clinical examination and laboratory tests are often altered during pregnancy, leading to a delay in diagnosis. US is often the first investigation used to diagnose acute appendicitis in the pregnant patient and the parameters for making the diagnosis include visualization of a blind-ending, dilated (>6–7 mm in diameter), aperistaltic, and noncompressible tubular structure arising from the cecum.[52] US of the appendix, with reported sensitivity and specificity values ranging from 50% to 100% and from 33% to 92%, respectively, is a highly operator-dependent examination and is limited by the pregnant body habitus, especially in the later stages of gestation.[8]

The multiplanar capacity and the excellent soft tissue contrast make MR imaging an excellent test for acute appendicitis if the appendix is not visualized by US. MR imaging features of a normal appendix include a diameter less than 6 mm, an appendiceal wall thickness less than 2 mm, low luminal signal intensity on T1- and T2-weighted images, and no periappendiceal fat stranding or fluid. MR imaging features of appendicitis include an appendiceal diameter greater than 7 mm, an appendiceal wall thickness greater than 2 mm, high signal intensity luminal contents on T2-weighted images caused by fluid or edema, and hyperintense periappendiceal fat stranding and fluid (**Fig. 7**).[2,53] MR imaging has a reported sensitivity of appendicitis during pregnancy of 100% and a 94% specificity.[2]

Oral contrast medium in not widely used in MR imaging clinical practice despite the evidence that the use of a negative intraluminal agent following a specific protocol[54] provides the highest rate of identification of normal appendix.

If MR imaging cannot be performed, because of absolute contraindications or it is not available, CT is an alternative. Positive CT findings are the same as in nonpregnant patients with high sensitivity and specificity of 92% and 99%, respectively.[52]

Intestinal obstruction

The incidence of intestinal obstruction in pregnancy ranges from 1 in 1500 to 1 in 66,000 deliveries. Causes of bowel obstruction in pregnant patients include adhesions, volvulus, intussusception, carcinoma, hernia, and acute appendicitis. Adhesions are the most common cause and the incidence of obstruction increases with the gestational age.[55] Presenting symptoms and signs are similar to those of nonpregnant patients including abdominal pain, vomiting, and tenderness to palpation. In long-standing or high-grade obstruction, US may show dilated loops of bowel with fluid levels and aperistalsis, but the point and the cause of bowel obstruction usually remain undetermined. MR imaging, using multiplanar T2-weighted single-shot fast spin echo imaging, confirmed the presence and identified the site of bowel obstruction in approximately 80% of cases (**Fig. 8**).[56,57]

If undiagnosed, this condition is associated with increased maternal and perinatal mortality. Correction of electrolyte disturbances, emergency laparotomy (midline), and resection and anastomosis or decompression of the bowel are the cornerstones of management.

Inflammatory bowel disease

Inflammatory bowel diseases (IBD) commonly affect young patients in the reproductive phase of their lives. However, the course of IBD is not adversely affected by pregnancy. These patients usually present abdominal pain, diarrhea, nausea, vomiting, and fever. The terminal ileum is the most commonly affected portion of the gastrointestinal tract (~80% of cases), making IBD a good mimic of appendicitis. MR imaging features of IBD include mural thickening, mural hyperenhancement, high signal intensity in the bowel wall on T2-weighted images, a narrowed bowel lumen, and free fluid and edema in the surrounding soft tissues. Potential complications of IBD include abscess, fistula, sinus tract formation, and bowel strictures, all of which are readily detected with MR imaging. In the general population, MR imaging has an overall sensitivity of 91% and specificity of 71% for active IBD (**Figs. 9** and **10**).[2,58] During pregnancy clinical exacerbations may have serious consequences to the pregnant woman and the fetus.

Hepatobiliary Causes

Hepatobiliary causes of abdominal pain in pregnant patients include cholelithiasis, choledocholithiasis, acute cholecystitis, pancreatitis, and hepatitis. These diseases are common in women of reproductive age. Pregnancy-specific entities include HELLP (hemolysis, elevated liver enzyme levels, and low platelet count) syndrome and acute fatty liver of pregnancy.

Acute cholecystitis

Gallbladder disease is the second most common nonobstetric indication for surgical intervention during pregnancy. The prevalence of gallstones in pregnant women is 5% to 12%.[58] A right upper quadrant US is the most appropriate initial

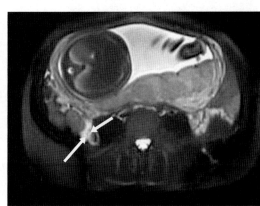

Fig. 7. Acute appendicitis in a 27-year-old woman at 34-weeks gestation presenting with right-sided abdominal pain. Axial T2-weighted HASTE fat-saturated image shows mural thickening of the appendix with high signal intensity of the periappendiceal fat caused by inflammatory changes (*arrows*).

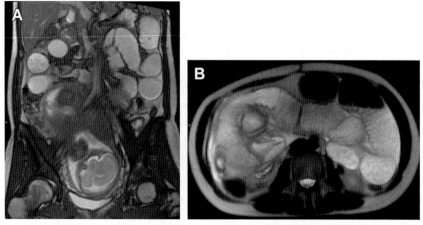

Fig. 8. A 34-year-old woman at 30-weeks gestation presenting with diffuse abdominal pain. Coronal true FISP (*A*) and axial HASTE (*B*) images show multiple dilated fluid-filled loops with the tapering of the bowel loops at the point of obstruction ("beak sign") indicating adhesion, the presence of which was confirmed at laparoscopy.

imaging study for the evaluation of acute cholecystitis in pregnancy. US findings of acute cholecystitis include gallbladder distention (>5 cm in diameter), wall thickening (>3 mm), pericholecystic fluid, and wall hyperemia. The sonographic Murphy sign is defined as the presence of maximal tenderness elicited by direct pressure of the transducer over a sonographically localized gallbladder. This sign has been shown to be present in 98.8% of 497 suspected cases of acute cholecystitis.[59,60] MR imaging is the most appropriate second-line imaging test to evaluate biliary disease during pregnancy. MR imaging findings include gallbladder wall thickening of greater than 3 mm, increased signal intensity in the gallbladder wall (edema) on T2-weighted images, increased signal intensity surrounding the gallbladder (pericholecystic fluid) on T2-weighted images, and a signal void in the cystic duct or gallbladder neck caused by an obstructing stone. Complications include perforation and pericholecystic abscess. MR imaging has a positive predictive value of up to 100% in accurate diagnosis of acute cholecystitis.[2]

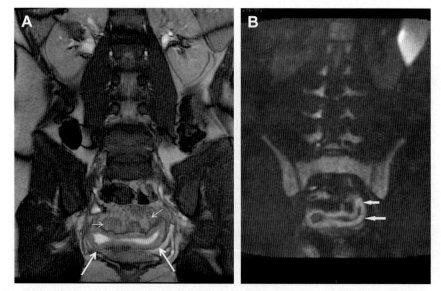

Fig. 9. Active Crohn disease in a 31-year-old woman at 13-weeks gestation presenting with acute abdominal pain. Coronal true FISP image (*A*) shows wall thickening of a distal ileal loop (*long arrows*) associated with extensive fibrofatty proliferation of mesentery (*short arrows*). Coronal diffusion-weighted image (*B*) shows restriction of the diffusion of bowel wall (*arrows*), indicating acute inflammation.

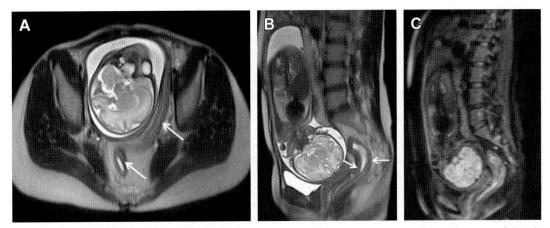

Fig. 10. Active ulcerative colitis in a 29-year-old woman at 34-weeks gestation presenting with acute pelvic pain. Axial (*A*) and sagittal (*B*) T2-weighted HASTE images show the presence of diffuse irregular circumferential wall thickening of the rectum and of the distal sigmoid colon (*arrows*). Sagittal diffusion-weighted sequence (*C*) shows increased signal intensity of the mucosa with submucosal sparing.

MR cholangiopancreatography is highly sensitive (98%) and specific (94%) for the detection of biliary disease and is more sensitive than US for the detection of choledocholithiasis (**Fig. 11**).

Management involves intravenous fluids to correct electrolyte imbalance, analgesics and anti-inflammatory agents, nasogastric suction, and the use of intravenous antibiotics. Recurrent attacks of cholecystitis and complications, such as empyema or perforation, warrant surgical or interventional radiology treatment. Percutaneous drainage of the abscess may be warranted. Laparoscopic cholecystectomy has been described during pregnancy.

Acute pancreatitis

The incidence of pancreatitis in pregnancy ranges from 1 in 1000 to 1 in 10,000. The annual incidence in the general population is 5 to 80 per 100,000. More than 70% of cases of acute pancreatitis during pregnancy are caused by gallstones.[61] Patients typically present with abdominal pain, nausea, vomiting, and elevated amylase or lipase levels. US of the right upper quadrant is a safe and inexpensive test. Although it has low diagnostic value for acute pancreatitis, it can reliably detect gallstones and biliary dilatation. The value of US is limited by intestinal gas or the patient body habitus.

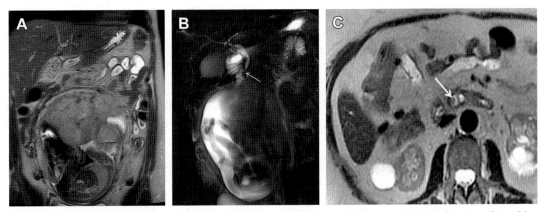

Fig. 11. A 27-year-old woman at 24-weeks gestation presenting with right-sided abdominal pain and vomiting. Coronal T2-weighted HASTE image (*A*) shows a dilated gallbladder with multiple small gallstones, seen at US examination. MR cholangiopancreatography image (*B*) shows a mildly dilated common bile duct with distal stenosis. Axial T2-weighted HASTE images (*C*) show a small distal common bile duct stone (*arrow*), missed by US examination. Endoscopic retrograde cholangiopancreatography confirmed a small stone that was extracted.

MR cholangiopancreatography should be considered when US findings are indeterminate. It enables the study of the pancreatic parenchyma and diagnosis of common bile duct stones with a sensitivity of more than 90% without exposure of the mother or the fetus to ionizing radiation.[62] At MR imaging, the peripancreatic fluid and edema associated with pancreatitis appear as high signal intensity surrounding the pancreas on T2-weighted images. Biliary and pancreatic ductal dilatation can also be seen. Complications of acute pancreatitis that are seen at MR imaging include abscess, pseudocyst, pancreatic necrosis, and splenic vein thrombosis.[2]

Although unrecognized and untreated pancreatitis may be associated with increased maternal and perinatal morbidity and mortality, it is generally a self-limiting illness. Supportive treatment with intravenous fluids, correction of electrolyte imbalance, glucose levels, serum calcium levels, and keeping the patient on nothing-by-mouth status forms the mainstay of treatment. In severe disease, nasogastric suction and total parenteral nutrition may need to be considered. Rarely, if the condition deteriorates, emergency surgery may be indicated to remove gallstones.

Hemolysis, elevated liver enzyme levels syndrome

The incidence is reported as 0.2% to 0.6% of all pregnancies, and 10% to 20% of women with co-morbid preeclampsia.[63] HELLP syndrome is characterized by three diagnostic laboratory criteria: hemolysis (H), elevated liver tests (EL), and low platelet count (LP). In some patients elevated liver function values are associated with right upper quadrant or epigastric pain. The main US imaging findings include hepatic edema, ascites, and hepatomegaly. Acute complications of HELLP syndrome that are better seen at MR imaging include intrahepatic and extrahepatic hematomas, hepatic edema caused by early ischemia, and hepatic necrosis.[2]

Management focuses on control of blood pressure, prevention of seizures, correction of coagulation abnormality, and delivery. The role of corticosteroids is controversial. Rarely, distention of the Glisson capsule of the liver may lead to hepatic rupture. Patients may present with acute upper abdominal pain and hemorrhagic shock. Emergency laparotomy with repair of liver laceration, packing to control bleeding, and correction of coagulation abnormalities with recombinant factor VII may need to be considered. Very rarely, resection of the hepatic lobe or hepatic artery ligation may need to be undertaken as lifesaving measures.

Vascular Causes

There are a variety of potentially painful vascular conditions that have a higher incidence during pregnancy, including venous thromboembolic disease and gonadal vein dilatation, which can be detected on MR imaging.

Venous thromboembolic disease

During pregnancy venous stasis and hypercoagulability increase the risk for venous thrombosis. Venous stasis is caused by a combination of progesterone-induced venodilation, pelvic venous compression by the gravid uterus, and pulsatile compression of the left iliac vein by the right iliac artery. Most venous thromboembolic events occur in the lower extremities. However, pregnant patients are also at increased risk for pelvic, hepatic (Budd-Chiari syndrome), mesenteric, and gonadal venous thrombi. Prompt diagnosis and treatment of venous thrombosis during pregnancy is essential to avoid potential complications, such as thrombophlebitis, occlusion of the inferior vena cava and renal veins, and pulmonary embolism. Mesenteric venous thrombosis, a possible cause of bowel infarction, is difficult to diagnose because patients typically present with nonspecific and poorly localized abdominal pain.

Although the preferred imaging examination for evaluating venous disease is contrast-enhanced CT or MR venography, venous disease during pregnancy can be detected with the more routine sequences of an MR imaging examination performed for suspected appendicitis. For example, a true FISP sequence can demonstrate the presence (high signal intensity) or absence (low signal intensity) of flow within veins. It can also demonstrate a luminal thrombus as a low-signal-intensity filling defect in an otherwise high-signal-intensity patent abdominal or pelvic vein. In contrast, thrombosis or lack of flow in a vein on T2-weighted images appears as absence of the normal low-signal-intensity flow void of a patent vessel. On T1-weighted images, a venous thrombus is of variable signal intensity, depending on the age of luminal blood products.[2] However, images from these unenhanced MR imaging sequences should be interpreted with caution because unenhanced sequences are limited by flow signal artifacts.[64]

Gonadal vein dilatation

Unenhanced true FISP, T2-weighted, and T1-weighted sequences can also demonstrate the caliber of abdominal and pelvic vessels. In particular, the MR images from a study performed for possible appendicitis should also be reviewed for enlargement of the gonadal veins as a potential cause of abdominal pain.

Although gonadal vein dilatation is a common and typically normal finding in pregnancy because the veins dilate to accommodate increased blood flow, dilatation of the gonadal vein itself or resulting extrinsic compression of the ureter by the enlarged gonadal vein has been referred to as right ovarian vein syndrome.[65] Rarely, rupture of the dilated right ovarian vein during pregnancy has been described.[66] However, ovarian vein dilatation is likely a diagnosis of exclusion when it is the only finding at MR imaging to account for the pregnant patient's abdominal pain.

SUMMARY

The cause of acute abdominal pain during pregnancy is often difficult to establish because of the presence of multiple confounding factors. Diagnostic imaging with US, the first-line diagnostic test in pregnant women, is limited because of the altered body habitus, the small field of view, and the presence of interfering overlying structures. MR imaging is usually used when US is inconclusive and represents an excellent modality for imaging abdominal pain in pregnancy, providing a systematic evaluation of the entire abdomen and pelvis with a high diagnostic accuracy.

REFERENCES

1. Chandraharan E, Arulkumaran S. Acute abdomen and abdominal pain in pregnancy. Obstet Gynaecol Reprod Med 2008;18:205–12.
2. Spalluto LB, Woodfield CA, DeBenedectis CM, et al. MRI imaging evaluation of abdominal pain during pregnancy: appendicitis and other nonobstetric causes. Radiographics 2012;32:317–34.
3. Masselli G, Brunelli R, Monti R, et al. Imaging for acute pelvic pain in pregnancy. Insights Imaging 2014;5:165–81.
4. Miller DL. Safety assurance in obstetrical ultrasound. Semin Ultrasound CT MR 2008;29:156–64.
5. American College of Radiology. ACR practice guideline for imaging pregnant or potentially pregnant adolescents and women with ionizing radiation. 2008. Available at: http://www.acr.org/Secondary MainMenuCategories/quality_safety/guidelines/dx/ Pregnancy.aspx. Accessed February 21, 2010.
6. Thomsen HS, Morcos SK, Almén T, et al. Nephrogenic systemic fibrosis and gadolinium-based contrast media: updated ESUR Contrast Medium Safety Committee guidelines. Eur Radiol 2013;23: 307–18.
7. Wallace GW, Davis MA, Semelka RC, et al. Imaging the pregnant patient with abdominal pain. Abdom Imaging 2012;37:849–60.
8. Masselli G, Derchi L, McHugo J, et al. Acute abdominal and pelvic pain in pregnancy: ESUR recommendations. Eur Radiol 2013;23:3485–500.
9. Moini A, Hosseini R, Jahangiri N, et al. Risk factors for ectopic pregnancy: a case-control study. J Res Med Sci 2014;19:844–9.
10. Petrides A, Dinglas C, Chavez M, et al. Revisiting ectopic pregnancy: a pictorial essay. J Clin Imaging Sci 2014;4:37.
11. Lipscomb GH, Stovall TG, Ling FW. Nonsurgical treatment of ectopic pregnancy. N Engl J Med 2000;343:1325–9.
12. Levine D. Ectopic pregnancy. Radiology 2007;245: 385–97.
13. Takahashi A, Takahama J, Marugami N, et al. Ectopic pregnancy: MRI findings and clinical utility. Abdom Imaging 2013;38:844–50.
14. Cacciatore B. Can the status of tubal pregnancy be predicted with transvaginal sonography? A prospective comparison of sonographic, surgical, and serum hCG findings. Radiology 1990;177:481–4.
15. Brown DL, Doubilet PM. Transvaginal sonography for diagnosing ectopic pregnancy: positivity criteria and performance characteristics. J Ultrasound Med 1994;13:259–66.
16. Nyberg DA, Mack LA, Jeffrey RB Jr, et al. Endovaginal sonographic evaluation of ectopic pregnancy: a prospective study. AJR Am J Roentgenol 1987;149: 1181–6.
17. Kao LY, Scheinfeld MH, Chernyak V, et al. Beyond ultrasound: CT and MRI of ectopic pregnancy. AJR Am J Roentgenol 2014;202:904–11.
18. Tamai K, Koyama T, Togashi K, et al. MR features of ectopic pregnancy. Eur Radiol 2007;17(12): 3236–46.
19. Leunen K, Hall DR, Odendaal HJ, et al. The profile and complications of women with placental abruption and intrauterine death. J Trop Pediatr 2003;49: 231–4.
20. Denis M, Enquobahrie DA, Tadesse MG, et al. Placental genome and maternal-placental genetic interactions: a genome-wide and candidate gene association study of placental abruption. PLoS One 2014;9:e116346.
21. Jaffe MH, Schoen WC, Silver TM, et al. Sonography of abruptio placentae. AJR Am J Roentgenol 1981; 137:1049–54.
22. Harris RD, Cho C, Wells WA. Sonography of the placenta with emphasis on pathological correlation. Semin Ultrasound CT MR 1996;17:66–89.
23. Yeo L, Ananth C, Vintzileos A. Placenta abruption. In: Sciarra J, editor. Gynecology and obstetrics. Hagerstown (MD): Lippincott Williams & Wilkins; 2004.

24. Nyberg DA, Cyr DR, Mack LA, et al. Sonographic spectrum of placental abruption. AJR Am J Roentgenol 1987;148:161–4.

25. Masselli G, Brunelli R, Di Tola M, et al. MR imaging in the evaluation of placental abruption: correlation with sonographic findings. Radiology 2011;259:222–30.

26. Verswijvel G, Grieten M, Gyselaers W, et al. MRI in the assessment of pregnancy related intrauterine bleeding: a valuable adjunct to ultrasound? JBR-BTR 2002;85:189–92.

27. Atlas SW, Thulborn KR. Intracranial hemorrhage. In: Atlas SW, editor. Magnetic resonance imaging of the brain and of the spine. 4th edition. Philadelphia: Lippincott Williams & Wilkins; 2009. p. 644–94.

28. Wu S, Kocherginsky M, Hibbard JU. Abnormal placentation: twenty-year analysis. Am J Obstet Gynecol 2005;192:1458–61.

29. Comstock CH, Love JJ, Bronsteen RA, et al. Sonographic detection of placenta accrete in the second and third trimesters of pregnancy. Am J Obstet Gynecol 2004;190:1135–40.

30. Comstock CH, Bronsteen RA. The antenatal diagnosis of placenta accreta. BJOG 2014;121:171–81.

31. Masselli G, Brunelli R, Casciani E, et al. Magnetic resonance imaging in the evaluation of placental adhesive disorders: correlation with color Doppler ultrasound. Eur Radiol 2008;18:1292–9.

32. Masselli G, Gualdi G. MR imaging of the placenta: what a radiologist should know. Abdom Imaging 2013;38:573–87.

33. Lim PS, Greenberg M, Edelson MI, et al. Utility of ultrasound and MRI in prenatal diagnosis of placenta accreta: a pilot study. AJR Am J Roentgenol 2011; 197:1506–13.

34. Derman AY, Nikac V, Haberman S, et al. MRI of placenta accreta: a new imaging perspective. AJR Am J Roentgenol 2011;197:1514–21.

35. Mavromatidis G, Karavas G, Margioula-Siarkou C, et al. Spontaneous postpartum rupture of an intact uterus: a case report. J Clin Med Res 2015;7:56–8.

36. Hruska KM, Coughlin BF, Coggins AA, et al. MRI diagnosis of spontaneous uterine rupture of an unscarred uterus. Emerg Radiol 2006;12:186–8.

37. Masselli G, Brunelli R, Casciani E, et al. Acute abdominal and pelvic pain in pregnancy: MR imaging as a valuable adjunct to ultrasound? Abdom Imaging 2011;36:596–603.

38. Cengiz H, Kaya C, Ekin M, et al. Management of incidental adnexal masses on caesarean section. Niger Med J 2012;53:132–4.

39. Anthoulakis C, Nikoloudis N. Pelvic MRI as the "gold standard" in the subsequent evaluation of ultrasound-indeterminate adnexal lesions: a systematic review. Gynecol Oncol 2014;132:661–8.

40. Yacobozzi M, Nguyen D, Rakita D. Adnexal masses in pregnancy. Semin Ultrasound CT MR 2012;33:55–64.

41. Chang SD, Yen CF, Lo LM, et al. Surgical intervention for maternal ovarian torsion in pregnancy. Taiwan J Obstet Gynecol 2011;50:458–62.

42. Lourenco AP, Swenson D, Tubbs RJ, et al. Ovarian and tubal torsion: imaging findings on US, CT, and MRI. Emerg Radiol 2014;21:179–87.

43. Chiou SY, Lev-Toaff AS, Masuda E, et al. Adnexal torsion: new clinical and imaging observations by sonography, computed tomography, and magnetic resonance imaging. J Ultrasound Med 2007;26: 1289–301.

44. Rothmund R, Taran FA, Boeer B, et al. Surgical and conservative management of symptomatic leiomyomas during pregnancy: a retrospective pilot study. Geburtshilfe Frauenheilkd 2013;73:330–4.

45. Muram D, Gillieson M, Walters JH. Myomas of the uterus in pregnancy: ultrasonographic follow-up. Am J Obstet Gynecol 1980;138:16–9.

46. Murase E, Siegelman ES, Outwater EK, et al. Uterine leiomyomas: histopathologic features, MR imaging findings, differential diagnosis, and treatment. Radiographics 1999;19:1179–97.

47. Masselli G, Brunelli R, Parasassi T, et al. Magnetic resonance imaging of clinically stable late pregnancy bleeding: beyond ultrasound. Eur Radiol 2011;21:1841–9.

48. Semins MJ, Matlaga BR. Management of urolithiasis in pregnancy. Int J Womens Health 2013;5:599–604.

49. Semins MJ, Matlaga BR. Kidney stones and pregnancy. Adv Chronic Kidney Dis 2013;20:260–4.

50. Masselli G, Derme M, Laghi F, et al. Imaging of stone disease in pregnancy. Abdom Imaging 2013;38: 1409–14.

51. Masselli G, Derme M, Bernieri MG, et al. Stone disease in pregnancy: imaging-guided therapy. Insights Imaging 2014;5:691–6.

52. Gilo NB, Amini D, Landy HJ. Appendicitis and cholecystitis in pregnancy. Clin Obstet Gynecol 2009;52: 586–96.

53. Dewhurst C, Beddy P, Pedrosa I. MRI evaluation of acute appendicitis in pregnancy. J Magn Reson Imaging 2013;37:566–75.

54. Pedrosa I, Levine D, Eyvazzadeh AD, et al. MR imaging evaluation of acute appendicitis in pregnancy. Radiology 2006;238:891–9.

55. Kalu E, Sherriff E, Alsibai MA, et al. Gestational intestinal obstruction: a case report and review of literature. Arch Gynecol Obstet 2006;274:60–2.

56. Masselli G, Gualdi G. MR imaging of the small bowel. Radiology 2012;264:333–48.

57. Juglard R, Rimbot A, Marty A, et al. Bowel obstruction in pregnancy: value of single shot fast spin echo MR sequence (SS-FSE). J Radiol 2003;84:1986–8.

58. Hahnemann ML, Nensa F, Kinner S, et al. Improved detection of inflammatory bowel disease by additional automated motility analysis in magnetic resonance imaging. Invest Radiol 2015;50:67–72.

59. Ellington SR, Flowers L, Legardy-Williams JK, et al. Recent trends in hepatic diseases during pregnancy in the United States, 2002-2010. Am J Obstet Gynecol 2015;212(4):524.e1–7.

60. Ralls PW, Halls J, Lapin SA, et al. Prospective evaluation of the sonographic Murphy sign in suspected acute cholecystitis. J Clin Ultrasound 1982;10:113–5.

61. Abdullah B, Kathiresan Pillai T, Cheen LH, et al. Severe acute pancreatitis in pregnancy. Case Rep Obstet Gynecol 2015;2015:239068.

62. Papadakis EP, Sarigianni M, Mikhailidis DP, et al. Acute pancreatitis in pregnancy: an overview. Eur J Obstet Gynecol Reprod Biol 2011;159:261–6.

63. Bennett M. Do not forget about HELLP! BMJ Case Rep 2011.

64. Pedrosa I, Morrin M, Oleaga L, et al. Is true FISP imaging reliable in the evaluation of venous thrombosis? AJR Am J Roentgenol 2005;185:1632–40.

65. Pedrosa I, Zeikus EA, Levine D, et al. MR imaging of acute right lower quadrant pain in pregnant and nonpregnant patients. Radiographics 2007;27:721–43.

66. Munir SI, Lo T, Seaton J. Spontaneous rupture of utero-ovarian vessels in pregnancy. BMJ Case Rep 2012;2012.

MR Evaluation of the Nontraumatic Acute Abdomen with CT Correlation

Peter Bannas, MD[a,b], Perry J. Pickhardt, MD[a,*]

KEYWORDS

• Acute abdomen • MR imaging • Computed tomography • CT

KEY POINTS

- MR imaging provides excellent image quality of the abdominal cavity in the setting of the nontraumatic acute abdomen.
- MR imaging allows diagnosis of a broad spectrum of diseases in the setting of the nontraumatic abdomen, comparable in many ways to CT.
- The practicing radiologist should be familiar with MR imaging techniques used for individual cases to establish the correct diagnosis.
- MR imaging protocols should to be tailored for each individual, to achieve optimal image quality and maximal diagnostic yield.
- MR imaging findings often parallel those of CT for most acute abdominal pathology, with each modality having relative strengths and weaknesses.

INTRODUCTION

Acute abdominal pain is a common complaint in patients examined in the emergency department (ED).[1] The causes of acute abdominal pain range from life-threatening to benign self-limiting disorders. Acute appendicitis, diverticulitis, cholecystitis, and bowel obstruction are common causes of acute abdominal pain requiring medical attention. For proper treatment, a diagnostic workup that enables the clinician to differentiate between the various causes of acute abdominal pain is important, and imaging plays a critical role in this process.[2] Many patients are referred without a clear pretest diagnosis, and imaging is warranted to determine the diagnosis and guide treatment in these patients.[2]

According to American College of Radiology (ACR) appropriateness criteria, contrast-enhanced computed tomography (CT) of the abdomen and pelvis is considered the most appropriate examination for patients with acute abdominal pain, including those with fever or suspected abdominal abscess.[3] However, exposure to ionizing radiation is a relative disadvantage of CT,[4] and the use of intravenous contrast medium is another drawback in patients with known allergy, renal insufficiency, or pregnancy. Ultrasound is often the second choice of imaging modality,[3] but lacks the ability to screen for a broad range of pathologies in the same manner as CT.

MR imaging is potentially an attractive alternative. Although MR currently plays only a limited role in the assessment of abdominal pain presenting to the ED in the nongravid population,[2,5] its utility in the pregnant and pediatric population has already been demonstrated.[6,7] Current evidence suggests that MR could be used for a broader

[a] Department of Radiology, University of Wisconsin-Madison, 600 Highland Avenue, Madison, WI 53792-3252, USA; [b] Department of Radiology, University Hospital Hamburg-Eppendorf, Martinistrasse 52, Hamburg 20246, Germany
* Corresponding author. Department of Radiology, University of Wisconsin School of Medicine & Public Health, E3/311 Clinical Science Center, 600 Highland Avenue, Madison, WI 53792-3252.
E-mail address: ppickhardt2@uwhealth.org

Radiol Clin N Am 53 (2015) 1327–1339
http://dx.doi.org/10.1016/j.rcl.2015.06.014
0033-8389/15/$ – see front matter © 2015 Elsevier Inc. All rights reserved.

range of indications in the general adolescent and adult population.[5]

A major advantage of MR imaging is the lack of ionizing exposure, allowing for its use in pregnancy. As physicians and patients become more aware of the potential risks associated with exposure to ionizing radiation, MR utilization in the ED is likely to also increase also in the nongravid population. The higher intrinsic contrast of soft tissues with MR imaging as compared with CT is another advantage, as intravenous contrast medium may not always be required. Although contrast-enhanced MR imaging is generally preferred, non–contrast-enhanced protocols are available and may be a good option for patients with impaired renal function or who have allergies to gadolinium-based contrast agents. MR imaging allows for additional opportunities that are not available to CT, such as diffusion-weighted imaging (DWI), which may prove valuable in the assessment of the acute abdomen.

Despite its apparent advantages, MR has not yet played a significant role in imaging of the acute abdomen in the ED. Requests for MR imaging for this indication are exceptional in most hospitals. In general, MR imaging tends to be thought of as an expensive and time-consuming examination that requires multiple breathhold acquisitions that may be problematic for patients with acute abdominal pain. However, with newer techniques, such as accelerated parallel imaging and free-breathing techniques, these limitations may become less relevant in the future. Indeed, time-efficient protocols can be currently performed within approximately 15 minutes. One drawback that should be considered on a case-by-case basis includes the patient's ability to both remain still during the examination and tolerate the claustrophobic confines of a conventional MR imaging bore. However, new wide-bore MR scanners will be more widely available in the future.

Another reason why MR imaging is not widely used in this acute clinical setting is the lower availability of MR imaging in the ED and the lack of around-the-clock availability of MR technologists at many hospitals.[8] The infrequent use of ED-based MR imaging in turn leads naturally to an unfamiliarity of radiologists with MR imaging findings in the setting of acute abdominal pain.[5] Consequently, even during office hours when MR imaging is available, radiologists may rather order a CT over MR simply because they are familiar with the typical imaging findings. However, the ED utilization of MR is expected to increase as its availability increases.[9]

In this review, we present the typical MR findings of the most frequent disease entities in the setting of the nontraumatic acute abdomen. Because of our unique institutional experience with a prospective MR-CT clinical trial in patients presenting to the ED with acute abdominal symptoms, we are able to show the direct CT correlate of these MR findings to familiarize the readers with their appearance.

MR IMAGING PROTOCOL

Patient comfort is of paramount importance to ensure a successful examination with minimal motion artifact, particularly in patients with acute abdominal pain. Feet-first supine imaging is recommended for all examinations, particularly for claustrophobic patients.

The appropriate MR imaging sequences should be used and tailored for each individual to achieve optimal image quality and maximize diagnostic yield. We routinely perform contrast-enhanced protocols. However, non–contrast-enhanced protocols may be used in patients with contraindications to gadolinium-based contrast agents, or in pregnancy.

Generally, all examinations should include and begin with a coronal and axial single-shot T2-weighted fast spin echo (SSFSE) sequence. The SSFSE technique provides motion-resistant high-contrast anatomic images, where blood, bile ducts, and pancreatic ducts appear bright. The acquired images generally already allow for a good overview of the abdominal cavity. In the event of an aborted examination, the acquired images may provide enough diagnostic information for further triage of the patient.

The next acquisitions are axial or coronal T2-weighted FSE sequences with fat saturation. The use of fat suppression is recommended to improve the conspicuity of subtle findings. The acquired images are very sensitive for detection of even small fluid collections that are indicative of inflammatory changes and may allow focusing subsequent (contrast-enhanced) sequences on a specific site of pathology.

Pre–contrast-enhanced and post–contrast-enhanced T1-weighted fat-saturated axial and coronal sequences should follow to improve detection and characterization of pathologic findings.

DWI is very sensitive for localization of inflammatory changes and can further help to identify inflammatory foci. Other optional techniques include in-phase and out-of-phase imaging for lesion characterization and MR cholangiopancreatography (MRCP) for excellent depiction of bile ducts, pancreatic ducts, and cystic structures.

MR IMAGING FINDINGS WITH COMPUTED TOMOGRAPHY CORRELATION
Acute Appendicitis

Acute appendicitis is the most common abdominal emergency requiring surgery.[10] The prevalence of appendicitis among patients who present with abdominal pain to the ED is approximately 14%.[10] Acute appendicitis has a slight male predisposition and has the highest incidence between the ages of 10 and 19, with a median age of 22 years.[11] Making an accurate and timely diagnosis of appendicitis is challenging but important. A false-positive diagnosis may lead to unnecessary surgical exploration and a false-negative diagnosis has the risk of further morbidity related to perforation. Compared with uncomplicated appendicitis, perforated appendicitis is associated with a 2-fold to 10-fold increase in mortality.[12] A combination of clinical features, including pain migration, abdominal rigidity, and elevated inflammatory parameters, has a relatively high predictive value for appendicitis but is present in only a small proportion of patients suspected of having appendicitis. This makes it difficult to clinically determine the diagnosis in most patients and emphasizes the added value of imaging in patients with suspected appendicitis.

CT is the preferred imaging technique for the diagnosis and assessment of acute appendicitis.[13] CT is the most accurate imaging technique for evaluating suspected acute appendicitis and alternative etiologies of right lower quadrant pain.[14,15] Drawbacks of CT include the use of ionizing radiation and the nephrotoxic potential of intravenous iodinated contrast agents. Ultrasound does not use ionizing radiation but is operator-dependent and has a significantly lower diagnostic accuracy.[16] MR imaging has demonstrated promising accuracy for the assessment and diagnosis of acute appendicitis in pregnancy.[17,18] Although fewer data are available for nonpregnant adult patients and pediatric cohorts, preliminary results have been encouraging.[19–21] In our experience to date, the diagnostic performance for appendicitis in nonpregnant adults is comparable to CT, although others have shown that an initial learning curve exists.[22,23]

The normal MR appearance of the appendix consists of a slender tubular structure with a diameter of less than 6 mm and a wall thickness of less than 2 mm.[24,25] The signal intensity of the normal appendiceal wall is intermediate on all sequences and parallels that of other bowel walls. The appendix typically has low luminal signal intensity on T1-weighted and T2-weighted images, with no periappendiceal inflammatory stranding or fluid.

MR imaging features of acute appendicitis include some combination of an increased appendiceal diameter greater than 7 mm, an appendiceal wall thickness greater than 2 mm, increased wall enhancement, high signal-intensity luminal contents on T2-weighted images due to fluid or edema, and hyperintense stranding and fluid in the periappendiceal fat (Figs. 1 and 2).[6,23] These edematous changes and periappendiceal stranding are best demonstrated on T2-weighted fat-suppressed (STIR) images.[9] After contrast injection, the inflamed appendix shows contrast enhancement that is stronger than that of nonaffected bowel walls. DWI images show restricted diffusion and may thereby pinpoint the site of the appendix (see Fig. 1C), being often complementary to T2-weighted and postcontrast T1-weighted series in our experience.[22,26]

An appendix with hyperintense luminal contents on T2-weighted images and a diameter between 6 and 7 mm without associated wall thickening or periappendiceal fat stranding or fluid is considered indeterminate for appendicitis and warrants close clinical follow-up.[6,27] DWI and postcontrast T1-weighted imaging may be helpful in these equivocal cases. We have observed cases with abnormal early wall enhancement on MR where the corresponding CT and clinical evaluation were deemed negative for appendicitis. It is unclear if these cases represent false-positive MR diagnoses or very early appendicitis that resolves, as there is no pathology-based reference standard in the absence of surgery.

Acute Diverticulitis

Acute colonic diverticulitis is another common cause of acute abdominal pain in the ED.[28] The incidence of colonic diverticulosis increases with age. Seventy-two percent of patients admitted to the hospital for diverticulitis have uncomplicated diverticulitis. Most patients with uncomplicated diverticulitis can follow a conservative treatment regimen of antibiotics and diet modification. Patients with sizable peridiverticular abscesses are treated with percutaneous drainage. If patients do not respond to or deteriorate while undergoing conservative treatment, they will generally undergo surgery.[29,30]

CT plays a major role in confirming the diagnosis and in staging complications of acute colonic diverticulitis as well as in the detection of alternative diseases.[29,30] However, MR also has been shown to be accurate in the diagnosis of acute diverticulitis.[31] The sensitivity and specificity of MR imaging in detection of diverticulitis are 86% to 94% and 88% to 92%, respectively.[32] The

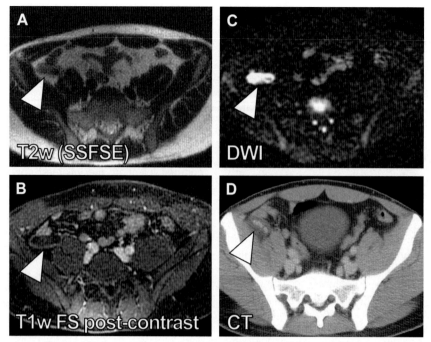

Fig. 1. Acute appendicitis in 26-year-old man. (*A*) Axial T2-weighted SSFSE and (*B*) postcontrast T1-weighted images show a dilated appendix (*arrowheads*) but minimal or no wall thickening, enhancement, or periappendiceal stranding. (*C*) DWI image (b-value = 500) shows markedly restricted diffusion of the appendix (*arrow*), indicative of inflammatory edema. (*D*) Contrast-enhanced CT shows a dilated appendix (*arrowhead*) with multiple dense appendicoliths, one of which may be suggested on MR by the low signal void on T2-weighted SSFSE image.

normal MR appearance of the colon shows a regular bowel wall thickness with intermediate signal intensity on all imaging sequences.

MR imaging findings of diverticulitis include an inflamed diverticulum with associated focal eccentric or segmental bowel wall thickening, increased signal intensity in the surrounding soft tissues (pericolonic fat stranding) on T2-weighted images, and inflammatory narrowing of the bowel lumen (**Fig. 3**).[6] Most cases of colonic diverticulitis involve the left colon (sigmoid > descending colon), but right-sided diverticulitis is not rare (see **Fig. 3**). Right-sided diverticulitis will often mimic appendicitis in terms of clinical presentation. Stranding of the pericolonic fat can be best appreciated on T2-weighted fat-suppressed images and there also may be pericolonic free fluid adjacent to the affected bowel segment. After contrast injection, the inflamed colonic segment shows contrast-enhancement that is stronger than that of nonaffected bowel loops. Complications of acute diverticulitis, such as abscess, colovesical fistula, and perforation, also can be seen with MR imaging.

Acute Cholecystitis

The prevalence of acute cholecystitis in patients who present with abdominal pain to the ED can

be up to 5%.[33] Most cases are caused by an impacted gallstone leading to obstruction of the cystic duct. Radiologic findings have an important influence on treatment management in patients with cholecystitis.[2] Treatment generally consists of (laparoscopic) cholecystectomy and should be performed with 96 hours after onset of symptoms. Imaging findings are therefore essential to allow for early decisions regarding timely treatment for cholecystitis.

Ultrasound is considered the most appropriate imaging modality when acute cholecystitis is the leading clinical concern.[34] CT or MR may be helpful in equivocal cases and may identify complications of acute cholecystitis. In cases in which the clinical presentation is more nonspecific, the patient may first undergo CT imaging evaluation; however, MR could potentially play a similar role. When ultrasound findings are inconclusive for biliary disease, MR imaging may be considered, and is the preferred imaging test in pregnant patients who present with suspected cholecystitis.[34] MR imaging has been shown to be more accurate than CT for the diagnosis of acute cholecystitis and the detection of common bile duct stones.[35] MR imaging has been shown to have a positive predictive value of up to 100% for acute cholecystitis.[36]

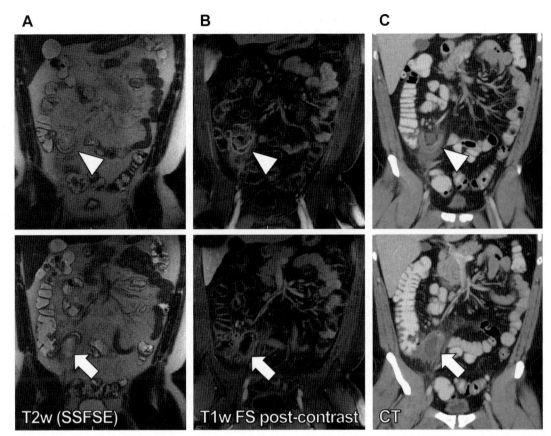

Fig. 2. Complicated acute appendicitis in a 26-year-old man. (*A*) Coronal T2-weighted SSFSE images show a fluid-filled enlarged and wall-thickened appendix (*arrowhead*) with a periappendiceal abscess (*arrow*) and surrounding inflammatory fat stranding. (*B*) Coronal contrast-enhanced T1-weighted images demonstrate enhancement of the inflamed appendix (*arrowhead*), the abscess wall (*arrow*), and inflammatory fat stranding. (*C*) The CT appearance follows that of MR imaging, demonstrating the enlarged and wall-thickened appendix (*arrowhead*), stranding of the adjacent fat, abscess (*arrow*), and contrast enhancement.

Fluid-sensitive T2-weighted fat-suppressed sequences should be performed to assess the size of the gallbladder and the presence of pericholecystic edema. MRCP imaging allows for excellent depiction of the biliary ducts, gallbladder, and pancreatic duct, and is highly sensitive for stone detection as hypointense signal voids. Contrast-enhanced T1-weighted fat-suppressed imaging is performed to assess for gallbladder hyperemia.

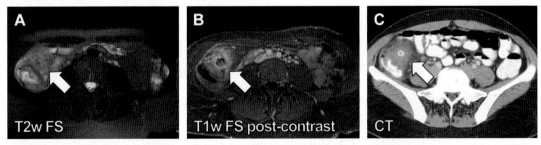

Fig. 3. Acute cecal diverticulitis in a 30-year-old woman. (*A*) Axial T2-weighted fat-suppressed image shows eccentric bowel wall thickening and pericolonic inflammation surrounding the right-sided diverticulitis (*arrow*). (*B*) Axial contrast-enhanced T1-weighted image demonstrates inflammatory enhancement surrounding the impacted and inflamed diverticulum (*arrow*) that is stronger than of nonaffected bowel loops. (*C*) CT appearance follows that of MR imaging, demonstrating the wall thickening and inflammation surrounding the involved diverticulum (*arrow*).

The normal MR appearance of the gallbladder shows variable size distention and is best identified on T2-weighted images. The normal gallbladder wall thickness is less than 3 mm and has intermediate signal intensity on T1-weighted images.[36] The normal gallbladder wall enhances uniformly after contrast injection.[36] Gallstones in the gallbladder or ducts appear as hypointense structures on both T1-weighted and T2-weighted images and are best appreciated on T2-weighted images against the hyperintense signal of the bile.

The obstructed and inflamed gallbladder shows hydropic distention, wall thickening of greater than 3 mm, and pericholecystic inflammatory changes (Fig. 4). The normal low T2 signal intensity wall of the gallbladder increases in signal, appearing ill-defined or stratified on non–fat-suppressed T2 imaging.[9] Obstructing gallstones are the most common cause and can be identified in many cases as a signal void in the cystic duct or gallbladder neck on T2-weighted images.[9,37] Choledocholithiasis is another feature that can be diagnosed with high accuracy using MRCP imaging, even if stones are small and distally located.[38] After contrast injection, the thickened gallbladder wall demonstrates increased enhancement. If ischemic necrosis is present, the resulting gangrene may result in foci of intramural hyperintensity on T2-weighted fat-suppressed images.[39,40] The gangrenous areas or the entire gallbladder shows little or no enhancement after contrast injection.[39–41] Complications include perforation and pericholecystic abscess.

Acute Pancreatitis

Acute pancreatitis is the leading cause of admission to hospital for nonsurgical gastrointestinal disorders.[42] Gallstones and alcohol misuse are the main etiologic risk factors. Patients typically present with abdominal pain, nausea, vomiting, and elevated amylase or lipase levels. Acute pancreatitis has 2 major categories: acute interstitial edematous pancreatitis and necrotizing acute pancreatitis.[42] Necrotizing acute pancreatitis affects 6% to 20% of patients with pancreatitis and is associated with increased morbidity and mortality.[43] As the incidence and admission rates of acute pancreatitis increase, so does the demand for effective management.

CT plays an important role in the management of patients with acute pancreatitis.[44] However, CT and MR are equally endorsed if pancreatitis is suspected and ultrasound is nondiagnostic.[44] Indeed, MR of the pancreas is useful as both a problem-solving tool and an initial imaging examination of choice.[45] MR imaging provides excellent visualization of the pancreatic parenchyma and the pancreatic duct, as well as the common bile duct, for offending stones.

The normal pancreas is best appreciated on T1-weighted fat-suppressed images.[9,46] The pancreatic duct can be best assessed on T2-weighted images as a hyperintense tubular structure with good contrast against the hypointense pancreas parenchyma. After contrast injection, the pancreas shows avid and early enhancement in the arterial phase before washing out in the late portal venous phase.[46]

In pancreatitis, proteolytic enzymes are released and locally disintegrate portions of the pancreatic parenchyma. This induces edema, fluid collections, and in some patients, necrosis. T1-weighted imaging demonstrates an enlarged pancreas with heterogeneously decreased signal intensity[9] due to the edema. T2-weighted fat-suppressed images best visualize the edema and peripancreatic fluid collections (Fig. 5).[46] Complications of acute pancreatitis that can be seen at MR imaging include pancreatic and peripancreatic fluid collection (with or without

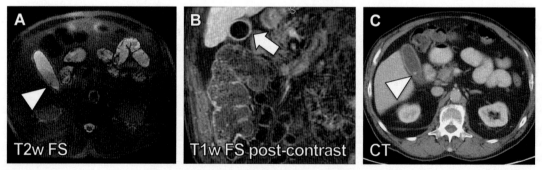

Fig. 4. Acute cholecystitis in a 65-year-old man. (*A*) Axial T2-weighted fat-suppressed image shows gallbladder wall thickening with intramural high signal indicating edema. A small calculus is seen in the gallbladder (*arrowhead*). (*B*) Coronal contrast-enhanced T1-weighted image demonstrates increased mucosal enhancement of the wall-thickened and acutely inflamed gallbladder (*arrow*). (*C*) CT appearance follows that of MR imaging, demonstrating the wall-thickened gallbladder, low-attenuation intramural edema, and a small calculus (*arrowhead*).

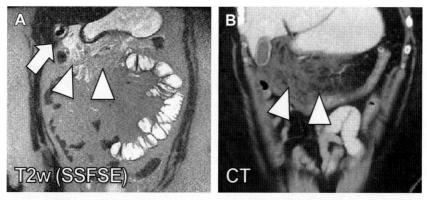

Fig. 5. Acute pancreatitis in a 47-year-old woman. (*A*) Coronal T2-weighted SSFSE image demonstrates fluid signal infiltrating the peripancreatic fat (*arrowheads*) related to the acute pancreatic inflammation. The examination was aborted after the acquisition of the T2-weighted SSFSE due to the patient experiencing extreme pain, but the limited acquired images provided enough diagnostic information for further triage of the patient. Note the large gallstones in the gallbladder (*arrow*) and reactive gastric wall thickening. (*B*) The CT appearance generally follows that of MR imaging, demonstrating peripancreatic infiltration (*arrowheads*) and gastric wall thickening, but note that the gallstones are not CT visible because of low attenuation.

superinfection) and pancreatic necrosis. Vascular complications such as arterial pseudoaneurysms and venous thrombosis can be best appreciated after contrast injection.[9]

Bowel Obstruction

Bowel obstruction is a relatively frequent cause of acute abdominal pain and ED presentation.[47] Most patients found to have bowel obstruction after they present to the ED have small bowel obstruction (SBO).[47] SBO can manifest as generalized vague abdominal pain often accompanied by nausea and vomiting. SBO is most frequently caused by postoperative adhesions. Patient characteristics and risk factors associated with bowel obstruction are previous abdominal surgery, age older than 50 years, and history of constipation.[48] In patients with SBO complicated by ischemia (eg, closed loop obstruction from strangulated hernia), immediate surgery is warranted, whereas many other patients with simple or low-grade obstruction can be treated conservatively. For appropriate treatment, it is important to identify the cause (eg, adhesion, inflammation, neoplasm, or hernia) and severity of the obstruction. Because clinical evaluation is limited in the diagnosis of bowel obstruction, imaging is routinely performed to identify the site, cause, and severity of the obstruction.[2]

CT has emerged as the preeminent imaging modality and should be considered in the initial evaluation of patients with suspected SBO.[49] Evidence supporting the accuracy of MR imaging in the diagnosis of SBO is limited, but results are promising. In some settings, MR is reported to have a sensitivity of 95% and a specificity of 100%[50]

and may even be superior to CT in the preoperative diagnosis of bowel obstruction.[51]

The MR appearance of high-grade SBO parallels that of CT, demonstrating dilated loops of proximal bowel with air fluid levels, which are best appreciated on axial T2-weighted images.[9,52] Because SBO is most often due to adhesions, which are usually not visible, a diagnosis of exclusion is often made at CT or MR. For other causes of mechanical SBO, a more specific diagnosis can be made (**Fig. 6**). The key finding that suggests SBO is a clear change in bowel diameter, or transition point. Loops proximal to the obstruction are distended, whereas loops distal to the obstruction are collapsed. Hence, the presence of adhesions can be inferred by a lack of focal mass or other abnormality, coupled with tethering or kinking of bowel loops at the transition point of abrupt bowel loop caliber change.[53,54] Occasionally, adhesions can be identified on T2-weighted sequences as hypointense bands traversing the hyperintense mesenteric fat.[53,54] Other benign causes of SBO include hernia, gallstone ileus, and inflammatory or fibrostenotic stricture in Crohn disease (see **Fig. 6**).[9] Malignant etiologies may demonstrate a focal mass and locoregional lymph node enlargement.[53]

Inflammatory Bowel Disease

Inflammatory bowel disease mainly consists of the idiopathic disorders of Crohn disease and ulcerative colitis.[55] Crohn disease not only affects the small intestine and large intestine, but can also affect the entire digestive tract, whereas ulcerative colitis primarily affects the colon and the rectum.[55] The peak incidence of initial presentation of Crohn

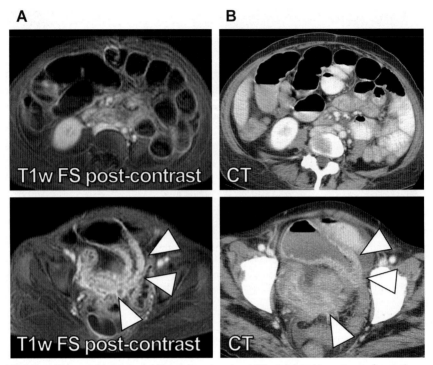

Fig. 6. Distal SBO in a 47-year-old woman. (*A*) Axial postcontrast T1-weighted images performed as part of an MR angiography protocol for suspected mesenteric ischemia shows a thickened and enhancing segment of inflamed distal ileum (*arrowheads*) causing small bowel obstruction with upstream dilatation. (*B*) Contrast-enhanced CT shows similar findings (*arrowheads*), which subsequently proved to be Crohn disease with combined acute inflammation and fibrostenotic disease.

disease is age 15 to 29[56] and occurs in approximately 0.1% of Western populations.[57] Patients present with abdominal pain, diarrhea, nausea, vomiting, and fever. The disease is characterized by transmural inflammation of the bowel wall. The terminal ileum is the most commonly affected portion of the gastrointestinal tract (~80% of cases), making initial presentation a good mimic of appendicitis.[6,58] MR has an overall sensitivity of 91% and specificity of 71% for active IBD[59]; however, it should be noted that the preferred method for imaging Crohn disease is CT or MR enteroclysis,[54] which is not typically performed in the emergency setting.[9]

The MR appearance of Crohn disease parallels that of CT and demonstrates inflammatory bowel wall thickening. Key MR imaging features of Crohn disease include the mural thickening, mural enhancement, intramural high signal intensity on T2-weighted images, a narrowed bowel lumen, and free fluid and edema in the surrounding soft tissues (**Fig. 7**).[6] The inflamed and thickened bowel wall can be best appreciated on fat-saturated T2-weighted images and may show ulcerations. Perienteric inflammation and reactive lymphadenopathy are common ancillary findings.

Mucosal hyperenhancement and mesenteric hypervascularity are typical findings after contrast injection.[9,54] In severe cases, MR may also demonstrate complications such as fistula, abscess, and bowel strictures with associated bowel obstruction (see **Fig. 6**).

Ovarian Torsion

Ovarian torsion is an uncommon gynecologic emergency that requires early diagnosis to allow ovary-sparing surgery.[60] Adnexal torsion most often occurs in women of child-bearing age, but is not rare in premenarchal girls or postmenopausal women.[61] Ovarian torsion is often associated with a cyst or a tumor, the most common being mature cystic teratoma, but torsion without an obvious lead point is also common.[61] The classic clinical presentation overlaps that of appendicitis and includes nausea, vomiting, and pelvic pain. The prevalence of ovarian torsion during pregnancy is 1 in 1800, similar to that of appendicitis. The ovary twists on its vascular pedicle, resulting in partial to complete obstruction of arterial inflow and venous outflow, which can lead to ischemia, edema, hemorrhage, and necrosis.

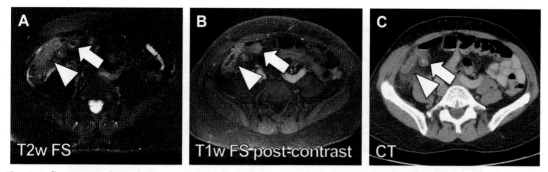

Fig. 7. Inflammatory bowel disease (Crohn) in a 54-year-old man. (*A*) Axial T2-weighted fat-suppressed image shows luminal narrowing, wall thickening (*arrow*), and pericolonic stranding (*arrowhead*). (*B*) Axial contrast-enhanced T1-weighted image also demonstrates wall thickening (*arrow*) plus mucosal enhancement (*arrowhead*). (*C*) CT appearance follows that of MR, demonstrating luminal narrowing, wall thickening (*arrow*), mucosal enhancement, and pericolonic fat stranding (*arrowhead*).

Ultrasound is the first-line imaging modality if a gynecologic abnormality is suspected.[62] If ultrasound is nondiagnostic, MR imaging is particularly useful, as the tissue contrast inherent to MR imaging permits excellent characterization of the abnormal ovary.[9] If MR becomes more widely available in the ED setting, it could potentially replace the common current combination of ultrasound and CT for acute lower abdominal/pelvic pain in women.

The normal ovary is almost always visible on MR imaging in the reproductive age and measures approximately $3 \times 3 \times 2$ cm.[63] The signal intensity of normal ovary is isointense to that of the uterine myometrium on T1-weighted images.[63,64] The T2-weighted imaging appearance is affected by the patient's menopausal status. The premenopausal ovary demonstrates a zonal anatomy with a low signal intensity cortex and high signal intensity medulla. Within the medulla, there are circumscribed rounded foci of fluid intensity signal, which correspond to follicles.[63,64] The normal ovary enhances less than or equal to that of the uterine myometrium after contrast injection.[63,64]

In ovarian torsion, T2-weighted images demonstrate an asymmetrically enlarged ovary with increased signal and peripherally arrayed hydropic follicles (**Fig. 8**).[9,65] The ischemia from torsion leads to central ovarian edema, which induces peripheral displacement of the follicles.[66] As ischemia progresses to hemorrhagic infarct, the appearance of the ovary also changes on T1-weighted images. Initially, the ovary is homogeneously hypointense and as the ischemia progresses to hemorrhagic infarction, the T1-signal of the ovary becomes hyperintense.[9,67] The twisted fallopian tube may be appreciated as a thickened and vascular pedicle.[6,68] The torsion reduces or completely occludes the vascular supply, resulting in decreased, minimal, or even absent enhancement after contrast injection and should be compared with the nontorsed contralateral ovary.[9]

Urolithiasis

Acute flank pain is a common presenting complaint to the ED, requiring a broad differential diagnosis and workup. Urolithiasis is the most frequent cause of acute, severe, unilateral flank pain, ultimately affecting 3% to 5% of the population in industrialized countries.[69,70]

Low-dose noncontrast CT is the imaging study of choice for accurate evaluation of patients with acute onset of flank pain and suspicion of stone disease.[71] CT has a high sensitivity (approaching 100%) and can reliably characterize the location and size of an offending ureteral calculus, identify complications, and diagnose alternative etiologies of abdominal pain, such as appendicitis. By comparison, the sensitivity of radiographs (59%) and ultrasound (24%–57%) for the detection of renal and ureteral calculi is relatively poor.[71]

Although MR would not be considered an imaging modality of choice, diagnosis of symptomatic urolithiasis can be made, largely through secondary signs of obstruction, as an alternative diagnosis in the case of other initially suspected diseases. Hence, a familiarity with the MR imaging features of urolithiasis and obstruction is useful in the setting of nonspecific abdominal pain. MR urography can be performed without contrast administration with static-fluid T2-weighted sequences or after intravenous contrast administration with excretory T1-weighted sequences.[72] MR urography can be used to thoroughly evaluate the renal parenchyma, the pelvicaliceal system, and the rest of the urinary tract in a single imaging study, as in CT urography.[72]

The MR appearance of obstructive urolithiasis parallels that of CT, with excellent delineation of

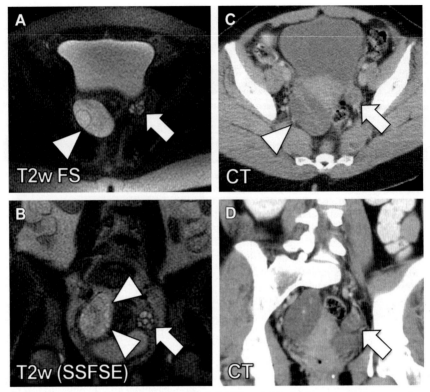

Fig. 8. Ovarian torsion in a 27-year-old woman. (*A*) Axial T2-weighted fat-suppressed image demonstrates an enlarged edematous right ovary (*arrowhead*) with increased signal intensity as compared with the unaffected left ovary (*arrow*). Note hydropic follicle. (*B*) Coronal T2-weighted SSFSE image demonstrates peripheral displacement of the follicles (*arrowheads*) and normal appearance of the follicles of the unaffected left ovary (*arrow*). (*C*) Axial and (*D*) coronal CT images demonstrate the asymmetric increase in size of the edematous right ovary (*arrowhead*) as compared to the unaffected left ovary (*arrow*).

the dilated collecting system and ureters (**Fig. 9**).[73] The dilated ureter can often be traced to the point of the obstruction. Features of obstructive hydronephrosis at MR imaging include renal enlargement, perinephric and periureteric fluid, and an abrupt change in ureteral caliber at the level of obstruction. MR imaging is also particularly helpful in demonstrating complications of

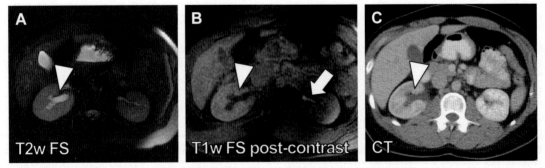

Fig. 9. Urolithiasis in a 22-year-old man with obstruction of the right ureter. (*A*) Axial T2-weighted fat-suppressed image demonstrates a mildly dilated right upper collecting system (*arrowhead*). (*B*) Axial contrast-enhanced T1-weighted image 3 minutes after injection demonstrates contrast excretion into the unaffected left collecting system (*arrow*), while there is no contrast excretion visible in the obstructed right kidney (*arrowhead*). (*C*) CT appearance follows that of MR and demonstrates the dilated collecting system (*arrowhead*) and delayed nephrogram for the obstructed right kidney when compared with the unaffected left kidney. A calculus was detected with CT in the distal ureter (not shown) that was not visible on MR imaging.

pyelonephritis, such as abscess formation. When visible at MR imaging, the obstructing ureteral calculus appears as a low signal intensity–filling defect in the ureter. Dynamic T1-weighted imaging can be performed after contrast injection to assess the dynamics of the obstruction. In the setting of obstruction, MR imaging has a high sensitivity (94%–100 %) for the detection of the obstructing calculus.[73] However, in the case of nonobstructive urolithiasis, MR imaging is limited in its ability to reliably depict small calculi.[72]

OTHER ALTERNATIVE DIAGNOSES

In addition to the more common entities causing acute abdominal pain discussed and demonstrated previously, we have observed many less common entities over the course of our recent CT-MR trial, allowing for direct comparison of findings. Examples of other bowel-centered disease have included both infectious and ischemic colitis, angiotensin-converting enzyme inhibitor–induced angioedema, and Meckels diverticulitis. Fat-based peritoneal conditions include epiploic appendagitis and omental infarction. Gynecologic conditions beyond ovarian torsion have included hemorrhagic and ruptured ovarian cysts, pelvic inflammatory disease, acute fibroid degeneration, and acute complication of ovarian cancer. In general, the CT and MR findings have been comparable, with certain advantages and disadvantages seen with each imaging modality, suggesting overall equivalence in diagnostic ability.

WHAT THE REFEREEING PHYSICIAN NEEDS TO KNOW

MR imaging is a safe, noninvasive imaging technique that uses no ionizing radiation. However, clinicians considering referral of patients with acute abdomen should be aware of certain risks.[74] The most obvious risk is created by the strong magnetic field, which is always on. Therefore, MR scanning may not be safe for patients with certain types of metal implants or electronic devices, such as cardiac pacemakers. MR-based contrast agents are very safe in general, and have a higher safety profile than iodinated contrast agents used for CT, with a lower rate of adverse events and no known nephrotoxicity. Contraindications of MR imaging and MR contrast agents are discussed in further detail at www.mrisafety.com or in the ACR white paper on MR imaging safety.[74]

SUMMARY

MR imaging provides for detailed evaluation in the setting of the nontraumatic acute abdomen that is comparable to CT, with certain advantages and disadvantages. MR imaging allows for diagnosis of a broad spectrum of acute diseases in the setting of the nontraumatic abdomen. As availability of MR in the ED setting increases, its use in this clinical scenario is expected to increase as well. The practicing radiologist should be familiar with the MR appearance of the typical acute pathologies seen in the setting of nontraumatic acute abdomen.

REFERENCES

1. Bhuiya FA, Pitts SR, McCaig LF. Emergency department visits for chest pain and abdominal pain: United States, 1999-2008. NCHS Data Brief 2010;(43):1–8.
2. Stoker J, van Randen A, Laméris W, et al. Imaging patients with acute abdominal pain. Radiology 2009;253(1):31–46.
3. ACR. ACR appropriateness criteria. American College of Radiology Web site 2012. Available at: https://acsearch.acr.org/docs/69467/Narrative/. Accessed February 21, 2015.
4. Brenner DJ, Hall EJ. Computed tomography–an increasing source of radiation exposure. N Engl J Med 2007;357(22):2277–84.
5. Stoker J. Magnetic resonance imaging and the acute abdomen. Br J Surg 2008;95(10):1193–4.
6. Spalluto LB, Woodfield CA, DeBenedectis CM, et al. MR imaging evaluation of abdominal pain during pregnancy: appendicitis and other nonobstetric causes. Radiographics 2012;32(2):317–34.
7. Israel GM, Malguria N, McCarthy S, et al. MRI vs. ultrasound for suspected appendicitis during pregnancy. J Magn Reson Imaging 2008;28(2):428–33.
8. Ginde AA, Foianini A, Renner DM, et al. Availability and quality of computed tomography and magnetic resonance imaging equipment in U.S. emergency departments. Acad Emerg Med 2008; 15(8):780–3.
9. Ditkofsky NG, Singh A, Avery L, et al. The role of emergency MRI in the setting of acute abdominal pain. Emerg Radiol 2014;21(6):615–24.
10. Humes DJ, Simpson J. Acute appendicitis. BMJ 2006;333(7567):530–4.
11. Buckius MT, McGrath B, Monk J, et al. Changing epidemiology of acute appendicitis in the United States: study period 1993-2008. J Surg Res 2012; 175(2):185–90.
12. Andersson RE. The natural history and traditional management of appendicitis revisited: spontaneous resolution and predominance of prehospital perforations imply that a correct diagnosis is more important than an early diagnosis. World J Surg 2007; 31(1):86–92.

13. Smith MP, Katz DS, Lalani T, et al. ACR appropriateness criteria(R) right lower quadrant pain—suspected appendicitis. Ultrasound Q 2014;31(2):85–91.

14. Pickhardt PJ, Lawrence EM, Pooler BD, et al. Diagnostic performance of multidetector computed tomography for suspected acute appendicitis. Ann Intern Med 2011;154(12):789–96. W-291.

15. Pooler BD, Lawrence EM, Pickhardt PJ. Alternative diagnoses to suspected appendicitis at CT. Radiology 2012;265(3):733–42.

16. Terasawa T, Blackmore CC, Bent S, et al. Systematic review: computed tomography and ultrasonography to detect acute appendicitis in adults and adolescents. Ann Intern Med 2004;141(7):537–46.

17. Oto A. MR imaging evaluation of acute abdominal pain during pregnancy. Magn Reson Imaging Clin N Am 2006;14(4):489–501, vi.

18. Oto A, Ernst RD, Shah R, et al. Right-lower-quadrant pain and suspected appendicitis in pregnant women: evaluation with MR imaging—Initial experience. Radiology 2005;234(2):445–51.

19. Leeuwenburgh MMN, Wiezer MJ, Wiarda BM, et al. Accuracy of MRI compared with ultrasound imaging and selective use of CT to discriminate simple from perforated appendicitis. Br J Surg 2014;101(1):E147–55.

20. Orth RC, Guillerman RP, Zhang W, et al. Prospective comparison of MR imaging and US for the diagnosis of pediatric appendicitis. Radiology 2014;272(1):233–40.

21. Thieme ME, Leeuwenburgh MM, Valdehueza ZD, et al. Diagnostic accuracy and patient acceptance of MRI in children with suspected appendicitis. Eur Radiol 2014;24(3):630–7.

22. Leeuwenburgh MMN, Wiarda BM, Bipat S, et al. Acute appendicitis on abdominal MR images: training readers to improve diagnostic accuracy. Radiology 2012;264(2):455–63.

23. Leeuwenburgh MMN, Wiarda BM, Jensch S, et al. Accuracy and interobserver agreement between MR-non-expert radiologists and MR-experts in reading MRI for suspected appendicitis. Eur J Radiol 2014;83(1):103–10.

24. Dewhurst C, Beddy P, Pedrosa I. MRI evaluation of acute appendicitis in pregnancy. J Magn Reson Imaging 2013;37(3):566–75.

25. Leeuwenburgh MMN, Jensch S, Gratama JW, et al. MRI features associated with acute appendicitis. Eur Radiol 2014;24(1):214–22.

26. Inci E, Kilickesmez O, Hocaoglu E, et al. Utility of diffusion-weighted imaging in the diagnosis of acute appendicitis. Eur Radiol 2011;21(4):768–75.

27. Pedrosa I, Levine D, Eyvazzadeh AD, et al. MR imaging evaluation of acute appendicitis in pregnancy. Radiology 2006;238(3):891–9.

28. Jacobs DO. Clinical practice. Diverticulitis. N Engl J Med 2007;357(20):2057–66.

29. Kaiser AM, Jiang JK, Lake JP, et al. The management of complicated diverticulitis and the role of computed tomography. Am J Gastroenterol 2005;100(4):910–7.

30. Feingold D, Steele SR, Lee S, et al. Practice parameters for the treatment of sigmoid diverticulitis. Dis Colon Rectum 2014;57(3):284–94.

31. Oh KY, Gilfeather M, Kennedy A, et al. Limited abdominal MRI in the evaluation of acute right upper quadrant pain. Abdom Imaging 2003;28(5):643–51.

32. Destigter KK, Keating DP. Imaging update: acute colonic diverticulitis. Clin Colon Rectal Surg 2009;22(3):147–55.

33. Strasberg SM. Clinical practice. Acute calculous cholecystitis. N Engl J Med 2008;358(26):2804–11.

34. Yarmish GM, Smith MP, Rosen MP, et al. ACR appropriateness criteria right upper quadrant pain. J Am Coll Radiol 2014;11(3):316–22.

35. Aube C, Delorme B, Yzet T, et al. MR cholangiopancreatography versus endoscopic sonography in suspected common bile duct lithiasis: a prospective, comparative study. AJR Am J Roentgenol 2005;184(1):55–62.

36. Catalano OA, Sahani DV, Kalva SP, et al. MR imaging of the gallbladder: a pictorial essay. Radiographics 2008;28(1):135–55 [quiz: 324].

37. Yeh BM, Liu PS, Soto JA, et al. MR imaging and CT of the biliary tract. Radiographics 2009;29(6):1669–88.

38. Tonolini M, Ravelli A, Villa C, et al. Urgent MRI with MR cholangiopancreatography (MRCP) of acute cholecystitis and related complications: diagnostic role and spectrum of imaging findings. Emerg Radiol 2012;19(4):341–8.

39. Gore RM, Yaghmai V, Newmark GM, et al. Imaging benign and malignant disease of the gallbladder. Radiol Clin North Am 2002;40(6):1307–23, vi.

40. O'Connor OJ, Maher MM. Imaging of cholecystitis. AJR Am J Roentgenol 2011;196(4):W367–74.

41. Loud PA, Semelka RC, Kettritz U, et al. MRI of acute cholecystitis: comparison with the normal gallbladder and other entities. Magn Reson Imaging 1996;14(4):349–55.

42. Lankisch PG, Apte M, Banks PA. Acute pancreatitis. Lancet 2015;386(9988):85–96.

43. Werner J, Feuerbach S, Uhl W, et al. Management of acute pancreatitis: from surgery to interventional intensive care. Gut 2005;54(3):426–36.

44. Baker ME, Nelson RC, Rosen MP, et al. ACR appropriateness criteria(R) acute pancreatitis. Ultrasound Q 2014;30(4):267–73.

45. O'Neill E, Hammond N, Miller FH. MR imaging of the pancreas. Radiol Clin North Am 2014;52(4):757–77.

46. Miller FH, Keppke AL, Dalal K, et al. MRI of pancreatitis and its complications: part 1, acute pancreatitis. AJR Am J Roentgenol 2004;183(6):1637–44.

47. Taylor MR, Lalani N. Adult small bowel obstruction. Acad Emerg Med 2013;20(6):528–44.

48. Bohner H, Yang Q, Franke C, et al. Simple data from history and physical examination help to exclude bowel obstruction and to avoid radiographic studies in patients with acute abdominal pain. Eur J Surg 1998;164(10):777–84.

49. Ros PR, Huprich JE. ACR appropriateness criteria on suspected small-bowel obstruction. J Am Coll Radiol 2006;3(11):838–41.

50. Beall DP, Fortman BJ, Lawler BC, et al. Imaging bowel obstruction: a comparison between fast magnetic resonance imaging and helical computed tomography. Clin Radiol 2002;57(8):719–24.

51. Matsuoka H, Takahara T, Masaki T, et al. Preoperative evaluation by magnetic resonance imaging in patients with bowel obstruction. Am J Surg 2002; 183(6):614–7.

52. Hammond NA, Miller FH, Yaghmai V, et al. MR imaging of acute bowel pathology: a pictorial review. Emerg Radiol 2008;15(2):99–104.

53. Masselli G, Gualdi G. MR imaging of the small bowel. Radiology 2012;264(2):333–48.

54. Fidler JL, Guimaraes L, Einstein DM. MR imaging of the small bowel. Radiographics 2009;29(6): 1811–25.

55. Baumgart DC, Sandborn WJ. Inflammatory bowel disease: clinical aspects and established and evolving therapies. Lancet 2007;369(9573): 1641–57.

56. Hovde O, Moum BA. Epidemiology and clinical course of Crohn's disease: results from observational studies. World J Gastroenterol 2012;18(15): 1723–31.

57. Baumgart DC, Sandborn WJ. Crohn's disease. Lancet 2012;380(9853):1590–605.

58. Furukawa A, Saotome T, Yamasaki M, et al. Cross-sectional imaging in Crohn disease. Radiographics 2004;24(3):689–702.

59. Koh DM, Miao Y, Chinn RJ, et al. MR imaging evaluation of the activity of Crohn's disease. AJR Am J Roentgenol 2001;177(6):1325–32.

60. Nair S, Joy S, Nayar J. Five year retrospective case series of adnexal torsion. J Clin Diagn Res 2014; 8(12):OC09–13.

61. Oelsner G, Shashar D. Adnexal torsion. Clin Obstet Gynecol 2006;49(3):459–63.

62. Andreotti RF, Lee SI, Dejesus Allison SO, et al. ACR appropriateness criteria(R) acute pelvic pain in the reproductive age group. Ultrasound Q 2011;27(3): 205–10.

63. Togashi K. MR imaging of the ovaries: normal appearance and benign disease. Radiol Clin North Am 2003;41(4):799–811.

64. Outwater EK, Mitchell DG. Normal ovaries and functional cysts: MR appearance. Radiology 1996; 198(2):397–402.

65. Duigenan S, Oliva E, Lee SI. Ovarian torsion: diagnostic features on CT and MRI with pathologic correlation. AJR Am J Roentgenol 2012;198(2):W122–31.

66. Kramer LA, Lalani T, Kawashima A. Massive edema of the ovary: high resolution MR findings using a phased-array pelvic coil. J Magn Reson Imaging 1997;7(4):758–60.

67. Lourenco AP, Swenson D, Tubbs RJ, et al. Ovarian and tubal torsion: imaging findings on US, CT, and MRI. Emerg Radiol 2014;21(2):179–87.

68. Pedrosa I, Zeikus EA, Levine D, et al. MR imaging of acute right lower quadrant pain in pregnant and nonpregnant patients. Radiographics 2007;27(3): 721–43 [discussion: 743–53].

69. Hiatt RA, Dales LG, Friedman GD, et al. Frequency of urolithiasis in a prepaid medical care program. Am J Epidemiol 1982;115(2):255–65.

70. Graham A, Luber S, Wolfson AB. Urolithiasis in the emergency department. Emerg Med Clin North Am 2011;29(3):519–38.

71. Coursey CA, Casalino DD, Remer EM, et al. ACR Appropriateness Criteria(R) acute onset flank pain–suspicion of stone disease. Ultrasound Q 2012; 28(3):227–33.

72. O'Connor OJ, McLaughlin P, Maher MM. MR urography. AJR Am J Roentgenol 2010;195(3):W201–6.

73. Kawashima A, Glockner JF, King BF Jr. CT urography and MR urography. Radiol Clin North Am 2003;41(5):945–61.

74. Expert Panel on MR Safety, Kanal E, Barkovich AJ, et al. ACR guidance document on MR safe practices: 2013. J Magn Reson Imaging 2013;37(3): 501–30.

Index

Note: Page numbers of article titles are in **boldface** type.

Radiol Clin N Am 53 (2015) 1341–1348
http://dx.doi.org/10.1016/S0033-8389(15)00175-X
0033-8389/15/$ – see front matter © 2015 Elsevier Inc. All rights reserved.

radiologic.theclinics.com

United States Postal Service

Statement of Ownership, Management, and Circulation
(All Periodicals Publications Except Requestor Publications)

1. Publication Title	2. Publication Number	3. Filing Date
Radiologic Clinics of North America	5 9 6 - 5 1 0	9/18/15

4. Issue Frequency	5. Number of Issues Published Annually	6. Annual Subscription Price
Jan, Mar, May, Jul, Sep, Nov	6	$460.00

7. Complete Mailing Address of Known Office of Publication (Not printer) (Street, city, county, state, and ZIP+4®)

Elsevier Inc.
360 Park Avenue South
New York, NY 10010-1710

Contact Person
Stephen R. Bushing

Telephone (Include area code)
215-239-3688

8. Complete Mailing Address of Headquarters or General Business Office of Publisher (Not printer)

Elsevier Inc., 360 Park Avenue South, New York, NY 10010-1710

9. Full Names and Complete Mailing Addresses of Publisher, Editor, and Managing Editor (Do not leave blank)

Publisher (Name and complete mailing address)

Linda Belfus, Elsevier Inc., 1600 John F. Kennedy Blvd., Suite 1800, Philadelphia, PA 19103

Editor (Name and complete mailing address)

John Vassallo, Elsevier Inc., 1600 John F. Kennedy Blvd., Suite 1800, Philadelphia, PA 19103-2899

Managing Editor (Name and complete mailing address)

Adrianne Brigido, Elsevier Inc., 1600 John F. Kennedy Blvd., Suite 1800, Philadelphia, PA 19103-2899

10. Owner (Do not leave blank. If the publication is owned by a corporation, give the name and address of the corporation immediately followed by the names and addresses of all stockholders owning or holding 1 percent or more of the total amount of stock. If not owned by a corporation, give the names and addresses of the individual owners. If owned by a partnership or other unincorporated firm, give its name and address as well as those of each individual owner. If the publication is published by a nonprofit organization, give its name and address.)

Full Name	Complete Mailing Address
Wholly owned subsidiary of	1600 John F. Kennedy Blvd., Ste. 1800
Reed/Elsevier, US holdings	Philadelphia, PA 19103-2899

11. Known Bondholders, Mortgagees, and Other Security Holders Owning or Holding 1 Percent or More of Total Amount of Bonds, Mortgages, or Other Securities. If none, check box ☐ None

Full Name	Complete Mailing Address
N/A	

12. Tax Status (For completion by nonprofit organizations authorized to mail at nonprofit rates) (Check one)
The purpose, function, and nonprofit status of this organization and the exempt status for federal income tax purposes:
☐ Has Not Changed During Preceding 12 Months
☐ Has Changed During Preceding 12 Months (Publisher must submit explanation of change with this statement)

13. Publication Title	14. Issue Date for Circulation Data Below
Radiologic Clinics of North America	July 2015

15. Extent and Nature of Circulation			Average No. Copies Each Issue During Preceding 12 Months	No. Copies of Single Issue Published Nearest to Filing Date
a. Total Number of Copies (Net press run)			2488	2177
b. Legitimate Paid and/Or Requested Distribution (By Mail and Outside the Mail)	(1)	Mailed Outside-County Paid/Requested Mail Subscriptions stated on PS Form 3541. (Include paid distribution above nominal rate, advertiser's proof copies and exchange copies)	1342	1013
	(2)	Mailed In-County Paid/Requested Mail Subscriptions stated on PS Form 3541. (Include paid distribution above nominal rate, advertiser's proof copies and exchange copies)		
	(3)	Paid Distribution Outside the Mails Including Sales Through Dealers And Carriers, Street Vendors, Counter Sales, and Other Paid Distribution Outside USPS®	470	477
	(4)	Paid Distribution by Other Classes of Mail Through the USPS (e.g. First-Class Mail®)		
c. Total Paid and/or Requested Circulation (Sum of 15b (1), (2), (3), and (4))			1812	1490
d. Free or Nominal Rate Distribution (By Mail and Outside the Mail)	(1)	Free or Nominal Rate Outside-County Copies included on PS Form 3541	54	45
	(2)	Free or Nominal Rate In-County Copies included on PS Form 3541		
	(3)	Free or Nominal Rate Copies mailed at Other classes Through the USPS (e.g. First-Class Mail®)		
	(4)	Free or Nominal Rate Distribution Outside the Mail (Carriers or Other means)		
e. Total Nonrequested Distribution (Sum of 15d (1), (2), (3) and (4))			54	45
f. Total Distribution (Sum of 15c and 15e)			1866	1535
g. Copies not Distributed (See instructions to publishers #4 (page #3))			622	642
h. Total (Sum of 15f and g)			2488	2177
i. Percent Paid and/or Requested Circulation (15c divided by 15f times 100)			97.11%	97.07%

* If you are claiming electronic copies go to line 16 on page 3. If you are not claiming Electronic copies, skip to line 17 on page 3

16. Electronic Copy Circulation	Average No. Copies Each Issue During Preceding 12 Months	No. Copies of Single Issue Published Nearest to Filing Date
a. Paid Electronic Copies		
b. Total paid Print Copies (Line 15c) + Paid Electronic copies (Line 16a)		
c. Total Print Distribution (Line 15f) + Paid Electronic Copies (Line 16a)		
d. Percent Paid (Both Print & Electronic copies) (16b divided by 16c X 100)		

☐ I certify that 50% of all my distributed copies (electronic and print) are paid above a nominal price

17. Publication of Statement of Ownership
If the publication is a general publication, publication of this statement is required. Will be printed in the __November 2015__ issue of this publication.

18. Signature and Title of Editor, Publisher, Business Manager, or Owner	Date
Stephen R. Bushing	September 18, 2015

Stephen R. Bushing – Inventory Distribution Coordinator

I certify that all information furnished on this form is true and complete. I understand that anyone who furnishes false or misleading information on this form or who omits material or information requested on the form may be subject to criminal sanctions (including fines and imprisonment) and/or civil sanctions (including civil penalties).

PS Form 3526, July 2014 (Page 3 of 3)

PS Form 3526, July 2014 (Page 1 of 3 (Instructions Page 3)) PSN 7530-01-000-9931 **PRIVACY NOTICE:** See our Privacy policy in www.usps.com

Moving?

Make sure your subscription moves with you!

To notify us of your new address, find your **Clinics Account Number** (located on your mailing label above your name), and contact customer service at:

Email: journalscustomerservice-usa@elsevier.com

800-654-2452 (subscribers in the U.S. & Canada)
314-447-8871 (subscribers outside of the U.S. & Canada)

Fax number: 314-447-8029

Elsevier Health Sciences Division
Subscription Customer Service
3251 Riverport Lane
Maryland Heights, MO 63043

*To ensure uninterrupted delivery of your subscription, please notify us at least 4 weeks in advance of move.

ELSEVIER